POCKET HANDBOOK
OF PRIMARY CARE
PSYCHIATRY

Senior Contributing Editor

ROBERT CANCRO, M.D., MED D.Sc.
Professor and Chairman, Department of Psychiatry,
New York University School of Medicine;
Director, Department of Psychiatry, Tisch Hospital,
the University Hospital of the New York University Medical Center,
New York, New York;
Director, Nathan S. Kline Institute for Psychiatric Research,
Orangeburg, New York

POCKET HANDBOOK
OF PRIMARY CARE
PSYCHIATRY

HAROLD I. KAPLAN, M.D.

Professor of Psychiatry, New York University School of Medicine;
Attending Psychiatrist, Tisch Hospital, the University Hospital of the
New York University Medical Center;
Attending Psychiatrist, Bellevue Hospital Center;
Consultant Psychiatrist, Lenox Hill Hospital; New York, New York

BENJAMIN J. SADOCK, M.D.

Professor and Vice Chairman, Department of Psychiatry,
New York University School of Medicine;
Attending Psychiatrist, Tisch Hospital, the University Hospital of the
New York University Medical Center;
Attending Psychiatrist, Bellevue Hospital Center;
Consultant Psychiatrist, Lenox Hill Hospital, New York, New York

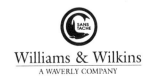

Williams & Wilkins
A WAVERLY COMPANY

BALTIMORE • PHILADELPHIA • LONDON • PARIS • BANGKOK
BUENOS AIRES • HONG KONG • MUNICH • SYDNEY • TOKYO • WROCLAW

Editor: Susan M. Gay
Managing Editor: Kathleen Courtney Millet
Production Coordinator: Barbara J. Felton
Copy Editor: Bonnie Montgomery
Designer: Wilma E. Rosenberger
Illustration Planner: Lorraine Wrzosek
Typesetter: Innodata Publishing Services Division
Printer/Binder: Vicks Lithograph

Rose Tree Corporate Center
1400 North Providence Road
Building II, Suite 5025
Media, Pennsylvania 19063-2043 USA

Printed in the United States of America

Library of Congress Cataloging-in-Publication Data
Kaplan, Harold I.
  Pocket handbook of primary care psychiatry / Harold I. Kaplan,
Benjamin J. Sadock.
    p.   cm.
  Includes index.
  ISBN 0-683-30017-2
  1. Psychiatry—Handbooks, manuals, etc.   2. Primary care
(Medicine)—Handbooks, manuals, etc.   I. Sadock, Benjamin J.
  II. Title.
  [DNLM: 1. Mental Disorders—handbooks.   2. Primary Health Care—
handbooks.   WM 34 K17pn 1997]
  RC456.K363   1997
  616.89—dc20
  DNLM/DLC
for Library of Congress   96-32243
                                                                              CIP

To purchase additional copies of this book, call our customer service department at **(800) 638-0672** or fax orders to **(800) 447-8438**. For other book services, including chapter reprints and large quantity sales, ask for the Special Sales department.

Canadian customers should call **(800) 268-4178**, or fax **(905) 470-6780**. For all other calls originating outside of the United States, please call **(410) 528-4223** or fax us at **(410) 528-8550**.

Visit Williams & Wilkins on the Internet: **http://www.wwilkins.com** or contact our customer service department at **custserv@wwilkins.com**. Williams & Wilkins customer service representatives are available from 8:30 am to 6:00 pm, EST, Monday through Friday, for telephone access.

                                                              98 99 00
                                                        4 5 6 7 8 9 10

Dedicated
to our wives,
Nancy Barrett Kaplan
and
Virginia Alcott Sadock,
without whose help and sacrifice
this book would not have been possible

Preface

The primary care physician is the foundation on which the current system of health delivery in the United States is based. Most Americans access health care via physicians trained in family medicine, general practice, general pediatrics, and general internal medicine. Primary care physicians deal not only with the physical complaints of their patients but also with their mental, emotional, and social concerns. It is those areas of concern that make up the field of primary care psychiatry.

The *Pocket Handbook of Primary Care Psychiatry* is geared to the needs of the generalist facing the challenge of evaluating and treating patients with psychiatric illness. Primary care psychiatry encompasses the full range of emotional disorders, and this book is designed to make that task easier. Most patients with psychiatric disorders are seen first by the generalist and not by the psychiatrist.

In addition to the primary care physician, this book will also be of use to others—clinical psychologists, clinical social workers, psychiatric nurses, and non-primary care physicians—professionals are frequently on the front-line of providing mental health services. Medical students, psychiatric residents and psychiatrists who require a brief overview of clinical psychiatry will also find this book helpful. As in all of our books, the humanistic aspects of medical care are emphasized. The qualities of compassion, empathy, and understanding are especially necessary when patients complain of emotional problems that may arouse fear, confusion, embarrassment, or guilt.

ORGANIZATION

This book is divided into three major areas. Area A consists of a series of succinctly written chapters that cover the field of primary care psychiatry. They include (1) an introduction to the role of the primary care physician in dealing with the patient with psychiatric problems, including interview techniques; (2) an overview of psychiatric signs and symptoms; (3) the evaluation of the patient, including the psychiatric history and the mental status examination; and (4) an overview of medical and surgical problems that are accompanied by or that cause psychiatric signs and symptoms.

Area B contains discussions of almost every psychiatric disorder that may be encountered in the office. Such conditions may present as a sign or a symptom of a major mental disorder, such as delusions in schizophrenia, or as the early manifestation of a potentially fatal illness, such as dementia in acquired immune deficiency syndrome (AIDS). The decision to include a particular psychiatric disorder in this book was based on many factors: frequency of presentation, incidence, prevalence, severity, and type of symptoms. Conditions that may constitute a psychiatric emergency are also covered, since such conditions often have a potential lethality and carry a risk of danger to self or others. Much of the content of Area B is derived from our *Pocket Handbook of Emergency Psychiatric Medicine*, which has been updated and revised.

Area C covers the treatment and management of psychiatric disorders. A section on drugs is included that is geared to the office practice of psychiatry. A chart of the drugs and the classes of drugs used in the treatment of major psychiatric disorders is also included; the chart indicates the various medications that are used to treat a particular disorder and is completely up-to-date. The section on movement disorders describes some of the more distressing side effects that may occur with neuroleptic medication and provides explicit directions on treatment. Finally, a brief description of the various types of psychotherapies is included for those primary care physicians interested in providing such therapy, or if not, making the appropriate referral to a professional who can do so.

For each psychiatric sign, symptom, or disorder covered in this book the reader will find (1) a definition of the condition; (2) the criteria used to diagnose the disorder, including the differential diagnosis; (3) interviewing guidelines to use with the patient and with friends or relatives who are in attendance; (4) practical guidelines about treatment and proper disposition; and (5) a discussion on drug treatment, including the specific drugs and dosages used to manage the situation.

Teaching System

Pocket Handbook of Primary Care Psychiatry is one in a series of concise practical guides that deal with specific issues in the treatment of psychiatric disorders. Other books in this series include *Pocket Handbook of Clinical Psychiatry* and *Pocket Handbook of Psychiatric Drug Treatment*. The handbooks form one part of a comprehensive system developed to facilitate the teaching of psychiatry and the behavioral sciences. The handbooks are compactly designed and concisely written to be carried in the pocket by the clinical clerk or practicing physician as a ready reference.

The keystone of the system is *Comprehensive Textbook of Psychiatry,* now in its sixth (1995) edition; that textbook is global in its depth and scope and encyclopedic in its breadth of information. *Kaplan and Sadock's Synopsis of Psychiatry,* another part of the system, is now in its seventh (1994) edition; it is designed for practicing psychiatrists, psychiatric residents, and medical students. Another part of the system, *Study Guide and Self-Examination Review for Kaplan and Sadock's Synopsis of Psychiatry,* is now in its fifth (1994) edition; it contains multiple-choice questions keyed to those books. Finally, the system includes *Comprehensive Glossary of Psychiatry and Psychology* (1991), which provides simply written definitions of terms of interest for psychiatrists and other physicians, psychologists, students, other mental health professionals, and the general public.

The teaching system is unique in that it provides a comprehensive library of psychiatry that can fulfill all the educational needs of the student and the practitioner.

Illustrated Drug Identification Guide

A unique aspect of this book is the inclusion of colored plates of all the major drugs used in psychiatry. Both the forms in which they are commercially available and their doses are indicated to help the physician recognize and prescribe the medications. The plates are completely up-to-date. Many emergencies are due to the misuse, abuse, or intentional overdose of drugs that can be identified by using the colored plates.

References

We have not included specific references at the end of each section; however, for further information, the reader is referred to the sixth (1995) edition of our standard work, *Comprehensive Textbook of Psychiatry,* or the seventh (1994) edition of *Synopsis of Psychiatry,* in which each of the topics included in this book is discussed in depth.

ACKNOWLEDGMENTS

We wish to thank several persons who helped in the preparation of parts of this text: Norman Sussman, M.D., James C.-Y. Chou, M.D., and Michael Allen, M.D.

Justin Hollingsworth served as project editor. He carried out his complex tasks with great skill. He was assisted by Justin Hartung and Jennifer Peters. We thank them all for their extraordinary efforts.

Virginia Sadock, M.D., Clinical Professor of Psychiatry and Director of Graduate Education in Human Sexuality at New York University Medical Center, deserves special mention and thanks for her help in every aspect of this book.

Finally, we thank Robert Cancro, M.D., Professor and Chairman of the Department of Psychiatry at New York University Medical Center, who served as senior contributing editor. We are deeply grateful for the inspiration and support he offers in all our academic endeavors.

Harold I. Kaplan, M.D.
Benjamin J. Sadock, M.D.

July 1996
New York University Medical Center
New York, New York

Contents

Area A

Psychiatry and Primary Care Medicine

1

The Primary Care Physician and Psychiatric Assessment

Primary care psychiatry is that branch of medicine concerned with the prevention, diagnosis, and treatment of mental disorders as provided by primary care physicians, who are trained as internists, family practitioners, pediatricians, obstetricians, and gynecologists. The range of care provided by primary care physicians includes the physical, mental, emotional, and social concerns of their patients. Ten times as many patients with psychiatric illness are seen by primary care physicians as are seen by psychiatrists, and primary care physicians prescribe more psychotropic drugs than psychiatrists do.

Primary care psychiatry encompasses many common psychiatric disorders and conditions, such as depression, anxiety, substance abuse, chronic pain syndromes, death, dying, and bereavement. Generalists also deal with the patients' reactions to acute and chronic illness and their reactions to illness in their family members.

A common psychiatric condition (5 to 10 percent of primary care patients) the physician must confront is somatization, in which the patient has many somatic symptoms that cannot be explained on the basis of physical examinations or laboratory results. Another similar condition is hypochondriasis. Hypochondriasis is characterized by the patient's unrealistic or inaccurate interpretation of physical symptoms or sensations. The hypochondriac patient fears that he or she has a serious disease with no medical evidence to support the fear. Approximately 5 percent of primary care patients have hypochondriasis, and 80 percent of those patients have an underlying anxiety or depressive disorder.

DOCTOR-PATIENT RELATIONSHIP

The development of an effective doctor-patient relationship requires the establishment of trust and rapport between the two persons. Rapport is facilitated by the doctor putting the patient at ease, listening to the patient, expressing compassion when appropriate, and demonstrating expertise.

Models of the Doctor-Patient Relationship

Models of the doctor-patient relationship emerge from the personalities of both the doctor and the patient. Often neither the doctor nor the patient is conscious of choosing a model, but because the expectations and the needs are largely unspoken and may be different for each person, disappointment develops in the relationship. The doctor must be conscious of the model in operation with each patient and be able to shift models, depending on the needs of the patient and on the treatment requirements of specific clinical situations.

Four relationship models are summarized in Table 1–1.

TABLE 1-1
MODELS OF THE PHYSICIAN-PATIENT RELATIONSHIP

Model	Role of Physician and Patient	Clinical Example
Active-passive	Physician assumes entire responsibility for patient's care; patient takes no part in treatment	Patient is unconscious, immobile, or delirious; patient has extremely passive personality structure
Teacher-student	Physician is authoritarian and controlling; patient is dependent and acceptant	Patient is recovering from surgery
Mutual participation	Equality between doctor and patient; both require and depend on each other's input	Treatment of chronic illnesses such as renal failure or diabetes
Intimate model	Most often represents a psychological need by the physician to turn the care of the patient into a relationship of mutual sharing of personal information and love	Generally considered dysfunctional and unethical; a sexual relationship may be subject to criminal prosecution

General Considerations

Gaining insight into the relationship between physicians and patients requires constant evaluation. Physicians who possess self-respect will feel secure enough to recognize and modify attitudes destructive to the relationship. Doctors need to empathize with their patients, but they should neither assume their patients' burdens nor believe that only they are their patients' saviors. Physicians should be able to leave the problems of their patients at the office or the hospital. Patients used as substitutes for an intimacy or a relationship in the physicians' personal lives will handicap the physicians' efforts to help ill persons. Patients need sympathy and understanding, but not sentimentality.

Doctors have been sued, attacked, and even killed, because the patients held their doctors responsible for an unsatisfactory outcome of the treatment. Consequently, the physician fearing the risks of treating those patients may assume a defensive or rigid attitude with all patients. A rigid manner may create the appearance of thoroughness and efficiency but may hamper the trust needed to establish rapport with the patient; whereas, a flexible approach leads to increased responsiveness in the subtle doctor-patient interplay. Uncertainty is present in all clinical situations, so doctors must accept that they cannot control everything in the care of a patient. Regardless of how conscientious, competent, or caring the physician is, in some situations diseases cannot be controlled and death cannot be prevented.

Physicians must also face difficult issues that, because of their own prepossessions or predilections, they would prefer to avoid, especially when the issues are important to the patient.

BIOPSYCHOSOCIAL MODEL

The biopsychosocial model of disease and health stresses a three-part approach to understanding the patient: the biological part emphasizes the anatomical, structural, and molecular substrates of disease; the psychological part examines the effects of psychodynamic factors, motivation, and personality on the experience of illness; and the social part explains how the cultural, environmental, and familial conditions or experiences influence the expression and the experience of illness. All those parts must be considered in assessing the symptoms of physical illness in patients.

Reaction to Illness

Illness behavior describes a patient's reactions to the experience of being ill. The *sick role* is the role that society ascribes to persons when they are ill. Two characteristics of the sick role are that the person is excused from normal or customary responsibilities and is expected to want help to get well.

Illness behavior and the sick role are affected by the psychological factors of personality type and the personal meaning attributed to the experience of being ill; the habitual modes of thinking, feeling, and behaving; the cultural beliefs, class status, and ethnic identity; and society's treatment of those persons who become dependent and helpless and the role society assigns to those persons. Some persons experience illness as an overwhelming loss, whereas others experience the same illness as a challenge to overcome or perhaps a punishment to be endured.

Table 1–2 lists essential areas to be addressed in the assessment of illness behavior and questions that are helpful in making that assessment.

INTERVIEWING

The ability to conduct an effective interview is an important tool for a physician. An interviewer needs the skills to gather the data necessary to competently treat the patient and to obtain the patient's compliance with the physician's advice.

Every interview has three main components, all of which demand specific techniques and skills: the beginning of the interview, the interview proper, and the closing of the interview. In general, an interviewer must convey a nonjudgmental

TABLE 1–2
ASSESSMENT OF INDIVIDUAL ILLNESS BEHAVIOR

Prior illness episodes, especially illnesses of standard severity (childbirth, renal stones, surgery)
Cultural degree of stoicism
Cultural beliefs concerning the specific problem
Personal meaning or beliefs about the particular problem

Specific questions to ask to elicit the patient's explanatory model:

1. What do you call your problem? What name does it have?
2. What do you think caused your problem?
3. Why do you think it started when it did?
4. What does your sickness do to you? How does it work?
5. How severe is it? Will it have a short or long course?
6. What do you fear most about your sickness?
7. What are the chief problems that your sickness has caused for you?
8. What kind of treatment do you think you should receive? What are the most important results you hope to receive from treatment?
9. What have you done so far to treat your sickness?

Table from M Lipkin Jr: Psychiatry and medicine. In *Comprehensive Textbook of Psychiatry*, ed 5, H I Kaplan, B J Sadock, editors, p 1280. Williams & Wilkins, Baltimore, 1989.

attitude, demonstrate interest, concern, and kindness, and use his or her empathic responses to develop rapport.

Beginning the Interview

The first communication between the doctor and the patient has the potential power to determine the success of the remainder of the interview. Patients often feel vulnerable, anxious, and intimidated when first meeting with physicians. A physician who quickly establishes rapport, puts the patient at ease, and demonstrates respect for the patient will elicit a productive exchange of information. That exchange is critical to formulating a correct diagnosis and to establishing treatment goals.

The physician should know the patient's name and should introduce themselves to the patient and any other persons who are present. The physician should ask the patient if he or she wishes any of the accompanying relatives or friends to be present during the interview. A request for the presence of another person during the interview should be respected. The presence of the other person may reduce the patient's anxiety and help to gain the trust of a significant person in the patient's life, a person who may be essential to the patient's acceptance of the doctor.

The physician should, however, speak to the patient alone. The patient may be hesitant to discuss certain topics in the presence of other family members or friends. To ensure that the patient has a chance to speak with the physician privately, after talking with the patient and the other persons present, the physician could say: "I appreciate speaking with all of you and getting your thoughts and input about what is going on with Mr. X. At this point I would like to speak to Mr. X alone, since he and I will be working together closely in the coming weeks. If you would like to meet with me again, I would be happy to arrange a meeting."

Opening Questions

Most patients do not speak freely unless they are assured of privacy. A physician who begins the interview in a private and quiet office, and restricts outside interruptions, conveys to the patient that the interview is important and that what the patient has to say is worthy of serious consideration.

After the introductions and initial assessments are concluded, possible opening questions are: "Can you tell me about the troubles that bring you in today?" or "Tell me about the problems you have been having." A second question or remark often elicits additional information that the patient was initially reluctant to give and suggests to the patient that the physician is interested in hearing more. The physician could then ask, "What other problems have you been experiencing?" A less directive approach to the opening questions is to ask the patient, "Where shall we start?" or "Where would you prefer to begin?"

A physician interviewing a patient referred by another doctor for consultation can indicate that he or she already knows something about the patient's condition or complaint. For example, the consulting doctor may say, "Your doctor has told me something about what is troubling you, but I'd like to hear what is troubling you in your own words."

A patient who appears frightened or resistant at the beginning of an interview should be encouraged, in a gentle and supportive way, to share his or her feelings about the interview. Acknowledging the patient's anxiety is frequently the first step to uncovering the origins of the anxiety and enables the physician to offer appropriate reassurance. For example, the physician could say, "I notice that you seem to be feeling anxious about talking with me, and I wonder if there is anything I can do, or any question I can answer, that will make it easier for you," or "I know that talking to a doctor can be difficult or frightening, especially one you have never met before, but I would like to make you feel as comfortable as possible. Is there anything you can put your finger on that is making it tough for you to talk to me?"

It is also important for the primary care physician to learn if there are any precipitant events in the patient's life that may have contributed to his or her stress. Precipitant events are often significant contributors to the patient's current problems; examples of those events include: real or symbolic losses (for example, death and separations); milestone events (for example, significant birthdays); and physical changes (for example, a new diet or medication). Physicians who are unaware of such stresses in a patient's life may fail to ask the questions that could extract crucial data.

Interview Proper

In the interview proper the physician discovers in detail what is troubling the patient, proceeding in a systematic way that facilitates the identification of relevant problems within the context of an ongoing, empathic working alliance with the patient.

Content versus Process.   The *content* of an interview is the oral conversation between the doctor and the patient: the topics discussed, the subjects mentioned. The *process* of the interview is the nonverbal communication between the doctor and the patient: what is happening in the interview beneath the surface appearances. Process involves feelings and reactions that are unacknowledged or unconscious. For example, patients may use body language to express feelings they cannot express verbally—a clenched fist or nervous tearing at a tissue while maintaining a calm outward demeanor. Patients may shift the interview away from an anxiety-provoking subject on to a neutral topic or return repeatedly to a particular topic, regardless of the direction the interview appeared to be taking. Trivial remarks or apparently casual asides may reveal serious underlying concerns—for example, "Oh, by the way, a neighbor of mine tells me that he knows someone with the same symptoms as my son, and that person has cancer."

Specific Interviewing Techniques.   Table 1–3 summarizes specific interviewing techniques.

Open-ended versus closed-ended questions.   Conducting a successful interview requires that the physician seek a fine balance between allowing the patient's story

TABLE 1-3
TECHNIQUES OF PHYSICIAN-PATIENT INTERVIEWING

Technique	Purpose
Reflection physician repeats or paraphrases in a supportive manner something the patient has said; emphatic response	Indicates the physician is listening and understands the patient's concerns
Facilitation physician provides verbal and nonverbal cues to encourage the patient to keep talking. Examples include leaning forward, and saying "Yes, and then?" or "Uh-huh, go on."	Helps the patient continue in the interview
Silence can be used in a constructive manner when the physician makes it clear that not every moment must be filled with talk	Allows the patient to contemplate, cry, or just sit in an accepting, supporting environment
Confrontation physician points out to the patient something the physician thinks the patient is not paying attention to, is missing, or is in some way denying	Helps the patient face whatever needs to be faced in a direct but respectful way; breaks through the defense of denial. Should be used cautiously
Clarification physician attempts to get details from the patient about what the patient has already said	Allows patient to expand upon complaints or symptoms
Interpretation the physician states something about the patient's behavior or thoughts about which the patient may not be aware; should be used after rapport has been established	Helps clarify conflicts or interrelationships of which the patient may not be aware
Summation periodically, the physician briefly summarizes what the patient has said	Assures both the patient and the physician that the information obtained is what the patient intends to communicate
Explanation physician explains the treatment plan in easily understandable language	Prevents confusion, and alleviates anxiety
Transition physician encourages the patient to move on to another subject	Allows the physician to gain more data on another topic
Self-revelation limited, discrete self-disclosure by the physician	Personal questions from the patient may mask hidden concerns or anxieties
Positive reinforcement physician encourages the patient to feel that the physician will not be upset by whatever the patient has to say	Facilitates an open exchange; allows the patient to feel comfortable with the physician
Reassurance an emphatic response by a concerned physician	Helps lead to increased patient trust and compliance; false reassurance is essentially lying and can impair the patient's confidence in the physician
Advice physician recommends a treatment plan or suggests a course of behavior; should not be offered without careful deliberation	Patient views physician as effective, concerned, and competent; if given too quickly may undermine patient's confidence

to unfold without direction or interruption and controlling the story flow by asking specific questions. In the ideal interview the interviewer begins with broad open-ended questions, continues to specific questions, and closes with detailed directive questions.

The first part of the interview is generally the most open-ended: The physician wants the patient to speak as much as possible in his or her own words. An example of an open-ended question is, "Can you tell me more about that?" A closed-ended question or directive question asks for specific information and allows the patient few options in answering. For example, if the patient says that he or she has been feeling depressed, the closed-ended question might be, "Your mother died recently, didn't she?" That question can be answered only by a "yes" or a "no," and the mother's death may or may not be the reason the patient is depressed. More information is likely to be obtained if the doctor responds with, "Tell me more about what you're feeling and what you think may be causing it." Closed-ended questions in the early part of an interview can lead to a restriction of the patient's responses. Directive questions are sometimes necessary to obtain important data, but, if overused will constrict the flow of information; the patient may believe that he or she is to respond only when directly questioned by the physician.

Closed-ended questions, however, can be effective in generating specific and quick responses on a clearly defined topic and are effective in eliciting information on the absence of certain symptoms (for example, auditory hallucinations and suicidal ideation). The closed-ended question is helpful in assessing such factors as the frequency, severity, and duration of symptoms.

Concluding the Interview

The doctor wants the patient to leave the interview feeling confident that all the pertinent information has been given to an informed, empathic listener. To bring the interview to a conclusion the doctor should tell the patient that the information shared has been helpful in clarifying the next steps in the treatment plan, and thank the patient. The physician should encourage the patient to ask questions before the interview is concluded and ascertain that the patient understands what to expect from any medication prescribed and how to take the medication.

The doctor should schedule another appointment or make a referral and explain how to get help quickly if it is necessary before the next appointment.

INTERVIEWS WITH SPECIAL PATIENT POPULATIONS

Difficult Patients

Effective management of the difficult patient requires skill on the part of any physician. The doctor must understand the overt emotions, the fears, and conflicts that direct the patients' behavior. Knowledge of the hidden motives of a patient's difficult behavior can diffuse the physician's anger, contempt, or anxiety, and direct the physician's energy toward helpful interventions.

Histrionic.   Histrionic patients act seductively with doctors because they have an unconscious need for reassurance that they are still attractive despite their illness, and because they fear that they will not be taken seriously unless they are found to be sexually desirable. They often appear overly emotional and intimate in their interactions with doctors. The patients do not really want to seduce the physician, but they may not know any other way to get what they feel they need. The physician needs to be calm, reassuring, firm, and nonflirtatious.

Demanding and Dependent. Demanding and dependent patients make repeated, urgent calls between scheduled appointments to demand that the doctor provide special attention. These patients need an inordinate supply of reassurance, but they often resist any such assurances. They frequently become angry or frightened if they believe the doctor is not taking their concerns seriously. The doctor must set the necessary limits while still expressing a willingness to listen and to care for the patient.

Demanding and Impulsive. Demanding and impulsive patients have difficulty delaying gratification and may demand that their discomfort be eliminated immediately. They are easily frustrated if satisfaction is hindered and may, if they feel thwarted by the doctor, act self-destructively. They may also appear manipulative and attention seeking. The surface manifestations—anger, petulance, aggression—conceal the patients' fear that their needs will go unmet unless they act in an aggressive manner. The doctor must calmly set firm limits, clearly define acceptable and unacceptable behavior, and hold patients responsible for their actions.

Narcissistic. Narcissistic patients have a tremendous need to appear perfect and are contemptuous of others, whom they perceive as imperfect. They may be rude, abrupt, arrogant, or demeaning. Initially they may overidealize the physician in their need to have a doctor who is as perfect as they believe they are. The patients' arrogant surface masks their feelings of inadequacy and helplessness and fear that others will discover the fallacy of their perfection.

Obsessive and Controlling. Obsessive and controlling patients are orderly, punctual, and overly concerned with detail. They often appear unemotional or aloof, especially when confronted with a potentially disturbing or frightening event. The patients are often afraid that, if they lose control of everything in their environment they will be dependent and helpless and thus may resist what they perceive to be control by the doctor. Physicians can strengthen the patients' sense of control by including the patients as much as possible in their own care and treatment and explaining in detail all aspects of the planned treatment.

Hypervigilant and Paranoid. Hypervigilant and paranoid patients are critical, evasive, and suspicious; they fear that other persons want to hurt them. They may misread the behavioral cues of other persons and see conspiracies in neutral events. They tend to blame others for any painful or harmful events in their lives. The patients are extremely mistrustful and may question the doctor's suggestions or treatment program. The doctor's expressions of warmth and empathy may be viewed with suspicion ("What does the doctor want from me?"), but the doctor must remain formal, respectful, and courteous. The doctor should be prepared to explain in detail each decision or planned procedure and to react nondefensively to the patients' suspicions.

Isolated and Solitary. Isolated and solitary patients are termed schizoid personalities. They appear detached and reclusive and need or want little human contact.

Intimate contact with a doctor is viewed with distaste; they would prefer to take care of themselves. The doctor should respect the patients' privacy as much as possible and expect little or no response to any overt concern or kindness.

Complaining, Martyrlike, and Passive-Aggressive.   Complaining, martyrlike, and passive-aggressive patients are unable to openly express angry feelings. They may express hostility indirectly or passively by being late for appointments or failing to make timely payments on their bills. The patients perceive themselves as self-sacrificing and unappreciated and see other persons as selfish and uncaring. They often secretly blame other persons for their problems and manage to make others, frequently family members, feel guilty for not doing or caring enough. The patients may unconsciously believe that the only way to be valued or loved is to be ill.

Doctors should take these patients' concerns seriously without encouraging the sick role. They should assure the patients that they will listen to them during regularly scheduled appointments but set firm limits on their availability to these patients. Doctors may also become involved with the patient's family members who deal with the patients' difficult style daily and who are likely to feel angry, frustrated, or guilty.

Sociopathic and Malingering.   Sociopathic patients are described as antisocial personalities: They do not appear to experience appropriate guilt and may not even be aware of what it means to feel guilty. Sociopathic persons may appear charming, socially adept, and intelligent, for they have perfected the appearance of appropriate behaviors; they are performing almost as an actor would in a scripted role. They survive by lies and manipulation and often have criminal histories; they are often self-destructive, harming others and themselves, in perhaps an unacknowledged expression of self-punishment.

Sociopathic patients often malinger, that is, consciously feign illness, for some clear secondary gain—for example, to obtain drugs, to gain a place to stay, or to hide from people pursuing them. Obviously, sociopathic persons do become ill and they need to be cared for in the same ways as other patients. Doctors must treat these patients with respect but with a heightened sense of vigilance. The patients, some with violent histories, can inspire legitimate fear in others. Doctors who feel threatened by patients should seek assistance and see the patients only when accompanied by another person. Firm limits must be set on the patients' behavior and the consequences of violation of these limits must be clearly stated. If inappropriate behavior occurs, the patients must be calmly but directly confronted, and held responsible for their actions.

Disliking a Patient

A physician who actively dislikes a patient is likely to be ineffective in treating that patient. If the physician keeps his or her feelings neutral, or as neutral as possible, and handles the patient with equanimity, the interpersonal relationship may shift from overt antagonism to an increased acceptance, or at least a grudging

TABLE 1–4
EXAMPLES OF DIFFICULT OR THREATENING PATIENTS

Patients who appear to repeatedly defeat attempts to help them, e.g., patients with severe heart disease who continue to smoke or drink

Patients who are perceived as uncooperative, e.g., patients who question or refuse treatments

Patients who fail to recover in response to treatment

Patients who use physical or somatic complaints to mask emotional problems, e.g., patients with somatization disorder, pain disorder, hypochondriasis, or factitious disorder

Patients with chronic cognitive disorders, e.g., patients with dementia of the Alzheimer's type

Patients who represent a professional failure, e.g., patients who are dying or in chronic pain

mutual respect. That process requires that the physician examine the intense counter-transferential reactions that are occurring and dispassionately explore the reasons the patient triggers the feelings of dislike. Doctors who have strong unconscious needs to appear superior and powerful may have problems with certain types of patients, but if the physician is cognizant of his or her own needs, capabilities, and limitations, then dealing with those patients seems less threatening.

Table 1–4 lists some examples of difficult or threatening patients.

Sexuality and the Physician

Physicians are likely at some point to feel a strong attraction to a patient. The doctor is a powerful figure in the culture of this country and may trigger many unconscious fantasies or needs—being rescued, being cared for, and being loved—in his or her patients. Doctors also may have their own unconscious needs or fantasies—being all-powerful, being able to rescue others, and being lovable. Those fantasies or needs are inherently unrealistic. A romantic or sexual relationship between the doctor and the patient can be destructive, especially for the patient.

Another aspect of sexuality and the physician is the countertransference between the doctor and patient when talking with patients about sexual issues or obtaining a sexual history. A reluctance to seek sexual information may reflect the physician's anxiety about his or her own sexuality or even an unconscious attraction to the patient. That reluctance may suggest to the patient that the physician is uncomfortable with the subject of sexuality, inhibiting the patient's willingness to discuss this issue and any number of other sensitive subjects.

A useful guide to monitor patients' attitudes is listed in Table 1–5.

SPECIFIC STRESSES ON THE PHYSICIAN

A trained physician learns the knowledge base and the techniques of the profession but he or she must also confront and resolve a number of significant attitudinal issues unique to the profession. Those issues include: balancing the ideals of compassionate concern with dispassionate objectivity; wishing to relieve pain and distress with making difficult and often painful decisions; and wanting to cure or control disease with accepting the realistic limits of the profession. Learning to balance those interrelated issues is critical to the prevention of depression and burn-out.

TABLE 1–5
CHECKLIST TO RATE SKILLS IN ESTABLISHING AND MAINTAINING RAPPORT

	YES	NO	N/A
1. I put the patient at ease.			
2. I recognized his state of mind.			
3. I addressed his distress.			
4. I helped him to warm up.			
5. I helped him to overcome suspiciousness.			
6. I curbed his intrusiveness.			
7. I stimulated his verbal production.			
8. I curbed his rambling.			
9. I understood his suffering.			
10. I expressed empathy for his suffering.			
11. I tuned in on his affect.			
12. I addressed his affect.			
13. I became aware of his level of insight.			
14. I assumed the patient's view of his disorder.			
15. I had a clear perception of the overt and the therapeutic goals of treatment.			
16. I stated the overt goal of treatment to him.			
17. I communicated to him that I am familiar with his illness.			
18. My questions convinced him that I am familiar with the symptoms of his disorder.			
19. I let him know that he is not alone with his illness.			
20. I expressed my intent to help him.			
21. The patient recognized my expertise.			
22. He respected my authority.			
23. He appeared fully cooperative.			
24. I recognized the patient's attitude toward his illness.			
25 The patient viewed his illness with distance.			
26. He presented himself as a sympathy-craving sufferer.			
27. He presented himself as a very important patient (VIP).			
28. He competed with me for leadership.			
29. He was submissive.			
30. I adjusted my role to the patient's role.			
31. The patient thanked me and made another appointment.			

Table from E Othmer, S L Othmer: *The Clinical Interview Using DSM-IV,* Vol 1, p 41. American Psychiatric Press, Washington, 1994. Used with permission.

The work of the physician involves constant contact with ill persons who are in pain, who are sad or fearful or suffering, and who will die. A feeling of futility and failure may permeate the physician's attitude, triggering feelings of anger or frustration directed toward one's profession, patients, and self. Unfortunately, the personality traits that draw many persons to the practice of medicine—for example, perfectionistic, controlling, obsessive—also place those persons at risk for maintaining a balanced outlook when coping with the stresses of the profession. Physicians who acquire self-knowledge, humor, and the traits of humility and kindness are likely to attain the balance necessary to meet the demands of their patients.

WHEN TO REFER TO THE PSYCHIATRIST

Primary care is a first-contact specialty, and primary care physicians are generally expected to deal with the mental and emotional concerns of their patients without psychiatric consultation. The primary care physician is an important resource for the psychiatrist. Physicians are often able to assess emotional illness early and, with timely and appropriate intervention, can reduce or eliminate the need for excessive psychiatric referral. In many situations, however, referral to the psychiatrist is advisable, and in some cases, essential.

Recognizing the many psychiatric disorders presented in the American Psychiatric Association's fourth edition of *Diagnostic and Statistical Manual of Mental Disorders* (DSM/IV), and possessing a detailed knowledge of drugs used in psychiatry, will enable the primary care physician to deal with most psychiatric problems. Skills in short-term psychodynamic psychotherapy, cognitive therapy, and family therapy will further expand the primary physician's therapeutic armamentarium.

A discussion of the psychotherapies is covered in Chapter 24.

Suicidal or Homicidal Patients

Suicidal or homicidal patients are perplexing persons to treat because determining whether the patient is likely to attempt suicide or homicide is difficult. Most patients with suicidal ideation suffer from depression, and treatment with an antidepressant drug can often reduce the risk of suicide. The patient should be referred to a psychiatrist to determine whether hospitalization is indicated if there are high risk factors for the patient attempting suicide or homicide, such as previous attempts, painful or disabling medical illness, recent stressors—for example, divorce, death of a loved one—or the patient has the means to carry out the act—for example, possesses a gun.

Physicians should have readily available a roster of psychiatrists to whom they can refer patients in emergencies. The patient must be accompanied by a responsible family member or friend during the interval between the time of the referral and the time of the scheduled psychiatric consultation, because it is dangerous to allow an actively suicidal patient to be unsupervised or to permit an unsupervised period to occur prior to psychiatric evaluation. Failure to discover a patient's suicidal or homicidal intent can result in harm to the patient or other persons, as well as a lawsuit against the primary care physician. An estimated one out of every two suicides leads to a malpractice action. Consultation with the psychiatrist provides a second opinion and timely intervention and protects the physician against liability.

Diagnostic Consultation

Diagnosis is a complex process and some clinicians are still grappling with the complexities of the various editions of DSM. The American Psychiatric Association has published a version of DSM/IV especially for primary care physicians which should prove more helpful in the diagnosis of patients.

A correct diagnosis of the disorder is critical in prescribing psychotropic medication. For example, the distinction between schizophrenia and bipolar disorders is often difficult, but the patient's disorder will only respond to a specific psychotropic medication: the schizophrenic condition responds to dopamine receptor antagonists antipsychotics; the bipolar disorder responds to lithium. When faced with a therapeutic nonresponse the primary care physician should reevaluate the diagnosis by obtaining a second opinion from the psychiatrist.

A patient who the primary care physician suspects is suffering from a psychotic disorder (characterized by hallucinations, delusions or generalized personality disorganization) should be referred to a psychiatrist. Psychotic disorders require complex management approaches that exceed the use of antipsychotic medication or lithium and include behavioral skills training, family-oriented therapies, and individual or group therapies; all are best coordinated by the psychiatrist.

Medication Management

The practice of pharmacotherapy encompasses: drug selection and prescription; administration of the drug; psychodynamic meaning of the drug to the patient; compliance of the patient; and family and environmental influences. A one-diagnosis-one-pill approach is rare.

Drugs must be used in effective doses for sufficient periods of time. The primary care physician may be excessively concerned with managing any adverse drug effects and thus may prescribe subtherapeutic doses and incomplete trials. Close continuing clinical observation is critical to the detection of the emergence of adverse effects and the evaluation of the patient's response to the drug. A referral to the psychiatrist should be made if the primary care physician notes the patient's response to treatment is inadequate or adverse effects are occurring. The psychiatrist will adjust the dosage and institute appropriate treatment for emergent adverse effects.

If drug treatment is ineffective, electroconvulsive therapy (ECT) may be needed, especially for catatonic patients and for elderly patients with major depression who are active suicidal risks. Psychiatrists are trained to administer those treatments.

Psychotherapy

The primary care physician is restrained from providing psychotherapy primarily because of time constraints. Some short-term therapies can be quickly learned (see Chapter 24), but effective patient outcomes are associated with a series of regularly

TABLE 1–6
GUIDELINES FOR PATIENT REFERRAL

It is important to exhibit confidence and enthusiasm when making a referral for psychiatric evaluation or psychotherapy. Patients will detect ambivalence and skepticism on the physician's part about the need for such treatment. It is usually helpful to recommend a psychiatrist or other mental health professional who is known *personally* by the physician.

Always present the psychiatric referral as part of the patient's ongoing medical care. Some patients view a psychiatric referral as a means to dump them onto another doctor or as a rejection. Patients should be reassured that any psychiatric treatment will be in parallel with their ongoing medical care.

Have the name and telephone number of your referral source readily available to give to the patient. Call the psychiatrist to personally explain the reason and need for the referral and what role you would like to continue to play in the patient's care.

Make the appointment for the psychiatric evaluation while the patient is still in the office or clinic.

Be sure to schedule a follow-up appointment after the date of the psychiatric evaluation to check on the patient's reaction to the referral and his or her response to the initial treatment.

Table from A Stoudemire: *Clinical Psychiatry for Medical Students,* p 457. Lippincott, Philadelphia, 1990. Used with permission.

scheduled sessions over a period of time. The primary care physician may have the experience and skill to treat a patient with one of the short-term techniques but, because of scheduling problems in a busy practice, could treat few patients. Although time-limited therapies are useful for some conditions, most emotional illnesses require a longer period of time for effective therapy. The primary care physician usually refers the patient to the psychiatrist who conducts the psychotherapy.

Guidelines for making the referral to the psychiatrist are listed in Table 1–6.

2
Psychiatric Signs and Symptoms

Psychiatry is concerned with phenomenology and the study of mental phenomena. Physicians must learn to be masters of precise observation and evocative description, and learning those skills involves the learning of a new language. Part of the language in psychiatry involves the recognition and the definition of behavioral and emotional signs and symptoms. *Signs* are objective findings observed by the clinician (for example, constricted affect and psychomotor retardation); *symptoms* are subjective experiences described by the patient (for example, depressed mood and decreased energy). A *syndrome* is a group of signs and symptoms that occur together as a recognizable condition that may be less specific than a clear-cut disorder or disease. Most psychiatric conditions are, in fact, syndromes. Becoming an expert in recognizing specific signs and symptoms allows the primary care physician to understandably communicate with psychiatrists and other clinicians, accurately make a diagnosis, effectively manage treatment, reliably predict a prognosis, and thoroughly explore pathophysiology, causes, and psychodynamic issues.

The outline that follows gives a comprehensive list of psychiatric signs and symptoms, each with a precise definition or description. Most of these signs and symptoms have their roots in essentially normal behavior and represent various points on the spectrum of behavior from normal to pathological.

I. Consciousness: state of awareness

Apperception: perception modified by one's own emotions and thoughts. Sensorium: state of cognitive functioning of the special senses (sometimes used as a synonym for consciousness). Disturbances of consciousness are most often associated with brain pathology.

A. Disturbances of consciousness
1. **Disorientation:** disturbance of orientation in time, place, or person
2. **Clouding of consciousness:** incomplete clear-mindedness with disturbances in perception and attitudes
3. **Stupor:** lack of reaction to and unawareness of surroundings
4. **Delirium:** bewildered, restless, confused, disoriented reaction associated with fear and hallucinations
5. **Coma:** profound degree of unconsciousness
6. **Coma vigil:** coma in which the patient appears to be asleep but ready to be aroused (also known as akinetic mutism)
7. **Twilight state:** disturbed consciousness with hallucinations
8. **Dreamlike state:** often used as a synonym for complex partial seizure or psychomotor epilepsy
9. **Somnolence:** abnormal drowsiness

B. Disturbances of attention: attention is the amount of effort exerted in focusing on certain portions of an experience; ability to sustain a focus on one activity; ability to concentrate

1. **Distractibility:** inability to concentrate attention; attention drawn to unimportant or irrelevant external stimuli
2. **Selective inattention:** blocking out only those things that generate anxiety
3. **Hypervigilance:** excessive attention and focus on all internal and external stimuli, usually secondary to delusional or paranoid states
4. **Trance:** focused attention and altered consciousness, usually seen in hypnosis, dissociative disorders, and ecstatic religious experiences

C. **Disturbances in suggestibility:** compliant and uncritical response to an idea or influence
   1. *Folie à deux* **(or** *folie à trois***):** communicated emotional illness between two (or three) persons
   2. **Hypnosis:** artificially induced modification of consciousness characterized by a heightened suggestibility

II. **Emotion:** a complex feeling state with psychic, somatic, and behavioral components that is related to affect and mood

   A. **Affect:** observed expression of emotion; may be inconsistent with patient's description of emotion
      1. **Appropriate affect:** condition in which the emotional tone is in harmony with the accompanying idea, thought, or speech; also further described as broad or full affect, in which a full range of emotions is appropriately expressed
      2. **Inappropriate affect:** disharmony between the emotional feeling tone and the idea, thought, or speech accompanying it
      3. **Blunted affect:** a disturbance in affect manifested by a severe reduction in the intensity of externalized feeling tone
      4. **Restricted or constricted affect:** reduction in intensity of feeling tone less severe than blunted affect but clearly reduced
      5. **Flat affect:** absence or near absence of any signs of affective expression; voice monotonous, face immobile
      6. **Labile affect:** rapid and abrupt changes in emotional feeling tone, unrelated to external stimuli

   B. **Mood:** a pervasive and sustained emotion, subjectively experienced and reported by the patient and observed by others; examples include depression, elation, anger
      1. **Dysphoric mood:** an unpleasant mood
      2. **Euthymic mood:** normal range of mood, implying absence of depressed or elevated mood
      3. **Expansive mood:** expression of one's feelings without restraint, frequently with an overestimation of one's significance or importance
      4. **Irritable mood:** easily annoyed and provoked to anger
      5. **Mood swings (labile mood):** oscillations between euphoria and depression or anxiety
      6. **Elevated mood:** air of confidence and enjoyment; a mood more cheerful than usual

    7. Euphoria: intense elation with feelings of grandeur

    8. Ecstasy: feeling of intense rapture

    9. Depression: psychopathological feeling of sadness

    10. Anhedonia: loss of interest in and withdrawal from all regular and pleasurable activities, often associated with depression

    11. Grief or mourning: sadness appropriate to a real loss

    12. Alexithymia: inability or difficulty in describing or being aware of one's emotions or mood

C. Other emotions

    1. Anxiety: feeling of apprehension caused by anticipation of danger, which may be internal or external

    2. Free-floating anxiety: pervasive, unfocused fear not attached to any idea

    3. Fear: anxiety caused by consciously recognized and realistic danger

    4. Agitation: severe anxiety associated with motor restlessness

    5. Tension: increased motor and psychological activity that is unpleasant

    6. Panic: acute, episodic, intense attack of anxiety associated with overwhelming feelings of dread and autonomic discharge

    7. Apathy: dulled emotional tone associated with detachment or indifference

    8. Ambivalence: coexistence of two opposing impulses toward the same thing in the same person at the same time

    9. Abreaction: emotional release or discharge after recalling a painful experience

    10. Shame: failure to live up to self-expectations

    11. Guilt: emotion secondary to doing what is perceived as wrong

D. Physiological disturbances associated with mood: signs of somatic (usually autonomic) dysfunction of the person, most often associated with depression (also called vegetative signs)

    1. Anorexia: loss of or decrease in appetite

    2. Hyperphagia: increase in appetite and intake of food

    3. Insomnia: lack of or diminished ability to sleep

        a. Initial: difficulty in falling asleep

        b. Middle: difficulty in sleeping through the night without waking up and difficulty in going back to sleep

        c. Terminal: early morning awakening

    4. Hypersomnia: excessive sleeping

    5. Diurnal variation: mood is regularly worst in the morning, immediately after awakening, and improves as the day progresses

    6. Diminished libido: decreased sexual interest, drive, and performance (increased libido is often associated with manic states)

    7. Constipation: inability or difficulty in defecating

III. Motor behavior (conation): the aspect of the psyche that includes impulses, motivations, wishes, drives, instincts, and cravings, as expressed by a person's behavior or motor activity.

1. **Echopraxia:** pathological imitation of movements of one person by another
2. **Catatonia:** motor anomalies in nonorganic disorders (as opposed to disturbances of consciousness and motor activity secondary to organic pathology)
   a. **Catalepsy:** general term for an immobile position that is constantly maintained
   b. **Catatonic excitement:** agitated, purposeless motor activity, uninfluenced by external stimuli
   c. **Catatonic stupor:** markedly slowed motor activity, often to a point of immobility and seeming unawareness of surroundings
   d. **Catatonic rigidity:** voluntary assumption of a rigid posture, held against all efforts to be moved
   e. **Catatonic posturing:** voluntary assumption of an inappropriate or bizarre posture, generally maintained for long periods of time
   f. *Cerea flexibilitas (waxy flexibility):* the person can be molded into a position that is then maintained; when the examiner moves the person's limb, the limb feels as if it were made of wax
3. **Negativism:** motiveless resistance to all attempts to be moved or to all instructions
4. **Cataplexy:** temporary loss of muscle tone and weakness precipitated by a variety of emotional states
5. **Stereotypy:** repetitive fixed pattern of physical action or speech
6. **Mannerism:** ingrained, habitual involuntary movement
7. **Automatism:** automatic performance of an act or acts generally representative of unconscious symbolic activity
8. **Command automatism:** automatic following of suggestions (also automatic obedience)
9. **Mutism:** voicelessness without structural abnormalities
10. **Overactivity**
    a. **Psychomotor agitation:** excessive motor and cognitive overactivity, usually nonproductive and in response to inner tension
    b. **Hyperactivity (hyperkinesis):** restless, aggressive, destructive activity, often associated with some underlying brain pathology
    c. **Tic:** involuntary, spasmodic motor movement
    d. **Sleepwalking (somnambulism):** motor activity during sleep
    e. **Akathisia:** subjective feeling of muscular tension secondary to antipsychotic or other medication, which can cause restlessness, pacing, repeated sitting and standing; can be mistaken for psychotic agitation
    f. **Compulsion:** uncontrollable impulse to perform an act repetitively
       i. **Dipsomania:** compulsion to drink alcohol
       ii. **Kleptomania:** compulsion to steal
       iii. **Nymphomania:** excessive and compulsive need for coitus in a woman
       iv. **Satyriasis:** excessive and compulsive need for coitus in a man
       v. **Trichotillomania:** compulsion to pull out one's hair

            vi. Ritual: automatic activity, compulsive in nature, anxiety-reducing in origin

       g. Ataxia: failure of muscle coordination; irregularity of muscle action

       h. Polyphagia: pathological overeating

11. Hypoactivity (hypokinesis): decreased motor and cognitive activity, as in psychomotor retardation; visible slowing of thought, speech, and movements

12. Mimicry: simple, imitative motor activity of childhood

13. Aggression: forceful goal-directed action that may be verbal or physical; the motor counterpart of the affect of rage, anger, or hostility

14. Acting out: direct expression of an unconscious wish or impulse in action; unconscious fantasy is lived out impulsively in behavior

15. Abulia: reduced impulse to act and think, associated with indifference about consequences of action; association with neurological deficit

IV. Thinking: goal-directed flow of ideas, symbols, and associations initiated by a problem or a task and leading toward a reality-oriented conclusion; when a logical sequence occurs, thinking is normal; parapraxis (unconsciously motivated lapse from logic is also called Freudian slip) considered part of normal thinking

A. General disturbances in form or process of thinking

1. Mental disorder: clinically significant behavior or psychological syndrome, associated with distress or disability, not just an expected response to a particular event or limited to relations between the person and society

2. Psychosis: inability to distinguish reality from fantasy; impaired reality testing, with the creation of a new reality (as opposed to neurosis: mental disorder in which reality testing is intact, behavior may not violate gross social norms, relatively enduring or recurrent without treatment)

3. Reality testing: the objective evaluation and judgment of the world outside the self

4. Formal thought disorder: disturbance in the form of thought, instead of the content of thought; thinking characterized by loosened associations, neologisms, and illogical constructs; thought process is disordered, and the person is defined as psychotic

5. Illogical thinking: thinking containing erroneous conclusions or internal contradictions; it is psychopathological only when it is marked and when not caused by cultural values or intellectual deficit

6. Dereism: mental activity not concordant with logic or experience

7. Autistic thinking: preoccupation with inner, private world; term used somewhat synonymously with dereism

8. Magical thinking: a form of dereistic thought; thinking that is similar to that of the preoperational phase in children (Jean Piaget), in which thoughts, words, or actions assume power (e.g., they can cause or prevent events)

    9. **Primary process thinking:** general term for thinking that is dereistic, illogical, magical; normally found in dreams, abnormally in psychosis

B. **Specific disturbances in form of thought**
    1. **Neologism:** new word created by the patient, often by combining syllables of other words, for idiosyncratic psychological reasons
    2. **Word salad:** incoherent mixture of words and phrases
    3. **Circumstantiality:** indirect speech that is delayed in reaching the point but eventually gets from original point to desired goal; characterized by an overinclusion of details and parenthetical remarks
    4. **Tangentiality:** inability to have goal-directed associations of thought; patient never gets from desired point to desired goal
    5. **Incoherence:** thought that, generally, is not understandable; running together of thoughts or words with no logical or grammatical connection, resulting in disorganization
    6. **Perseveration:** persisting response to a prior stimulus after a new stimulus has been presented, often associated with cognitive disorders
    7. **Verbigeration:** meaningless repetition of specific words or phrases
    8. **Echolalia:** psychopathological repeating of words or phrases of one person by another; tends to be repetitive and persistent, may be spoken with mocking or staccato intonation
    9. **Condensation:** fusion of various concepts into one
    10. **Irrelevant answer:** answer that is not in harmony with question asked (patient appears to ignore or not attend to question)
    11. **Loosening of associations:** flow of thought in which ideas shift from one subject to another in a completely unrelated way; when severe, speech may be incoherent
    12. **Derailment:** gradual or sudden deviation in train of thought without blocking; sometimes used synonymously with loosening of associations
    13. **Flight of ideas:** rapid, continuous verbalizations or plays on words produce constant shifting from one idea to another; the ideas tend to be connected, and in the less severe form a listener may be able to follow them
    14. **Clang association:** association of words similar in sound but not in meaning; words have no logical connection, may include rhyming and punning
    15. **Blocking:** abrupt interruption in train of thinking before a thought or idea is finished; after a brief pause, the person indicates no recall of what was being said or was going to be said (also known as thought deprivation)
    16. **Glossolalia:** the expression of a revelatory message through unintelligible words (also known as speaking in tongues); not considered a disturbance in thought if associated with practices of specific Pentecostal religions

C. **Specific disturbances in content of thought**
    1. **Poverty of content:** thought that gives little information because of vagueness, empty repetitions, or obscure phrases

2. **Overvalued idea:** unreasonable, sustained false belief maintained less firmly than a delusion
3. **Delusion:** false belief, based on incorrect inference about external reality, not consistent with patient's intelligence and cultural background, that cannot be corrected by reasoning
   a. **Bizarre delusion:** an absurd, totally implausible, strange false belief (e.g., invaders from space have implanted electrodes in the patient's brain)
   b. **Systematized delusion:** false belief or beliefs united by a single event or theme (e.g., patient is being persecuted by the CIA, the FBI, the Mafia, or the boss)
   c. **Mood-congruent delusion:** delusion with mood-appropriate content (e.g., a depressed patient believes that he or she is responsible for the destruction of the world)
   d. **Mood-incongruent delusion:** delusion with content that has no association to mood or is mood-neutral (e.g., a depressed patient has delusions of thought control or thought broadcasting)
   e. **Nihilistic delusion:** false feeling that self, others, or the world is nonexistent or ending
   f. **Delusion of poverty:** false belief that one is bereft or will be deprived of all material possessions
   g. **Somatic delusion:** false belief involving functioning of one's body (e.g., belief that one's brain is rotting or melting)
   h. **Paranoid delusions:** includes persecutory delusions and delusions of reference, control, and grandeur (distinguished from paranoid ideation, which is suspiciousness of less than delusional proportions)
      i. **Delusion of persecution:** false belief that one is being harassed, cheated, or persecuted; often found in litigious patients who have a pathological tendency to take legal action because of imagined mistreatment
      ii. **Delusion of grandeur:** exaggerated conception of one's importance, power, or identity
      iii. **Delusion of reference:** false belief that the behavior of others refers to oneself; that events, objects, or other people have a particular and unusual significance, usually of a negative nature; derived from idea of reference, in which one falsely feels that one is being talked about by others (e.g., belief that people on television or radio are talking to or about the patient)
   i. **Delusion of self-accusation:** false feeling of remorse and guilt
   j. **Delusion of control:** false feeling that one's will, thoughts, or feelings are being controlled by external forces
      i. **Thought withdrawal:** delusion that one's thoughts are being removed from one's mind by other people or forces
      ii. **Thought insertion:** delusion that thoughts are being implanted in one's mind by other people or forces
      iii. **Thought broadcasting:** delusion that one's thoughts can be heard by others, as though they were being broadcast into the air

    iv. Thought control: delusion that one's thoughts are being controlled by other people or forces

  k. Delusion of infidelity (delusional jealousy): false belief derived from pathological jealousy that one's lover is unfaithful

  l. Erotomania: delusional belief, more common in women than in men, that someone is deeply in love with them (also known as Clérambault-Kandinsky complex)

  m. *Pseudologia phantastica:* a type of lying, in which the person appears to believe in the reality of his or her fantasies and acts on them; associated with Munchausen syndrome, repeated feigning of illness

4. Trend or preoccupation of thought: centering of thought content on a particular idea, associated with a strong affective tone, such as a paranoid trend or a suicidal or homicidal preoccupation

5. Egomania: pathological self-preoccupation

6. Monomania: preoccupation with a single object

7. Hypochondria: exaggerated concern about one's health that is based not on real organic pathology but, rather, on unrealistic interpretations of physical signs or sensations as abnormal

8. Obsession: pathological persistence of an irresistible thought or feeling that cannot be eliminated from consciousness by logical effort, which is associated with anxiety (also termed rumination)

9. Compulsion: pathological need to act on an impulse that, if resisted, produces anxiety; repetitive behavior in response to an obsession or performed according to certain rules, with no true end in itself other than to prevent something from occurring in the future

10. Coprolalia: compulsive utterance of obscene words

11. Phobia: persistent, irrational, exaggerated, and invariably pathological dread of some specific type of stimulus or situation; results in a compelling desire to avoid the feared stimulus

  a. Specific phobia: circumscribed dread of a discrete object or situation (e.g., dread of spiders or snakes)

  b. Social phobia: dread of public humiliation, as in fear of public speaking, performing, or eating in public

  c. Acrophobia: dread of high places

  d. Agoraphobia: dread of open places

  e. Algophobia: dread of pain

  f. Ailurophobia: dread of cats

  g. Erythrophobia: dread of red (refers to a fear of blushing)

  h. Panphobia: dread of everything

  i. Claustrophobia: dread of closed places

  j. Xenophobia: dread of strangers

  k. Zoophobia: dread of animals

12. Noesis: a revelation in which immense illumination occurs in association with a sense that one has been chosen to lead and command

13. Unio mystica: an oceanic feeling, one of mystic unity with an infinite power; not considered a disturbance in thought content if congruent with patient's religious or cultural milieu

V. Speech: ideas, thoughts, feelings as expressed through language; communication through the use of words and language

A. Disturbances in speech
1. **Pressure of speech:** rapid speech that is increased in amount and difficult to interrupt
2. **Volubility (logorrhea):** copious, coherent, logical speech
3. **Poverty of speech:** restriction in the amount of speech used; replies may be monosyllabic
4. **Nonspontaneous speech:** verbal responses given only when asked or spoken to directly; no self-initiation of speech
5. **Poverty of content of speech:** speech that is adequate in amount but conveys little information because of vagueness, emptiness, or stereotyped phrases
6. **Dysprosody:** loss of normal speech melody (called prosody)
7. **Dysarthria:** difficulty in articulation, not in word finding or in grammar
8. **Excessively loud or soft speech:** loss of modulation of normal speech volume; may reflect a variety of pathological conditions ranging from psychosis to depression to deafness
9. **Stuttering:** frequent repetition or prolongation of a sound or syllable, leading to markedly impaired speech fluency
10. **Cluttering:** erratic and dysrhythmic speech, consisting of rapid and jerky spurts

B. Aphasic disturbances: disturbances in language output
1. **Motor aphasia:** disturbance of speech caused by a cognitive disorder in which understanding remains but ability to speak is grossly impaired; speech is halting, laborious, and inaccurate (also known as Broca's, nonfluent, and expressive aphasia)
2. **Sensory aphasia:** organic loss of ability to comprehend the meaning of words; speech is fluid and spontaneous but incoherent and nonsensical (also known as Wernicke's, fluent, and receptive aphasia)
3. **Nominal aphasia:** difficulty in finding correct name for an object (also termed anomia and amnestic aphasia)
4. **Syntactical aphasia:** inability to arrange words in proper sequence
5. **Jargon aphasia:** words produced are totally neologistic; nonsense words repeated with various intonations and inflections
6. **Global aphasia:** combination of a grossly nonfluent aphasia and a severe fluent aphasia

VI. Perception: process of transferring physical stimulation into psychological information; mental process by which sensory stimuli are brought to awareness

A. Disturbances of perception
1. **Hallucination:** false sensory perception not associated with real external stimuli; there may or may not be a delusional interpretation of the hallucinatory experience

a. **Hypnagogic hallucination:** false sensory perception occurring while falling asleep; generally considered nonpathological phenomenon

b. **Hypnopompic hallucination:** false perception occurring while awakening from sleep; generally considered nonpathological

c. **Auditory hallucination:** false perception of sound, usually voices but also other noises, such as music; most common hallucination in psychiatric disorders

d. **Visual hallucination:** false perception involving sight consisting of both formed images (e.g., people) and unformed images (e.g., flashes of light); most common in medically determined disorders

e. **Olfactory hallucination:** false perception of smell; most common in medical disorders

f. **Gustatory hallucination:** false perception of taste, such as unpleasant taste caused by an uncinate seizure; most common in medical disorders

g. **Tactile (haptic) hallucination:** false perception of touch or surface sensation, as from an amputated limb (phantom limb), crawling sensation on or under the skin (formication)

h. **Somatic hallucination:** false sensation of things occurring in or to the body, most often visceral in origin (also known as cenesthesic hallucination)

i. **Lilliputian hallucination:** false perception in which objects are seen as reduced in size (also termed micropsia)

j. **Mood-congruent hallucination:** hallucination in which the content is consistent with either a depressed or a manic mood (e.g., a depressed patient hears voices saying that the patient is a bad person; a manic patient hears voices saying that the patient is of inflated worth, power, and knowledge)

k. **Mood-incongruent hallucination:** hallucination in which the content is not consistent with either depressed or manic mood (e.g., in depression, hallucinations not involving such themes as guilt, deserved punishment, or inadequacy; in mania, hallucinations not involving such themes as inflated worth or power)

l. **Hallucinosis:** hallucinations, most often auditory, that are associated with chronic alcohol abuse and that occur within a clear sensorium, as opposed to delirium tremens (DTs), hallucinations that occur in the context of a clouded sensorium

m. **Synesthesia:** sensation or hallucination caused by another sensation (e.g., an auditory sensation is accompanied by or triggers a visual sensation; a sound is experienced as being seen, or a visual experience is heard)

n. **Trailing phenomenon:** perceptual abnormality associated with hallucinogenic drugs in which moving objects are seen as a series of discrete and discontinuous images

2. **Illusion:** misperception or misinterpretation of real external sensory stimuli

B. **Disturbances associated with cognitive disorder:** agnosia—an inability to recognize and interpret the significance of sensory impressions
   1. **Anosognosia (ignorance of illness):** inability to recognize a neurological deficit as occurring to oneself
   2. **Somatopagnosia (ignorance of the body):** inability to recognize a body part as one's own (also called autopagnosia)
   3. **Visual agnosia:** inability to recognize objects or persons
   4. **Astereognosis:** inability to recognize objects by touch
   5. **Prosopagnosia:** inability to recognize faces
   6. **Apraxia:** inability to carry out specific tasks
   7. **Simultagnosia:** inability to comprehend more than one element of a visual scene at a time or to integrate the parts into a whole
   8. **Adiadochokinesia:** inability to perform rapid alternating movements.

C. **Disturbances associated with conversion and dissociative phenomena:** somatization of repressed material or the development of physical symptoms and distortions involving the voluntary muscles or special sense organs; not under voluntary control and not explained by any physical disorder
   1. **Hysterical anesthesia:** loss of sensory modalities resulting from emotional conflicts
   2. **Macropsia:** state in which objects seem larger than they are
   3. **Micropsia:** state in which objects seem smaller than they are (both macropsia and micropsia can also be associated with clear organic conditions, such as complex partial seizures)
   4. **Depersonalization:** a subjective sense of being unreal, strange, or unfamiliar to oneself
   5. **Derealization:** a subjective sense that the environment is strange or unreal; a feeling of changed reality
   6. **Fugue:** taking on a new identity with amnesia for the old identity; often involves travel or wandering to new environments
   7. **Multiple personality:** one person who appears at different times to be two or more entirely different personalities and characters (called dissociative identity disorder in the fourth edition of *Diagnostic and Statistical Manual of Mental Disorders* [DSM-IV])

VII. **Memory:** function by which information stored in the brain is later recalled to consciousness

A. **Disturbances of memory**
   1. **Amnesia:** partial or total inability to recall past experiences; may be organic or emotional in origin
      a. **Anterograde:** amnesia for events occurring after a point in time
      b. **Retrograde:** amnesia prior to a point in time
   2. **Paramnesia:** falsification of memory by distortion of recall
      a. *Fausse reconnaissance:* false recognition
      b. **Retrospective falsification:** memory becomes unintentionally

(unconsciously) distorted by being filtered through patient's present emotional, cognitive, and experiential state

   c. Confabulation: unconscious filling of gaps in memory by imagined or untrue experiences that patient believes but that have no basis in fact; most often associated with organic pathology

   d. Déjà vu: illusion of visual recognition in which a new situation is incorrectly regarded as a repetition of a previous memory

   e. *Déjà entendu:* illusion of auditory recognition

   f. *Déjà pensé:* illusion that a new thought is recognized as a thought previously felt or expressed

   g. *Jamais vu:* false feeling of unfamiliarity with a real situation one has experienced

  3. Hypermnesia: exaggerated degree of retention and recall

  4. Eidetic image: visual memory of almost hallucinatory vividness

  5. Screen memory: a consciously tolerable memory covering for a painful memory

  6. Repression: defense mechanism characterized by unconscious forgetting of unacceptable ideas or impulses

  7. Lethologica: temporary inability to remember a name or a proper noun

B. Levels of memory

  1. Immediate: reproduction or recall of perceived material within seconds to minutes

  2. Recent: recall of events over past few days

  3. Recent past: recall of events over past few months

  4. Remote: recall of events in distant past

VIII. Intelligence: the ability to understand, recall, mobilize, and constructively integrate previous learning in meeting new situations

A. Mental retardation: lack of intelligence to a degree in which there is interference with social and vocational performance: mild (I.Q. of 50 or 55 to approximately 70), moderate (I.Q. of 35 or 40 to 50 or 55), severe (I.Q. of 20 or 25 to 35 or 40), or profound (I.Q. below 20 or 25); obsolete terms are idiot (mental age less than 3 years), imbecile (mental age of 3 to 7 years), and moron (mental age of about 8)

B. Dementia: organic and global deterioration of intellectual functioning without clouding of consciousness

  1. Dyscalculia (acalculia): loss of ability to do calculations not caused by anxiety or impairment in concentration

  2. Dysgraphia (agraphia): loss of ability to write in cursive style; loss of word structure

  3. Alexia: loss of a previously possessed reading facility; not explained by defective visual acuity

C. Pseudodementia: clinical features resembling a dementia not caused by an organic condition; most often caused by depression (dementia syndrome of depression)

D. Concrete thinking: literal thinking; limited use of metaphor without understanding of nuances of meaning; one-dimensional thought

E. Abstract thinking: ability to appreciate nuances of meaning; multidimensional thinking with ability to use metaphors and hypotheses appropriately

IX. Insight: ability of the patient to understand the true cause and meaning of a situation (such as a set of symptoms)

A. Intellectual insight: understanding of the objective reality of a set of circumstances without the ability to apply the understanding in any useful way to master the situation

B. True insight: understanding of the objective reality of a situation, coupled with the motivation and the emotional impetus to master the situation

C. Impaired insight: diminished ability to understand the objective reality of a situation

X. Judgment: ability to assess a situation correctly and to act appropriately within that situation

A. Critical judgment: ability to assess, discern, and choose among various options in a situation

B. Automatic judgment: reflex performance of an action

C. Impaired judgment: diminished ability to understand a situation correctly and to act appropriately

---

For a more detailed discussion of this topic, see H I Kaplan, B J Sadock: Typical Signs and Symptoms of Psychiatric Illness, Sec 9.3, p 535; J Yager, M J Gitlin: Clinical Manifestations of Psychiatric Disorders, Chap 10, p 637; Classification of Mental Disorders, Chap 11, pp 671–703, in CTP/VI.

3
Psychiatric History and Mental Status Examination

PSYCHIATRIC HISTORY

The psychiatric history is a life story told to the physician in the patient's own words. Many times the history also includes information from persons such as a parent or a spouse. A comprehensive patient history allows the physician to understand who the patient is, where the patient has come from, and where the patient is likely to go in the future—it is essential for a correct diagnosis and an effective treatment plan. The functions and objectives of the psychiatric history differ little from the medical interview (Table 3–1).

Doctors strive to glean from the psychiatric history insight into the patients' personality traits; their personal strengths and weaknesses; their closest personal relationships, both past and present; and their developmental history. This information is best elicited by allowing patients to tell their stories in their own words. Skillful interviewers recognize where to introduce additional questions so that all relevant areas are covered (Table 3–2).

MENTAL STATUS EXAMINATION

A patient's history remains stable; however, mental status can change daily or hourly. The mental status examination is a description of the patient's appearance, speech, actions, and thoughts during the interview. Even mute, incoherent, or uncooperative patients can communicate volumes to physicians who make careful observations. Although practitioners differ in how they organize the mental status examination, the format must contain certain categories of information (Table 3–3).

MEDICAL AND NEUROLOGICAL EXAMINATION

Psychiatric disorders that have an organic or medical cause (for example, depression secondary to meningioma) require a neurological or medical examination. Chapter 4 discusses these examinations in more detail.

RECORDING RESULTS

By the end of the examination, the physician decides whether psychosis is present, diagnoses any organic or medical disorders, and judges if the patient is suicidal or homicidal. Diagnostic classification is made according to the fourth edition of the American Psychiatric Association's *Diagnostic and Statistical Manual for Mental Disorders* (DSM-IV). DSM-IV uses a multiaxial classification scheme consisting of five axes, each of which should be covered in the diagnosis:

TABLE 3–1
THE THREE FUNCTIONS OF THE MEDICAL INTERVIEW

Functions	Objectives	Skills
I. Determining the nature of the problem	1. To enable the clinician to establish a diagnosis or recommend further diagnostic procedures, suggest a course of treatment, and predict the nature of the illness.	1. Knowledge base of diseases, disorders, problems, and clinical hypotheses from multiple conceptual domains: biomedical, sociocultural, psychodynamic, and behavioral. 2. Ability to elicit data for the above conceptual domains (encouraging the patient to tell his or her story, organizing the flow of the interview, the form of questions, the characterization of symptoms, the mental status examination). 3. Ability to perceive data from multiple sources (history, mental status exam, physician's subjective response to patient, nonverbal cues, listening at multiple levels.) 4. Hypothesis generation and testing. 5. Developing a therapeutic relationship (function II).
II. Developing and maintaining a therapeutic relationship	1. The patient's willingness to provide diagnostic information. 2. Relief of physical and psychological distress. 3. Willingness to accept treatment plan or a process of negotiation. 4. Patient satisfaction. 5. Physician satisfaction.	1. Defining the nature of the relationship. 2. Allowing the patient to tell his or her story. 3. Hearing, bearing, and tolerating the patient's expression of painful feelings. 4. Appropriate and genuine interest, empathy, support, and cognitive understanding. 5. Attending to common patient concerns over embarrassment, shame, and humiliation. 6. Elicitation of the patient's perspective. 7. Determining the nature of the problem (function I). 8. Communicating information and recommending treatment (function III).
III. Communicating information and implementing a treatment plan	1. The patient's understanding of the nature of the illness. 2. The patient's understanding of suggested diagnostic procedures. 3. The patient's understanding of the treatment possibilities. 4. Achievements of consensus between physician and patient over the above items 1–3. 5. Achievement of informed consent. 6. Improve coping mechanisms. 7. Lifestyle change.	1. Determining the nature of the problem (function I). 2. Developing a therapeutic relationship (function II). 3. Establishing the differences in perspective between physician and patient. 4. Educational strategies. 5. Clinical negotiations for conflict resolutions.

Table from A Lazare, I Bird, M Lipkin Jr, S Putnam: Three functions of the medical interview: An integrative conceptual framework. In *The Medical Interview*, M Lipkin Jr, S Putnam, A Lazare, editors. Springer-Verlag. New York, 1989. Used with permission.

TABLE 3–2
PSYCHIATRIC HISTORY

Topics	Questions/Comments
Identifying data: Name, age, race, sex, marital status, religion, education, address, phone number, occupation, source of referral, source of information if patient cannot cooperate.	This may be recorded while writing up the interview.
Chief complaint (CC): Brief statement in patient's own words of why patient is in the hospital or is being seen in consultation.	"Why are you coming to see a psychiatrist?" "What brought you to the hospital?" "What seems to be the problem?" Record answers verbatim.
History of present illness (HPI): Development of symptoms from time of onset to present; relation of life events, conflicts, stressors; drugs; change from previous level of functioning.	Record in patient's own words as much as possible. Get history of previous hospitalizations and treatment.
Previously psychiatric and medical disorders: Psychiatric disorders; psychosomatic, medical, neurological illnesses (craniocerebral trauma, convulsions).	Ascertain extent of illness, treatment, medications, outcomes, hospitals, doctors. Determine whether illness serves some additional purpose (secondary gain).
Personal history:	
Birth and infancy	To the extent known by the patient, ascertain mother's pregnancy and delivery, planned or unwanted pregnancy, developmental landmarks—standing, walking, talking, temperament.
Childhood	Feeding habits, toilet training, personality (shy, outgoing), general conduct and behavior, relationship with parents or caregivers, peers. Separations, nightmares, bedwetting, fears.
Adolescence	Peer and authority relationships, school history, grades, emotional problems, drug use, age of puberty.
Adulthood	Work history, choice of career, marital history, children, education, finances, military history, religion.
Sexual history: Sexual development, masturbation, anorgasmia, impotence, premature ejaculation, paraphilia, sexual orientation, general attitudes and feelings.	"Are there or have there been any problems or concerns about your sex life?" "How did you learn about sex?"
Family history: Psychiatric, medical, and genetic illnesses in mother, father, siblings; age of parents and occupations; if deceased, date and cause. Feelings about each family member, finances.	Get medication history of family (medications effective in family members for similar disorders may be effective in patient). "Describe your living conditions." "Did you have your own room?"

- **Axis I: Clinical syndromes**—Mental disorders (e.g., schizophrenia, bipolar disorder); other conditions that may be a focus of clinical attention but are not sufficiently severe to warrant a psychiatric diagnosis (e.g., relational problems, bereavement); borderline intellectual functioning is not listed here.
- **Axis II: Personality disorders and mental retardation**—Mental retardation and personality disorders; defense mechanisms and personality traits. Diagnoses on Axis I and Axis II can coexist. The Axis I or Axis II condition that is responsible for bringing the patient to the psychiatrist or hospital is called the principal or main diagnosis.
- **Axis III: Physical disorders or conditions**—Physical disorders (e.g., cirrhosis).
- **Axis IV: Psychosocial and environmental problems**—Stress in the patient's life (e.g., divorce, injury, death of a loved one).

TABLE 3–3
MENTAL STATUS EXAMINATION

Topics	Questions
General appearance: Note appearance, gait, dress, grooming (neat or unkempt), posture, gestures, facial expressions. Does patient appear older or younger than stated age?	Introduce yourself and direct patient to take a seat. In the hospital, bring your chair to bedside, do not sit on the bed. *Suggestions:* Unkempt and disheveled in organic or medical disorder; pinpoint pupils in narcotic addiction; withdrawal and stooped posture in depression.
Motoric behavior: Level of activity—psychomotor agitation or psychomotor retardation—tics, tremors, automatisms, mannerisms, grimacing, stereotypes, negativism, apraxia, echopraxia, waxy flexibility; emotional appearance—anxious, tense, panicky, bewildered, sad, unhappy; voice—faint, loud, hoarse; eye contact.	You may ask about obvious mannerisms, e.g. "I notice that your hand still shakes; can you tell me about that?" *Suggestions:* Fixed posturing, odd behavior in schizophrenia. Hyperactive with stimulant (cocaine) abuse and in mania. Psychomotor retardation in depression; tremors with anxiety. Eye contact is normally made approximately half the time during the interview.
Attitude during interview: How patient relates to examiner—irritable, aggressive, seductive, guarded, defensive, indifferent, apathetic, cooperative, sarcastic.	Comment about attitude. "You seem irritated about something; is that an accurate observation?" *Suggestions:* Suspiciousness in paranoia; seductive in hysteria; apathetic in medical illness or dementia.
Mood: Steady or sustained emotional state—gloomy, tense, hopeless, ecstatic, resentful, happy, bashful, sad, exultant, elated, euphoric, depressed, apathetic, anhedonic, fearful, suicidal, grandiose, nihilistic.	"How do you feel?" "How are your spirits?" "Do you have thoughts that life is not worth living or that you want to harm yourself?" "Do you have plans to take your own life?" "Do you want to die?" *Suggestions:* Suicidal ideas in 25% of depressives; elation in mania.
Affect: Feeling tone associated with idea—labile, blunt, appropriate to content, inappropriate, flat, *la belle indifférence*.	Observe nonverbal signs of emotion, body movement, facies, rhythm of voice (prosody). *Suggestions:* Changes in affect usual with schizophrenia; loss of prosody in organic or medical disorder, catatonia.
Speech: Slow, fast, pressured, garrulous, spontaneous, taciturn, stammering, stuttering, slurring, staccato. Pitch, articulation, aphasia, coprolalia, echolalia, incoherent, logorrhea, mute, paucity, stilted.	Ask patient to say "Methodist Episcopalian" to test for dysarthria. *Suggestions:* Manic patients show pressured speech; paucity of speech in depression; uneven or slurred speech in organic illness.
Perceptual disorders: Hallucinations—olfactory, auditory, haptic (tactile), gustatory, visual; illusions; hypnopompic or hypnagogic experiences; feelings of unreality, déjà vu, *déjà entendu*, macropsia.	"Do you ever see things or hear voices?" "Do you have strange experiences as you fall asleep or upon awakening?" "Has the world changed in any way?" *Suggestions:* Visual hallucinations suggest schizophrenia. Tactile hallucinations suggest cocainism, delirium tremens (DTs).

Continued

TABLE 3-3—*continued*

Topics	Questions
Thought content: Delusions—persecutory (paranoid), grandiose, infidelity, somatic, sensory, thought broadcasting, thought insertion, ideas of reference, ideas of unreality, phobias, obsessions, compulsions, ambivalence, autism, dereism, blocking, suicidal or homicidal preoccupation, conflicts, nihilistic ideas, hypochondriasis, depersonalization, derealization, flight of ideas, *idée fixe*, magical thinking, neologisms.	"Do you feel people want to harm you?" "Do you have special powers?" "Is anyone trying to influence you?" "Do you have strange body sensations?" "Are there thoughts that you can't get out of your mind?" "Do you think about the end of the world?" Ask about fantasies and dreams. *Suggestions:* Are delusions congruent with mood (grandiose delusions with elated mood) or incongruent? Mood, incongruent delusions point to schizophrenia. Illusions are common in delirium.
Thought process: Goal-directed ideas, loosened associations, illogical, tangential, relevant, circumstantial, rambling, ability to abstract, flight of ideas, clang associations, perseveration.	Ask meaning of proverbs to test abstraction, e.g., "People in glass houses should not throw stones." Concrete answer is, "Glass breaks." Abstract answers deal with projection, morality, criticism. Ask similarity between bird and butterfly (both alive), bread and cake (both food). *Suggestions:* Loose associations point to schizophrenia; flight of ideas, to mania; inability to abstract, to schizophrenia, brain damage.
Sensorium: Level of consciousness—alert, clear, confused, clouded, comatose, stuporous; orientation to time, place, person; cognition.	"What place is this?" "What is today's date?" "Do you know who I am?" "Do you know who you are?" *Suggestions:* Delirium or dementia shows clouded or wandering sensorium. Orientation to person remains intact longer than orientation to time or place.
Memory: **Remote memory (long-term memory)**	"Where were you born?" "Where did you go to school?" "Date of marriage?" "Birthdays of children?" "What were last week's newspaper headlines?" *Suggestions:* Patients with dementia of the Alzheimer's type retain remote memory longer than recent memory. Hypermnesia is seen in paranoid personality. Gaps in memory may be localized or filled in with confabulatory details.
Recent memory	"Where were you yesterday?" "What did you eat at your last meal?" In organic brain disease, recent memory loss (amnesia) usually occurs before remote memory loss.
Immediate memory **(short-term memory)**	Ask patient to repeat six digits forward, then backward (normal response). Ask patient to try to remember three nonrelated items; test patient after 5 minutes. *Suggestions:* Loss of memory occurs with organicity, dissociative disorder, conversion disorder. Anxiety can impair immediate retention and recent memory. Anterograde memory loss (amnesia) occurs after taking certain drugs, e.g., benzodiazepines.

Continued

TABLE 3–3—*continued*

Topics	Questions
Concentration and calculation: Ability to pay attention, distractibility, ability to do simple math.	Ask patient to count from 1 to 20 rapidly; do simple calculations (2 × 3, 4 × 9); do serial 7 test, i.e., subtract 7 from 100 and keep subtracting 7. "How many nickels in $1.35?" *Suggestions:* Rule out organic cause versus anxiety or depression (pseudodementia).
Information and intelligence: Use of vocabulary, level of education, fund of knowledge.	"Distance from New York City to Los Angeles." "Name some vegetables." "What is the largest river in the United States?" *Suggestions:* Check educational level to judge results. Rule out mental retardation, borderline intellectual functioning.
Judgment: Ability to understand relationships between facts and to draw conclusions; response in social situations.	"What is the thing to do if you find an envelope in the street that is sealed, stamped, and addressed?" *Suggestions:* Impaired in organic brain disease, schizophrenia, borderline intellectual functioning, intoxication.
Insight level: Realizing that there is physical or mental problem; denial of illness, ascribing blame to outside factors; recognizing need for treatment.	"Do you think you have a problem?" "Do you need treatment?" "What are your plans for the future?" *Suggestions:* Impaired in delirium, dementia, frontal lobe syndrome, psychosis, borderline intellectual functioning.

- **Axis V: Global assessment of functioning (GAF)**—The patient's highest level of social, occupational, and psychological functioning according to the GAF scale (Table 3–4). Examiners should use the 12 months prior to the current evaluation as a reference point and rate from 0 (inadequate information) to 1 (lowest) to 100 (highest).

Table 3–5 shows the DSM-IV multiaxial evaluation form, which can serve as a useful template to record the diagnosis. Primary care physicians may prefer to use the alternative nonaxial format (Table 3–6).

A sample DSM-IV diagnosis could look like this:

Axis I	Schizophrenia, catatonic type
Axis II	Borderline personality disorder
Axis III	Hypertension
Axis IV	Psychosocial problem: death of mother
Axis V	Current global assessment of functioning: 30 (behavior influenced by dementia)

After diagnosis, there are four other areas to be covered:

1. **Psychodynamic formulation**—Describe the defense mechanism used to control anxiety and summarize psychological factors, including precipitating events that account for illness. Table 3–7 presents a glossary of defense mechanisms and coping styles.
2. **Differential diagnosis**—List other mental and physical disorders to rule out.

TABLE 3–4
GLOBAL ASSESSMENT OF FUNCTIONING (GAF) SCALE

Consider psychological, social, and occupational functioning on a hypothetical continuum of mental health-illness. Do not include impairment in functioning due to physical (or environmental) limitations.

Code   (Note: Use intermediate codes when appropriate, e.g., 45, 68, 72)

91–100   Superior functioning in a wide range of activities, life's problems never seem to get out of hand, is sought out by others because of his or her many positive qualities. No symptoms.

81–90   Absent or minimal symptoms (e.g., mild anxiety before an exam), good functioning in all areas, interested and involved in a wide range of activities, society effective, generally satisfied with life, no more than everyday problems or concerns (e.g., an occasional argument with family members).

71–80   If symptoms are present, they are transient and expectable reactions to psychosocial stressors (e.g., difficulty concentrating after family argument): no more than slight impairment in social, occupational, or school functioning (e.g., temporarily falling behind in schoolwork).

61–70   Some mild symptoms (e.g., depressed mood and mild insomnia) OR some difficulty in social, occupational, or school functioning (e.g., occasional truancy or theft within the household), but generally functioning pretty well, has some meaningful interpersonal relationships.

51–60   Moderate symptoms (e.g., flat affect and circumstantial speech, occasional panic attacks) OR moderate difficulty in social, occupational, or school functioning (e.g., few friends, conflicts with peers or coworkers).

41–50   Serious symptoms (e.g., suicidal ideation, severe obsessional rituals, frequent shoplifting) OR any serious impairment in social, occupational, or school functioning (e.g., no friends, unable to keep a job).

31–40   Some impairment in reality testing or communication (e.g., speech is at times illogical, obscure, or irrelevant) OR major impairment in several areas, such as work or school, family relations, judgment, thinking, or mood (e.g., depressed man avoids friends, neglects family, and is unable to work; child frequently beats up younger children, is defiant at home, and is failing at school).

21–30   Behavior is considerably influenced by delusions or hallucinations OR serious impairment in communication or judgment (e.g., sometimes incoherent, acts grossly inappropriately, suicidal preoccupation) OR inability to function in almost all areas (e.g., stays in bed all day; no job, home, or friends).

11–20   Some danger of hurting self or others (e.g., suicide attempts without clear expectation of death; frequently violent; manic excitement) OR occasionally fails to maintain minimal personal hygiene (e.g., smears feces) OR gross impairment in communication (e.g., largely incoherent or mute).

0–10   Persistent danger of severely hurting self or others (e.g., recurrent violence) OR persistent inability to maintain minimal personal hygiene OR serious suicidal act with clear expectation of death.

0   Inadequate information.

Table from DSM-IV, *Diagnostic and Statistical Manual of Mental Disorders*, ed 4. Copyright American Psychiatric Association, Washington, 1994. Used with permission.

3. **Prognosis**—Describe the course of the illness and expected outcome based on history, mental status, and prognostic factors.
4. **Treatment plan**—Describe the treatment (i.e., psychotherapy, drug therapy, behavior modification, or hospitalization); note referrals to a psychiatrist, psychologist, or social worker; and include an assessment of the patient's cooperativeness, reliability, judgment, insight, and intelligence.

TABLE 3–5
MULTIAXIAL EVALUATION REPORT FORM

The following form is offered as one possibility for reporting multiaxial evaluations. In some settings, this form may be used exactly as is; in other settings, the form may be adapted to satisfy special needs.

AXIS I: Clinical Disorders
    Other Conditions That May Be a Focus of Clinical Attention

Diagnostic code   DSM-IV name

——— ——— ——— . ——— ———   _____
——— ——— ——— . ——— ———   _____
——— ——— ——— . ——— ———   _____

AXIS II: Personality Disorders
    Mental Retardation

Diagnostic code   DSM-IV name

——— ——— ——— . ——— ———   _____
——— ——— ——— . ——— ———   _____

AXIS III: General Medical Conditions

ICD-9-CM code   ICD-9-CM name

——— ——— ——— . ——— ———   _____
——— ——— ——— . ——— ———   _____
——— ——— ——— . ——— ———   _____

AXIS IV: Psychosocial and Environmental Problems

Check:
□ Problems with primary support group   *Specify:* _____
□ Problems related to the social environment   *Specify:* _____
□ Educational problems   *Specify:* _____
□ Occupational problems   *Specify:* _____
□ Housing problems   *Specify:* _____
□ Economic problems   *Specify:* _____
□ Problems with access to health care services   *Specify:* _____
□ Problems related to interaction with the legal system/crime   *Specify:* _____
□ Other psychosocial and environmental problems   *Specify:* _____

AXIS V: Global Assessment of Functioning Scale   Score: ——— ——— ———
                                                          Time frame: _____

Table from DSM-IV, *Diagnostic and Statistical Manual of Mental Disorders,* ed 4. Copyright American Psychiatric Association, Washington, 1994. Used with permission.

TABLE 3–6
NONAXIAL FORMAT

Clinicians who do not wish to use the multiaxial format may simply list the appropriate diagnoses. Those choosing this option should follow the general rule of recording as many coexisting mental disorders, general medical conditions, and other factors that are relevant to the care and treatment of the individual. The principal diagnosis or the reason for visit should be listed first. The examples listed below illustrate the reporting of diagnosis in a format that does not use the multiaxial system.

Example 1:
  Major depressive disorder, single episode, severe without psychotic features
  Alcohol abuse
  Dependent personality disorder
    Frequent use of denial

Example 2:
  Dysthymic disorder
  Reading disorder
  Otitis media, recurrent

Example 3:
  Mood disorder due to hypothyroidism, with depressive features
  Hypothyroidism
  Chronic angle-closure glaucoma
    Histrionic personality features

Example 4:
  Partner relational problems

TABLE 3–7
GLOSSARY OF SPECIFIC DEFENSE MECHANISMS AND COPING STYLES

acting out The individual deals with emotional conflict or internal or external stressors by actions rather than reflections or feelings. This definition is broader than the original concept of the acting out of transference feelings or wishes during psychotherapy and is intended to include behavior arising both within and outside the transference relationship. Defensive acting out is not synonymous with "bad behavior" because it requires evidence that the behavior is related to emotional conflicts.

affiliation The individual deals with emotional conflict or internal or external stressors by turning to others for help or support. This involves sharing problems with others but does not imply trying to make someone else responsible for them.

altruism The individual deals with emotional conflict or internal or external stressors by dedication to meeting the needs of others. Unlike the self-sacrifice sometimes characteristic of reaction formation, the individual receives gratification either vicariously or from the response of others.

anticipation The individual deals with emotional conflict or internal or external stressors by experiencing emotional reactions in advance of, or anticipating consequences of, possible future events and considering realistic, alternative responses or solutions.

autistic fantasy The individual deals with emotional conflict or internal or external stressors by excessive daydreaming as a substitute for human relationships, more effective action, or problem solving.

denial The individual deals with emotional conflict or internal or external stressors by refusing to acknowledge some painful aspect of external reality or subjective experience that would be apparent to others. The term *psychotic denial* is used when there is gross impairment in reality testing.

devaluation The individual deals with emotional conflict or internal or external stressors by attributing exaggerated negative qualities to self or others.

displacement The individual deals with emotional conflict or internal or external stressors by transferring a feeling about, or a response to, one object onto another (usually less threatening) substitute object.

dissociation The individual deals with emotional conflict or internal or external stressors with a breakdown in the usually integrated functions or consciousness, memory, perception of self or the environment, or sensory/motor behavior.

help-rejecting complaining The individual deals with emotional conflict or internal or external stressors by complaining or molding repetitious requests for help that disguise covert feelings of hostility or reproach toward others, which are then expressed by rejecting the suggestions, advice, or help that others offer. The complaints or requests may involve physical or psychological symptoms or life problems.

Continued

TABLE 3–7—*continued*

humor The individual deals with emotional conflict or external stressors by emphasizing the amusing or ironic aspects of the conflict or stressor.

idealization The individual deals with emotional conflict or internal or external stressors by attributing exaggerated positive qualities to others.

intellectualization The individual deals with emotional conflict or internal or external stressors by the excessive use of abstract thinking or the making of generalizations to control or minimize disturbing feelings.

isolation of affect The individual deals with emotional conflict or internal or external stressors by the separation of ideas from the feelings originally associated with them. The individual loses touch with the feelings associated with a given idea (e.g., a traumatic event) while remaining aware of the cognitive elements of it (e.g., descriptive details).

omnipotence The individual deals with emotional conflict or internal or external stressors by feeling or acting as if he or she possesses special powers or abilities and is superior to others.

passive aggression The individual deals with emotional conflict or internal or external stressors by indirectly and unassertively expressing aggression toward others. There is a facade of overt compliance masking covert resistance, resentment, or hostility. Passive aggression often occurs in response to demands for independent action or performance or the lack of gratification of dependent wishes but may be adaptive for individuals in subordinate positions who have no other way to express assertiveness more overtly.

projection The individual deals with emotional conflict or internal or external stressors by falsely attributing to another his or her own acceptable feelings, impulses, or thoughts.

projective identification As in projection, the individual deals with emotional conflict or internal or external stressors by falsely attributing to another his or her own unacceptable feelings, impulses, or thoughts. Unlike simple projection, the individual does not fully disavow what is projected. Instead, the individual remains aware of his or her own affects or impulses but misattributes them as justifiable reactions to the other person. Not infrequently, the individual induces the very feelings in others that were first mistakenly believed to be there, molding it difficult to clarify who did what to whom first.

rationalization The individual deals with emotional conflict or internal or external stressors by concealing the true motivations for his or her own thoughts, actions, or feelings through the elaboration of reassuring or self-serving but incorrect explanations.

reaction formation The individual deals with emotional conflict or internal or external stressors by substituting behavior, thoughts, or feelings that are diametrically opposed to his or her own unacceptable thoughts or feelings (this usually occurs in conjunction with their repression).

repression The individual deals with emotional conflict or internal or external stressors by expelling disturbing wishes, thoughts, or experiences from conscious awareness. The feeling component may remain conscious, detached from its associated ideas.

self-assertion The individual deals with emotional conflict or stressors by expressing his or her feelings and thoughts directly in a way that is not coercive or manipulative.

self-observation The individual deals with emotional conflict or stressors by reflecting on his or her own thoughts, feelings, motivation, and behavior, and responding appropriately.

splitting The individual deals with emotional conflict or internal or external stressors by compartmentalizing opposite affect states and failing to integrate the positive and negative qualities of the self or others into cohesive images. Because ambivalent affects cannot be experienced simultaneously, more balanced views and expectations of self or others are excluded from emotional awareness. Self and object images tend to alternate between polar opposites: exclusively loving, powerful, worthy, nurturant, and kind—or exclusively bad, hateful, angry, destructive, rejecting, or worthless.

sublimation The individual deals with emotional conflict or internal or external stressors by channeling potentially maladaptive feelings or impulses into socially acceptable behavior (e.g., contact sports to channel angry impulses).

suppression The individual deals with emotional conflict or internal or external stressors by intentionally avoiding thinking about disturbing problems, wishes, feelings, or experiences.

undoing The individual deals with emotional conflict or internal or external stressors by words or behavior designed to negate or to make amends symbolically for unacceptable thoughts, feelings, or actions.

Table from DSM-IV, *Diagnostic and Statistical Manual of Mental Disorders*, ed 4. Copyright American Psychiatric Association, Washington, 1994. Used with permission.

For a more detailed discussion of this topic, see G D Strauss: The Psychiatric Interview, History, and Mental Status Examination, Sec 9.1, p 521; H I Kaplan, B J Sadock: Psychiatric Report, Sec 9.2, p 531, in CTP/VI.

4

Primary Care Psychiatry and Medical Signs and Symptoms

Medical assessment consists of a thorough medical history, review of systems, general observation, physical examination, and diagnostic laboratory studies. The primary care physician should recognize the complex interplay between somatic illness and psychiatric illness: physical diseases may mimic psychiatric illnesses and vice versa. Also, the presenting symptoms of some physical illnesses may be psychiatric signs or symptoms; for example, a chief complaint of anxiety may be associated with mitral valve prolapse, which is revealed by cardiac auscultation. A complete medical workup, including an initial mental status examination, is essential for every patient.

MEDICAL HISTORY

During the examination, the physician should gather information about (1) known bodily diseases or dysfunctions, (2) hospitalizations and operative procedures, (3) medications taken recently or at present, (4) personal habits and occupational history, (5) family history of illnesses, and (6) specific physical complaints. Both the patient and the referring physician can contribute needed information about medical illnesses.

Information about previous episodes of illness may provide valuable clues about the nature of the present disorder. For example, if the present disorder is distinctly delusional, the patient has a history of several similar episodes, and each responded promptly to diverse treatments, this strongly suggests a substance-induced psychotic disorder. To pursue that lead, the physician should order a drug screen. The surgical history may also be useful; for example, a thyroidectomy suggests hypothyroidism as the cause of depression.

The physician must inquire about prescription drugs, as well as over-the-counter remedies, since medication side effects or intoxication may result in psychiatric signs and symptoms. Three examples suffice to highlight the importance of this inquiry: (1) a side effect of some hypertension medications is depression; (2) digitalis intoxication, causing impaired mental functioning, may occur when the drugs therapeutic dosage reaches high blood levels; (3) proprietary drugs may cause or contribute to an anticholinergic delirium.

An occupational history may provide essential information. Exposure to mercury may result in complaints suggesting a psychosis. Exposure to lead, may produce a cognitive disorder. Patients commonly encounter high lead levels near smelters, but also may risk exposure from imbibing moonshine with a high lead content.

REVIEW OF SYSTEMS

An inventory by systems should follow the open-ended inquiry. The review may be organized according to organ systems (for example, liver, pancreas), functional systems (for example, cardiovascular, gastrointestinal), or a combination of the two (as organized here), but the review should be comprehensive and thorough.

Head

Many patients give a history of headache; its duration, frequency, character, location, and severity should be ascertained. Headaches often result from substance abuse, including alcohol, nicotine, and caffeine. Vascular (migraine) headaches are precipitated by stress. Temporal arteritis causes unilateral throbbing headaches and may lead to blindness. Brain tumors and their accompanying increases in intracranial pressure may cause headaches.

A history of head injury may underlie a number of signs or symptoms, including headache. Subdural hematoma secondary to head injury can cause headaches; in boxers, repeated injuries can cause progressive dementia with extrapyramidal symptoms. The headache of subarachnoid hemorrhage is sudden, severe, and associated with changes in the sensorium. Normal pressure hydrocephalus may follow a head injury or encephalitis and may be associated with dementia and a shuffling gait.

Eye, Ear, Nose, and Throat

Visual acuity, diplopia, hearing problems, tinnitus, glossitis, and bad taste are covered in this area. A patient taking antipsychotics who gives a history of twitching about the mouth or disturbing movements of the tongue may be in the early and potentially reversible stage of tardive dyskinesia. Impaired vision may occur with thioridazine (Mellaril) in high dosages. A history of glaucoma contraindicates drugs with anticholinergic side effects. Aphonia may be hysterical in nature. The late stage of cocaine abuse can result in perforations of the nasal septum and difficulty in breathing. A transitory episode of diplopia may herald multiple sclerosis. Delusional disorder is more common in hearing-impaired persons than in those with normal hearing.

Respiratory System

Cough, asthma, pleurisy, hemoptysis, dyspnea, and orthopnea are considered in this section. Hyperventilation is suggested if the patient's symptoms include all or a few of the following: onset at rest, sighing respirations, apprehension, anxiety, depersonalization, palpitations, inability to swallow, numbness of the feet and hands, and carpopedal spasm. Dyspnea and breathlessness may occur in depression. In pulmonary or obstructive airway disease the onset of symptoms is usually insidious, whereas in depression it is sudden. In depression, breathlessness is experienced at rest, shows little change with exertion, and may fluctuate within a matter of minutes; the onset of breathlessness coincides with the onset of a mood disorder and is often accompanied by attacks of dizziness, sweating, palpitations, and paresthesias. In obstructive airway disease, only the patients with the most advanced respiratory incapacity experience breathlessness at rest. Most striking and of greatest assistance in making a differential diagnosis is the emphasis placed on the difficulty in inspiration experienced by patients with depression and on the difficulty in expiration experienced by patients with pulmonary disease. Bronchial asthma has sometimes been associated with childhood histories of extreme dependence on the mother. Patients with bronchospasm should not receive propranolol (Inderal) because it may block catecholamine-induced bronchodilation; propranolol is specifically contraindicated for patients with bronchial asthma because epinephrine given to such patients in an emergency will not be effective.

Cardiovascular System

Tachycardia, palpitations, and cardiac arrhythmia are among the most common signs of anxiety. Pheochromocytoma usually produces symptoms that mimic anxiety disorders, such as rapid heart beat, tremors, and pallor. Increased urinary catecholamines are diagnostic of pheochromocytoma. Patients taking guanethidine (Ismelin) for hypertension should not receive tricyclic drugs, which reduce or eliminate the antihypertensive effect of guanethidine. A history of hypertension may preclude the use of monoamine oxidase inhibitors (MAOIs) because of the risk of a hypertensive crisis if hypertensive patients inadvertently consume foods high in tyramine. Patients with a suspected cardiac disease should have an electrocardiogram before lithium (Eskalith) or tricyclics are prescribed. A history of substernal pain should be evaluated, keeping in mind that psychological stress can precipitate anginal-type chest pain in the presence of normal coronary arteries.

Gastrointestinal System

This area covers such topics as appetite, distress before or after meals, food preferences, diarrhea, vomiting, constipation, laxative use, and abdominal pain. A history of weight loss is common in depressive disorders, but depression may accompany the weight loss caused by ulcerative colitis, regional enteritis, and cancer. Anorexia nervosa is accompanied by severe weight loss in the presence of normal appetite. Avoidance of certain foods may be a phobic phenomenon or part of an obsessive ritual. Laxative abuse and induced vomiting is common in bulimia nervosa. Constipation is caused by opioid dependence and by psychotropic drugs with anticholinergic side effects. Cocaine abuse and amphetamine abuse cause a loss of appetite and weight loss. Weight gain occurs under stress. Polyphagia, polyuria, and polydipsia are the triad of diabetes mellitus. Polyuria, polydipsia, and diarrhea are signs of lithium toxicity.

Genitourinary System

Urinary frequency, nocturia, pain or burning on urination, and changes in the size and the force of the stream are some of the signs and symptoms in this area. Anticholinergic side effects associated with antipsychotics and tricyclic drugs may cause urinary retention in men with prostate hypertrophy. Erectile difficulty and retarded ejaculation are also common side effects of those drugs, and retrograde ejaculation occurs with thioridazine. A baseline level of sexual responsivity before using pharmacological agents should be obtained. A history of venereal diseases—for example, gonorrheal discharge, chancre, herpes, and pubic lice—may indicate sexual promiscuity. In some cases the first symptom of acquired immune deficiency syndrome (AIDS) is the gradual onset of mental confusion leading to dementia. If a psychotic patient remains incontinent after several days' treatment with a psychotropic medication, some cause other than a mental disorder should be suspected.

Menstrual System

A menstrual history should include the age of the onset of menarche and menopause; the periods' interval, regularity, duration, and amount of flow; irregular bleeding; dysmenorrhea; and abortions. Amenorrhea is characteristic of anorexia nervosa and also occurs in women who are psychologically stressed. Women who are afraid of becoming pregnant or who have a wish to be pregnant may have delayed periods. Pseudocyesis is false pregnancy with complete cessation of the menses. Perimenstrual mood changes (for example, irritability, depression, and dysphoria) should be noted. Painful menstruation can result from uterine disease (for example, myomata), from psychological conflicts about the menses, or from a combination of the two. Many women report an increase in sexual desire premenstrually. The emotional distress that some women experience after an abortion is usually mild and self-limited.

GENERAL OBSERVATION

An important part of the medical examination is subsumed under the broad head of general observation—using the examiner's visual, auditory, and olfactory senses. Such nonverbal clues as posture, facial expression, and mannerisms should also be noted.

Visual Evaluation

The visual scrutiny of the patient begins at the first encounter. When the patient goes from the waiting room to the interview room, the physician should observe the patient's gait. Is the patient unsteady? Ataxia suggests diffuse brain disease, alcohol or other substance intoxication, chorea, spinocerebellar degeneration, weakness based on a debilitating process, and an underlying disorder, such as myotonic dystrophy. Does the patient walk without the usual associated arm movements and turn in a rigid fashion, like a toy soldier, as is seen in early Parkinson's disease? Does the patient have an asymmetry of gait—turning one foot outward, dragging a leg, or not swinging one arm—suggesting a focal brain lesion?

As soon as the patient is seated, the physician should direct attention to grooming. Is the patient's hair combed, are the nails clean, and are the teeth brushed? Has clothing been chosen with care, and is it appropriate? Although inattention to dress and hygiene is common in mental disorders—in particular, depressive disorders—it is also a hallmark of cognitive disorders. Lapses—such as mismatching socks, stockings, or shoes—may suggest a cognitive disorder.

The physician should observe the patient's posture and any automatic movements should be noted. A stooped, flexed posture with a paucity of automatic movements may be due to Parkinson's disease, diffuse cerebral hemispheric disease, or the side effects of antipsychotics. An unusual tilt of the head may be adopted to avoid eye contact, but it can also result from diplopia, a visual field defect, or focal cerebellar dysfunction. Frequent quick, purposeless movements are characteristic of anxiety disorders, but they are equally characteristic of chorea and hyperthyroidism. Tremors, although commonly seen in anxiety disorders, may point to Parkinson's disease, essential tremor, or side effects of psychotropic medication. Unilateral paucity or excess of movement suggests focal brain disease.

The patient's appearance is then scrutinized to assess general health. Does the patient appear to be robust, or is there a sense of ill health? Does looseness of clothing indicate recent weight loss? Is the patient short of breath or coughing? Does the patient's general physiognomy suggest a specific disease? For example, men with Klinefelter's syndrome have a feminine fat distribution and lack the development of secondary male sex characteristics. Acromegaly is usually immediately recognizable.

What is the patient's nutritional status? Recent weight loss, although often seen in depressive disorders and schizophrenia, may be due to gastrointestinal disease, diffuse carcinomatosis, Addison's disease, hyperthyroidism, and many other somatic disorders. Obesity may result from either emotional distress or organic disease. Moon facies, truncal obesity, and buffalo hump are striking findings in Cushing's syndrome. The puffy, bloated appearance seen in hypothyroidism and the massive obesity and periodic respiration seen in Pickwickian syndrome are easily recognized.

The skin frequently provides valuable information. The yellow discoloration of hepatic dysfunction and the pallor of anemia are reasonably distinctive. Intense reddening may be due to carbon monoxide poisoning or to photosensitivity resulting from porphyria or phenothiazines. Eruptions may be manifestations of such disorders as systemic lupus erythematosus, tuberous sclerosis with adenoma sebaceum, and sensitivity to drugs. A dusky purplish cast to the face, plus telangiectasia, is almost pathognomonic of alcohol abuse.

Careful observation may reveal clues that lead to the correct diagnosis in patients who create their own skin lesions. For example, the location and the shape of the lesions and the time of their appearance may be characteristic of dermatitis factitia.

The patient's face and head should be scanned for evidence of disease. Premature whitening of the hair occurs in pernicious anemia, and thinning and coarseness of the hair occurs in myxedema. Pupillary changes are produced by various drugs—constriction by opioids and dilation by anticholinergic agents and hallucinogens. The combination of dilated and fixed pupils and dry skin and mucous membranes should immediately suggest the likelihood of atropine use or atropinelike toxicity. Diffusion of the conjunctiva suggests alcohol abuse, cannabis abuse, or obstruction of the superior vena cava. Flattening of the nasolabial fold on one side or weakness of one side of the face—as manifested in speaking, smiling, and grimacing—may be the result of focal dysfunction of the contralateral cerebral hemisphere.

The patient's state of alertness and responsiveness should be carefully evaluated. Drowsiness and inattentiveness may be due to a psychological problem, but they are more likely to result from an organic brain dysfunction, whether secondary to an intrinsic brain disease or to an exogenous factor, such as substance intoxication.

Auditory Evaluation

Listening intently is just as important as looking intently for evidence of somatic disorders.

Slowed speech is characteristic not only of depression but also of diffuse brain dysfunction and subcortical dysfunction; unusually rapid speech is characteristic not only of manic episodes and anxiety disorders but also of hyperthyroidism. A weak voice with monotony of tone may be clues to Parkinson's disease in patients who complain mainly of depression. A slow, low-pitched, hoarse voice should suggest the possibility of hypothyroidism; that voice quality has been described as sounding like a bad record of a drowsy, slightly intoxicated person with a bad cold and a plum in the mouth.

Difficulty in initiating speech may be due to anxiety or stuttering, or it may be indicative of Parkinson's disease or aphasia. Easy fatigability of speech may sometimes be a manifestation of an emotional problem, but it is also characteristic of myasthenia gravis.

Word production, as well as the quality of speech, is important. When words are mispronounced or incorrect words are used, aphasia, caused by a lesion of the dominant hemisphere, should be considered. The same possibility exists if the patient perseverates, has trouble finding a name or a word, or describes an object or an event in an indirect fashion (paraphasia). When not consonant with the patient's socioeconomic and educational level, coarseness, profanity, or inappropriate disclosures may indicate loss of inhibition caused by dementia.

Olfactory Evaluation

Much less is learned through the sense of smell than through the senses of sight and hearing, but occasionally smell provides useful information. The unpleasant odor of a patient who fails to bathe suggests an organic brain dysfunction and a depressive disorder. The odor of alcohol or an attempt to mask it is revealing in a patient concealing a drinking problem. Occasionally, a uriniferous odor calls attention to bladder dysfunction secondary to a nervous system disease. Characteristic odors are also noted in patients with diabetic acidosis, uremia, and hepatic coma.

PHYSICAL EXAMINATION

Selection of Patients

The nature of the patient's complaints is critical in determining if a complete physical examination is required. Complaints fall into three categories: (1) the body, (2) the mind, and (3) social interactions.

Bodily symptoms—such as headaches, erectile disorder, and palpitations—call for a thorough medical examination to determine what part, if any, somatic processes play in causing the distress. The same can be said for mental symptoms—such as depression, anxiety, hallucinations, and persecutory delusions—because they can be expressions of somatic processes. If the problem is clearly limited to the social sphere—as in long-standing difficulties in interactions with teachers, employers, parents, or a spouse—there may be no special indication for a physical examination.

Psychological Considerations

Even a routine physical examination may evoke adverse reactions; instruments, procedures, and the examining room may be frightening. A simple running account of what is being done can prevent much needless anxiety. Moreover, if the patient is consistently forewarned of the next step, the dread of being suddenly and painfully surprised recedes. Comments such as, "There's nothing to this" and "You don't have to be afraid because this won't hurt" leave the patient uninformed and are much less reassuring than a few words about what actually will be done.

Although the physical examination is likely to engender or intensify a reaction of anxiety, it can also generate sexual feelings. Some women with fantasies of being seduced may misinterpret an ordinary movement in the physical examination as a sexual advance. Similarly, a delusional man with homosexual fears may perceive a rectal examination as a sexual attack.

Lingering over the examination of a particular organ because an unusual but normal variation has aroused the physician's scientific curiosity is likely to raise concern in the patient that a serious pathological process has been discovered. Such a reaction in an anxious or hypochondriacal patient may be profound.

The physical examination is occasionally psychotherapeutic. An anxious patient may be relieved to learn that, in spite of troublesome symptoms, there is no evidence of the feared serious illness. The young person who complains of chest pain and is certain that the pain heralds a heart attack can usually be reassured by the report of normal findings after a physical examination and electrocardiogram. However, the reassurance relieves only the worry occasioned by the immediate episode. Unless treatment succeeds in dealing with the determinants of the reaction, recurrent episodes are likely. Sending a patient who has a deeply rooted fear of malignancy for still another test intended as reassuring is usually unrewarding.

During the performance of the physical examination, an observant physician may note indications of emotional distress. For instance, during genital examinations, patients' behavior may reveal information about their sexual attitudes and problems, and their reactions may be used later to open that area for discussion.

Deferring the Physical Examination

Occasionally, circumstances make it desirable or necessary to defer a complete medical assessment. For example, a delusional or manic patient may be combative or resistive or both. In that instance a medical history should be elicited from a family member if possible, but, unless there is a pressing reason to proceed with the examination, it should be deferred until the patient is tractable.

For psychological reasons it may be ill-advised to recommend a medical assessment at the time of an initial office visit. For example, with today's increased sensitivity and openness about sexual matters and a proneness to turn quickly to medical help, young men may complain about their failure in an initial attempt to consummate a sexual relationship. After taking a detailed history, the physician may conclude that the failure has been prematurely defined as a problem. If that is the case, neither a physical examination nor psychotherapy should be recommended, because they would have the undesirable effect of reinforcing the notion of pathology. Education, reassurance, and support may suffice.

Neurological Examination

During the history-taking process, the patient's level of awareness, attentiveness to the details of the examination, understanding, facial expression, speech, posture, and gait are noted. It is also assumed that a thorough mental status examination will be performed. The neurological examination should then be performed with two objectives in mind: (1) to elicit signs pointing to focal, circumscribed cerebral dysfunction and (2) to elicit signs suggesting diffuse, bilateral cerebral disease. The first objective is met by the routine neurological examination, which is designed primarily to reveal asymmetries in the motor, perceptual, and reflex functions of the two sides of the body caused by focal hemispheric disease. The second objective is met by seeking to elicit signs that have been attributed to diffuse brain dysfunction and to frontal lobe disease. Those signs include the sucking, snout, palmomental, and grasp reflexes and the persistence of the glabella tap response.

Incidental Findings

Primary care physicians should be able to evaluate the significance of psychological findings uncovered during evaluations. With a patient who complains of a lump in the throat (globus hystericus) and who is found on examination to have hypertrophied lymphoid tissue, it is tempting to wonder about cause-and-effect. How can one be sure that the finding is not incidental? Has the patient been known to have hypertrophied lymphoid tissue at a time when no complaint was made? Are there many persons with hypertrophied lymphoid tissue who never experience the sensation of a lump in the throat?

With a patient with multiple sclerosis who complains of an inability to walk but, on neurological examination, has only mild spasticity and a unilateral Babinski's sign, it is tempting to ascribe the symptom to the neurological disorder. However, in that instance the evidence of a neurological abnormality is out of keeping with manifest dysfunction. The same holds true for a patient with profound dementia in whom a small frontal meningioma is seen on a computed tomography (CT) scan. The knowledgeable physician should recognize that profound dementia may not result from such a small lesion so situated.

Often, a lesion is found that may account for a symptom, but the physician should make every effort to separate an incidental finding from a causative one, to separate a lesion merely found in the area of the symptom from a lesion producing the symptom.

PATIENT IN PSYCHIATRIC TREATMENT

While patients are being treated for psychiatric disorders, the primary care physician should be alert to the possibility of intercurrent illnesses that call for diagnosis studies. Patients in psychotherapy, particularly those in psychoanalysis, may be all too willing to ascribe their new symptoms to emotional causes. Attention should be given to the possible use of denial, especially if the symptoms seem to be unrelated to the conflicts currently in focus.

Symptoms such as drowsiness and dizziness and signs such as a skin eruption and a gait disturbance, common side effects of psychotropic medication, call for a medical reevaluation if the patient fails to respond in a reasonable time to changes in the dosage or the kind of medication prescribed. Patients receiving tricyclic or antipsychotic drugs who complain of blurred vision, usually an anticholinergic side effect, warrant reevaluation if the condition does not recede with a reduction in dosage or a change in medication. The absence of other anticholinergic side effects, such as a dry mouth and constipation, is an additional clue alerting the physician to a possible concomitant medical illness.

Early in an illness, few, if any, positive physical or laboratory results may be found. In such instances, especially if the evidence of psychic trauma or emotional conflicts is glaring, all symptoms are likely to be regarded as psychosocial in origin and new symptoms may also be seen in that light. Physicians may miss indications for repeating portions of the medical workup unless they are alert to clues suggesting that some symptoms do not fit the original diagnosis and point, instead, to a medical illness. Occasionally, a patient with an acute illness, such as encephalitis, is hospitalized with the diagnosis of schizophrenia; or a patient with a subacute illness, such as carcinoma of the pancreas, is treated in a private office or clinic with the diagnosis of a depressive disorder. Although it may not be possible to make the correct diagnosis at the time of the initial evaluation, continued surveillance and attention to clinical details usually provide clues leading to the recognition of the cause.

The likelihood of intercurrent illness is greater with some psychiatric disorders than with others. Substance abusers, for example, because of their life patterns, are susceptible to infection and are likely to suffer from the adverse effects of trauma, dietary deficiencies, and poor hygiene.

When somatic and psychological dysfunctions are known to coexist, the primary care physician should be thoroughly conversant with the patient's medical status. In cases of cardiac decompensation, peripheral neuropathy, and other disabling disorders, the nature and the degree of the impairment attributable to the physical disorder should be assessed. It is important to answer the question: Does the patient exploit a disability, or is it ignored or denied with resultant overexertion? To answer that question, the physician must assess the patient's capabilities and limitations, rather than make sweeping judgments based on a diagnostic label.

Special vigilance regarding medical status is required for some patients in treatment for somatoform or eating disorders, especially those with ulcerative colitis who are bleeding profusely and those with anorexia nervosa who are losing appreciable weight. Those disorders may become life-threatening.

Importance of Medical Illness

Among identified psychiatric patients, anywhere from 24 to 60 percent have been shown to suffer from associated physical disorders. In a survey of 2,090 psychiatric clinic patients, 43 percent were found to have associated physical disorders; of those, almost half the physical disorders had not been diagnosed by the referring sources. (In that study, 69 patients were found to have diabetes mellitus, but only 12 of the cases of diabetes had been diagnosed before referral.)

Psychiatric symptoms are nonspecific; they can herald both medical illness, and psychiatric illness. Moreover, psychiatric symptoms often precede the appearance of definitive medical symptoms. Some psychiatric symptoms—such as visual hallucinations, distortions, and illusions—should arouse a high level of suspicion.

The medical literature abounds with case reports of patients whose disorders were initially considered emotional but ultimately proved to be organic in origin. The data in most of the reports revealed features pointing toward organicity. Diagnostic errors arose because such features were accorded too little weight.

For a more detailed discussion of this topic, see Neuropsychiatry and Behavioral Neurology, Chap 2, pp 167–275; E D Caine, H Grossman, J M Lyness: Delirium, Dementia, and Amnestic and Other Cognitive Disorders and Mental Disorders Due to a General Medical Condition, Chap 12, p 705, in CTP/VI.

Area B

Clinical Problems in Psychiatry

5

Disorders Usually First Diagnosed in Infancy, Childhood, or Adolescence

5.1 Adolescent Crisis

Adolescent crisis is defined as turmoil in an adolescent leading to significant behavioral, academic, social, or psychiatric problems. Adolescents make up much of the caseload of the primary care physician, especially the pediatrician. Many of those adolescents are in crisis.

CLINICAL FEATURES AND DIAGNOSIS

An estimated 30 percent of hospital emergency room visits involve patients under 18 years of age, and about 15 percent of all general hospital psychiatric emergencies involve adolescents. Most researchers agree that the two most frequently encountered adolescent emergencies are (1) suicide or severe depressions and (2) violence or other antisocial manifestations. Suicide and homicide account for the greatest number of deaths in adolescence. Teenage girls are reportedly seen more frequently in psychiatric emergency rooms than are boys, in a ratio of 3 to 2; that ratio is attributed to the increased frequency of suicidal behavior in adolescent girls, especially those who are 12 to 14 years of age. The most common method of completed suicides in adolescents is the use of firearms. Chronic separations and losses, including suicide in the family, are common features in suicidal adolescents' backgrounds. Runaway teenagers account for up to 13 percent of adolescent psychiatric emergency assessments, and the vast majority run away to escape an abusive or destructive home life.

Important questions include the following: What is the patient's baseline behavior? How does the adolescent's present behavior compare with adolescents of the same age and background? How is the patient doing in school? How are the patient's parents doing? How does the patient socialize? What is the patient's history of sexual activity and violence? What are the patient's peer relationships like?

Depression in children and adolescents more often presents with behavioral problems, than with symptoms typically found in depressed adults. For example, acting out behavior and a decline in school performance may be signs of depression in an adolescent who sleeps well and has neither a change in weight nor anhedonia.

Other diagnostic questions and concerns include the following:

1. Is the patient psychotic?
2. Is there a history of drug or alcohol use?

3. Is the history consistent with a chronic psychotic disorder, a mood disorder, a substance abuse disorder, or a behavioral disorder, such as conduct disorder? Has there been a clear-cut change in mood recently?
4. Is there a childhood history of attention-deficit/hyperactivity disorder? This disorder often presages other mental disorders in adolescence and adulthood.
5. Is there a history of truancy, fire setting, cruelty to animals, stealing, fighting, temper tantrums, the use of a weapon, robbery, burglary, running away, forcing sexual activity, destruction of property, or other antisocial acts? If so, the patient may have a conduct disorder or an antisocial personality disorder. Homicide risk is greatly increased by any evidence of an organic mental syndrome, abnormal results on electroencephalograms (EEGs), childhood psychoses (especially schizophrenia), conduct disorders, severe mental retardation, compulsive fire setting, and a marked history of abuse or deprivation. A close association is reported between homicidal behavior and depressive phenomena.
6. Is there a history of temporal lobe or psychomotor epilepsy? A reported 18 percent of adolescents incarcerated for violent acts had probable temporal lobe epilepsy, compared with 0.5 percent of adolescents in the general population.
7. Has a recent or ongoing stressor precipitated the crisis? Is there an acute family problem? Has there been a recent loss? Has there been a change in the school or family environment? Is there an implicit or explicit family endorsement of violence?
8. Is the adolescent a victim of physical or sexual abuse? If so, the presenting problems may be those of depression, suicidal ideation and gestures, sexual acting out, truancy, running away, and alcohol and drug abuse.
9. Has the child been a participant in or a witness of any especially extreme, sudden, violent, or unusual event?
10. Is the adolescent involved with a cult?
11. Are there increased complaints of multiple vague medical symptoms, such as stomachaches, headaches, nausea, and eye problems?

INTERVIEWING AND PSYCHOTHERAPEUTIC GUIDELINES

Try to engage the patient in a nonthreatening way, and give the patient a chance to talk freely and to complain or ventilate. Many adolescents are threatened by the possibility of psychiatric intervention or hospitalization and do not know how to react.

It is often necessary to interview an adolescent alone, without the parents. The parents then may be seen separately or in conjunction with the adolescent. It may be helpful to reassure the patient that the interview is confidential and to convey that the focus is on what the patient perceives as problems. Some adolescents open up at the opportunity to speak with a supportive professional in safe conditions.

Sometimes adolescents refuse to participate in interviews in an attempt to exhibit some control over a situation into which they feel they have been placed against their wishes. In such a situation, directly confronting the adolescent's defiance is usually not helpful. A common and useful technique is to reframe the defiance in positive terms, such as a need for privacy or autonomy. A typical statement is, "I can understand your need for privacy. After all, coming here was not your idea, and you don't know me from Adam. Please, only talk when you feel it is safe to do so; I want to be able to respect your needs."

EVALUATION AND MANAGEMENT

1. Adolescent crisis is often a complex interaction of individual, family, psychoso-cial, biological, and medical problems; these patients can require time-consuming emergency evaluations. It is important to obtain information from corroborating sources, including the parents, other family members, a school counselor, and an outpatient therapist. It is also essential to rule out the presence of any underlying medical condition.
2. Try to avoid hospitalizing adolescents unless no other alternatives are possible. Hospitalization often stigmatizes the adolescent and interferes with school atten-dance. Furthermore, within the family structure, hospitalization identifies the patient as the one with the disorder when there may also be significant family pathology. Clear treatments and expected benefits of needed hospitalization should be delineated. For example, some violent patients with conduct disorders may receive only behavioral control and detention in the hospital. Often, finding an alternative living arrangement (with a relative or a friend) or arranging placement in a group home can resolve an acute crisis. However, in certain situations, such as active suicidal behavior, admission to a hospital may be the only responsible recourse.
3. Handling referrals is important: The compliance rate for referrals from an emer-gency setting to a clinic is reportedly less than 50 percent. The parents must be given the names of the clinic and the therapist. Make a follow-up call to the parents to determine if the appointment was kept.
4. Know the legal requirements for adolescents in your community regarding competence to consent to treatment and requirements for parental consent.
5. Consult the parents and the patient's school.
6. If an adolescent patient is psychotic, be aware of suicidal and violent behavior. In a psychotic adolescent, suicidal ideation, even without suicide attempts, is extremely serious and almost always necessitates hospitalization.
7. The potential for suicide and suicidal behavior must be monitored closely in adolescents who are acutely homicidal or violent, as the conjunction of the two behaviors is high.
8. Pay particular attention to the management of violent eruptions in the office, especially if the adolescent has a history of violence or is under the influence of alcohol or drugs.

DRUG TREATMENT

Specific treatment depends on the diagnosis. If the adolescent is found to be suffering from an identifiable diagnosis that responds to medication, treat accordingly. For instance, a psychotic, agitated adolescent could be treated with an antipsy-chotic drug, such as haloperidol (Haldol) 1 to 2 mg by mouth or intramuscularly (IM) every 30 to 60 minutes, until the agitation is controlled. The treatment of an adolescent with psychotropic medication is a decision that needs to be made by a psychiatrist experienced in the treatment of adolescent disorders. The decision depends on a high level of clinical acumen and sensitivity.

For a more detailed discussion of this topic, see J E Schowalter: Normal Adolescent Development, Sec 33.3, p 2161; C S Pataki: Child or Adolescent Antisocial Behavior, Sec 47.6, p 2477, in CTP/VI.

5.2 Bed-Wetting

Bed-wetting (enuresis) is pathological if it (1) occurs repeatedly in a patient at least 5 years old and (2) is not caused by a medical condition or a drug. Although bed-wetting is usually a self-limited condition, it may cause significant distress to affected children and their families. Frustrated parents often seek assistance from pediatricians and primary care physicians in treating this condition.

CLINICAL FEATURES AND DIAGNOSIS

Enuresis is the repeated voiding of urine into the patient's clothes or bed. The behavior may be intentional or involuntary and typically occurs both during daytime and at night. The duration, the course, and the precipitants of the disorder should be identified.

Organic causes, including anatomical defects in the urinary tract, infections, diabetes mellitus, diabetes insipidus, drug intoxication, epilepsy, sleepwalking, and the side effects of medication, such as antipsychotics, must be considered. The presence of urinary frequency, urgency, pain, or residual urine suggests an organic cause.

Boys, children in institutions, and children with a low socioeconomic status are at greatest risk for the disorder. Genetic factors exist. Bed-wetting is often precipi-tated by psychosocial stressors (for example, the birth of a sibling, moving, and marital discord between the parents).

INTERVIEWING AND PSYCHOTHERAPEUTIC GUIDELINES

Be supportive and reassuring in dealing with a child. Children often feel guilty and blamed, and they need empathy. Punitive or humiliating parental behaviors may be revealed when speaking with the parents, who should be educated about nonpunitive behavioral approaches to enuresis.

EVALUATION AND MANAGEMENT

For enuresis not due to a general medical condition, counsel the parents regarding appropriate toilet training, including record keeping and rewards for improvement.

Behavioral therapy with a bed pad attached to an alarm that sounds on wetness is often effective.

DRUG TREATMENT

Drugs are seldom indicated. Imipramine (Tofranil) has been used effectively, but only on a short-term basis. Tolerance often develops after six weeks, and relapse usually occurs within a few months after discontinuation of the drug. Desmopressin (DDAVP), an antidiuretic compound administered as a nasal spray, has shown initial success.

For a more detailed discussion of this topic, see E J Mikkelsen: Elimination Disorders, Chap 42, p 2337, in CTP/VI.

5.3 Fire Setting

Fire setting is pathological when it is planned and recurrent. It must be distinguished from the fascination of many young children with matches, lighters, and fire as part of the normal investigation of their environments. According the Federal Bureau of Investigation (FBI), youths account for over one third of the arrests for arson.

CLINICAL FEATURES AND DIAGNOSIS

Pathological fire setting occurs more often as part of conduct disorder or antisocial personality disorder than it does as a failure of impulse control (that is, pyromania). The essential features of pyromania are deliberate and purposeful fire setting on more than one occasion; tension or affective arousal before setting the fires; fascination with activities and equipment associated with fire fighting; and pleasure, gratification, or relief when setting fires. Fires can also be set in response to the hallucinations or delusions of schizophrenia or a manic episode.

INTERVIEWING AND PSYCHOTHERAPEUTIC GUIDELINES

Any underlying psychiatric disorder, such as conduct disorder, attention-deficit/hyperactivity disorder, mental retardation, substance-related disorder, should be treated. Fire setting as the primary behavior problem can be treated with specifically developed psychotherapies, including individual psychotherapy, family therapy, and many behavioral techniques.

Pyromania is extremely rare. In adults any possible psychiatric disorder, such as schizophrenia, dementia, bipolar I disorder, delusional disorder, substance intoxication, and antisocial personality disorder, should be ruled out. Monetary gain, revenge, and other motives must be considered.

Because pyromaniacs compulsively repeat their acts, law enforcement authorities should be notified.

INTERVIEWING AND PSYCHOTHERAPEUTIC GUIDELINES

Fire setting in children must be treated with the utmost seriousness. Intensive interventions should be undertaken as therapeutic and preventive measures, rather than as punishment.

Because of the recurrent nature of pyromania and pathological fire setting, any treatment program should include supervision of the patient to prevent a repeated episode of fire setting.

DRUG TREATMENT

No pharmacotherapy is available for pyromania or pathological fire setting, except for any underlying mental disorder.

For a more detailed discussion of this topic, see V K Burt: Impulse-Control Disorders Not Elsewhere Classified, Sec 24.1, p 1409; B Vitiello, P S Jensen: Disruptive Behavior Disorders, Chap 39, p 2311; C S Pataki: Child or Adolescent Antisocial Behavior, Sec 47.6, p 2477, in CTP/VI.

5.4 Mutism

Mutism is the absence of speech in a person capable of speaking. Selective mutism is an uncommon childhood disorder in which the child refuses to speak in certain settings. However, a common presentation of mutism is in adults, in whom it can be symptomatic of a wide range of psychiatric conditions, including malingering.

CLINICAL FEATURES AND DIAGNOSIS

The diagnosis of selective mutism in children is relatively straightforward, as the parents report that the child is able to talk normally at home. The child may follow directions or give other evidence of comprehension in the clinical setting, even if the child remains mute with the examiner.

The onset of mutism in children is usually between ages 5 and 6 years. Girls are affected more often than boys. The children typically talk only with the nuclear family at home.

In adults, mutism may be one aspect of severe psychomotor retardation in depression. The mute patients often visibly struggle to produce responses, then seemingly tire and abandon the effort. When the attempted interview is terminated, they may cling imploringly to the examiner and try again. They may lack the energy to express thoughts or have slowed thinking.

Schizophrenia may also present with mutism. As with depression, the patients may exhibit poverty of thought or a lack of energy or motivation. Schizophrenic persons may be too frightened of others to speak, may be completely preoccupied by internal stimuli, may have bizarre grandiose beliefs about themselves that entail silence, or may be paralyzed by ambivalence.

Other involuntary causes include certain drug intoxications, notably phencyclidine (PCP) and hallucinogens. Mutism may also occur as a symptom of a conversion disorder.

Mutism may be voluntarily produced to gain admission to a hospital. Particularly with patients from other cultures, the combination of a language barrier, unusual behavior in public, mistrust, the wish to avoid psychiatric attention or labeling, and perhaps personality factors may result in mutism with no other mental disorder.

INTERVIEWING AND PSYCHOTHERAPEUTIC GUIDELINES

The mute patient is likely to be frustrating. Time and patience is the key to obtaining data from mute patients. It may take hours or days to identify a patient, contact collateral sources of information, or otherwise obtain a history. Try a variety of approaches to find something about which the patient is able or willing to converse. Frequent brief contacts may be more useful than long, frustrating interviews. In general, simple, concrete questions yield more information than do complex, open-ended questions. Providing food or fluids gives the opportunity for social contact, a demonstration of concern, and observation. The nursing and social work staff members may be less threatening and more successful than the physicians. Surreptitious observation is important, as patients often socialize with peers, seeming to be normal until the examiner appears.

EVALUATION AND MANAGEMENT

1. The management of mutism depends on the cause. Depressed patients require support for nourishment and hydration. Schizophrenic patients may require encouragement for basic self-care. Catatonic patients should be closely observed, as dangerous periods of excitement may suddenly occur. Hospitalization may be necessary in such cases.
2. If mute patients require admission to a hospital, they usually require involuntary admission, as competence cannot be established. For patients who are voluntarily mute, the condition usually ceases to be a problem at some point simply because of the difficulty of remaining mute.

DRUG TREATMENT

Mute depressed patients may be psychotically depressed. Psychotic depression often requires both antipsychotic and antidepressant medications. The antipsychotic drugs, such as fluphenazine (Prolixin), trifluoperazine (Stelazine), or haloperidol (Haldol), all given at 2 to 5 mg a day, may be used. Explain the prescribed treatment, even if the patient is unresponsive. If the patient passively accepts treatment, that is probably adequate. If the patient actively refuses medication, involuntary treatment may be necessary.

Drug-induced psychoses may also be managed with benzodiazepines; lorazepam (Ativan) 1 to 2 mg by mouth or intramuscularly (IM) or oxazepam (Serax) 10 to 30 mg by mouth may be given at one-hour intervals.

If no progress is made with other techniques and sufficient time has elapsed to reduce the likelihood of malingering, an amobarbital (Amytal) interview may yield results.

For a more detailed discussion of this topic, see Substance-Related Disorders, Chap 13, pp 755–888; A A Lipton, R Cancro: Schizophrenia: Clinical Features, Sec 14.7, p 968; J E Mezzich, K-M Lin: Acute and Transient Psychotic Disorders and Culture-Bound Syndromes, Sec 15.3, p 1049; M J Mills, M S Lipian: Malingering, Sec 28.2, p 1614; L Baker, D P Cantwell: Selective Mutism, Sec 43.2, p 2351, in CTP/VI.

5.5 School Phobia and Refusal

School phobia is a form of separation anxiety in which children are afraid of school. They may refuse to go to school or endure school with great difficulty because of the overwhelming anxiety that occurs when they are faced with separation from parental figures.

School refusal may occur for a variety of reasons and under some circumstances may provoke a crisis. Anxiety may contribute to the refusal and may be related to separation from a parent or important caretaker, as in separation anxiety disorder, or anxiety about meeting future expectations, as in generalized anxiety disorder.

CLINICAL FEATURES AND DIAGNOSIS

Anxiety in children often does not appear in a pure form. Overanxious children may also suffer from separation anxiety disorder, social phobia, depression, panic disorder, learning disabilities, and enuresis. Each of those problems may contribute to school phobia and refusal in different ways. Children with generalized anxiety disorder are persistently concerned about future events and competence in a variety of areas, including athletic, academic, and social performance. Psychophysiological complaints are common in both separation anxiety disorder and overanxious disorder. Children may present with multiple somatic complaints given as the reason for absenteeism. Somatic symptoms secondary to school phobia generally disappear during vacations, holidays, and weekends. True medical illness may result in school refusal. Other causes include family dynamics (such as a dependent parent or caretaker who covertly encourages school refusal), realistic fear caused by victimization at school, and truancy. Children with school phobia have great difficulty in leaving for school; truant children leave readily, claiming to go to school. Truancy is often accompanied by other behavioral problems (for example, fighting and rule breaking). Children with separation anxiety disorder fear that something will happen to them or to their parents or caretakers while they are in school. Depression reduces energy and motivation and results in clinging behavior and school phobia in children.

INTERVIEWING AND PSYCHOTHERAPEUTIC GUIDELINES

The overanxious child may attempt to hide behind the parent and converses with great difficulty. The depressed child may also cling to the parent but may be more easily engaged than the overanxious child. A child with physical complaints should be given a thorough physical examination. The parent provides most of the history. Observation of the family dynamics can help to determine whether the parents are encouraging the school phobia because of their own dependence needs.

It is important for the pediatrician to explain to both that a return to school is extremely important. The child can be told that he or she need not attend class but that being in the school building itself is part of the therapy. The physician should find out if there is any area of the school (for example, principal's office, gym teacher's office) where the student feels comfortable.

EVALUATION AND MANAGEMENT

The pediatrician should perform a thorough medical evaluation to rule out organic illness as the cause of the school refusal. Demonstrating a lack of organic disease helps the clinician confront the child and the family with the psychological origin of the symptoms.

A full psychiatric evaluation is needed to rule out other psychiatric disorders, such as depression and psychosis, that can cause severe absenteeism.

A history should be obtained of the child's experience at school. Is the child being teased or bullied? The child's fears may be realistic and amenable to manipulation of the school environment.

If school phobia is diagnosed, give the family an explanation of the fear and instructions regarding the implementation of a structured, consistent treatment plan designed to get the child back into school as quickly as possible. It is imperative that the child return to school. The school can be enlisted to aid in the process, which should be carried out with an outpatient therapist. Strategies include having an adult take the child to school and sit in on classes for steadily decreasing amounts of time. A caretaker can telephone the child once daily at school. Any plan needs to address contributing family dynamics. Family therapy or individual psychotherapy for the parents may be needed.

DRUG TREATMENT

Imipramine (Tofranil) can be considered if other treatment modalities are unsuccessful. The medication should be implemented as part of an ongoing psychotherapeutic relationship and should not be initiated by the primary care physician.

For a more detailed discussion of this topic, see R E Mattison: Separation Anxiety Disorder and Anxiety in Children, Sec 43.1, p 2345, in CTP/VI.

5.6 Separation Anxiety

Separation anxiety is a type of phobic anxiety that occurs in children during
separation or while anticipating separation from a parent or important caretaker.
The child's reaction may approach terror or panic. Violence against the person
enforcing the separation is possible. Separation anxiety may precipitate a psychiatric
emergency. The age at onset is preschool through adolescence. Cases beginning
up to 12 years of age are common, but new cases in the teen years are rare.

CLINICAL FEATURES AND DIAGNOSIS

The diagnostic criteria for separation anxiety disorder are listed in Table 5.6–1.
Morbid fears, preoccupations, and ruminations are characteristic of the disorder.
Children become fearful that someone close to them will be hurt or that something
terrible will happen to them while they are away from important figures. Fears of
getting lost and of being kidnapped and never reunited with their parents are
common.

INTERVIEWING AND PSYCHOTHERAPEUTIC GUIDELINES

Parents provide most of the history. The parents and the child should be interviewed separately, if possible, and the child's reactions to separation efforts for the

TABLE 5.6–1
DIAGNOSTIC CRITERIA FOR SEPARATION ANXIETY DISORDER

A. Developmentally inappropriate and excessive anxiety concerning separation from home or
   from those to whom the individual is attached, as evidenced by three (or more) of
   the following:
   (1) recurrent excessive distress when separation from home or major attachment figures occurs
       or is anticipated
   (2) persistent and excessive worry about losing, or about possible harm befalling, major
       attachment figures
   (3) persistent and excessive worry that an untoward event will lead to separation from a major
       attachment figure (e.g., getting lost or being kidnapped)
   (4) persistent reluctance or refusal to go to school or elsewhere because of fear of separation
   (5) persistently and excessively fearful or reluctant to be alone or without major attachment
       figures at home or without significant adults in other settings
   (6) persistent reluctance or refusal to go to sleep without being near a major attachment figure
       or to sleep away from home
   (7) repeated nightmares involving the theme of separation
   (8) repeated complaints of physical symptoms (such as headaches, stomachaches, nausea,
       or vomiting) when separation from major attachment figures occurs or is anticipated
B. The duration of the disturbance is at least 4 weeks.
C. The onset is before age 18 years.
D. The disturbance causes clinically significant distress or impairment in social, academic
   (occupational), or other important areas of functioning.
E. The disturbance does not occur exclusively during the course of a pervasive developmental
   disorder, schizophrenia, or other psychotic disorder and, in adolescents and adults, is not better
   accounted for by panic disorder with agoraphobia.

Specify if:
   Early onset: if onset occurs before age 6 years

Table from DSM-IV, *Diagnostic and Statistical Manual of Mental Disorders*, ed. 4. Copyright American
Psychiatric Association, Washington, 1994. Used with permission.

interview should be noted. If the child is present during the parents' interviews, the child may accuse the parents of not loving him or her and may make it difficult for the parents to express their concerns. The child may argue the facts and minimize the problems, fearing that consultation has been sought to curtail the relationships with the parents. However, insisting on separation during early contacts may be both impractical and damaging to the nascent therapeutic relationship.

EVALUATION AND MANAGEMENT

1. Develop a comprehensive treatment plan, particularly in the case of school refusal. Planning should involve the child, the parents, the child's peers, and the school. Encourage the child to attend school, but, if a return to a full school day is overwhelming, arrange a program for the child to gradually increase the time at school.
2. Provide psychotherapy directed at increasing the child's autonomy by exploring the unconscious fears underlying the symptoms. Family therapy helps the parents be consistent and supportive and prepares the child for important changes in life.
3. Occasionally, the child and the family are enmeshed to a degree that frustrates any intervention. Such cases may require hospitalization to interrupt the operation of the family system and to allow for the development of new behavior.

DRUG TREATMENT

Tricyclic and tetracyclic antidepressants effectively reduce panic symptoms. A child psychiatrist can start imipramine (Tofranil) at a dosage of 25 mg daily and increase it in 25-mg increments up to a total of 150 to 200 mg a day. (Electrocardiographic [ECG] monitoring is needed.) If the child shows no response at that dosage, determine the plasma concentrations of imipramine and its active metabolite desmethylimipramine. The medication should be initiated as part of an ongoing treatment plan and therapeutic relationship. In most cases, the imipramine should not be started by the pediatrician. Diphenhydramine (Benadryl) in dosages of 10 to 25 mg by mouth at bedtime can be used for associated insomnia.

For a more detailed discussion of this topic, see R E Mattison: Separation Anxiety Disorder and Anxiety in Children, Sec 43.1, p 2345, in CTP/VI.

5.7 Tics

Tics are rapid, brief involuntary movements, vocalizations, or sensations. When they begin suddenly in school, the child may be brought to a pediatrician or the emergency room.

TABLE 5.7-1
TIC DISORDERS

	Age of Onset (years)		Tics		Duration
Tourette's disorder	<18		1 or more motor *and* at least 1 vocal		>12 mo
Chronic motor or vocal tic disorder	<18		1 or more vocal *or* motor (but not both)		>12 mo
Transient tic disorder	<18		1 or more vocal or motor		>4 wk and <12 mo
Tic disorder not otherwise specified (NOS)	18+	**or**	1 motor *and* 1 vocal	**or**	<4 wk

CLINICAL FEATURES AND DIAGNOSIS

Tics may be single or multiple, simple or complex, transient or long-term. Tourette's disorder is marked by the combination of motor and vocal tics. The onset is in childhood. Tics are usually not disabling in and of themselves, but are significant if they elicit comment or curiosity from others. Occasionally, particular tics are disruptive or result in orthopedic or dermatological complications.

Tic disorders (Table 5.7–1) as a group are (1) involuntary; (2) rapid, brief, sudden, and ejaculatory; (3) recurrent, repetitive, and stereotypical; (4) nonrhythmic, occurring at irregular intervals; (5) purposeless, inappropriate, and an end in themselves; and (6) irresistible but able to be suppressed for varying periods.

Simple motor tics, such as eye and head movements, are the most common initial symptoms. Complex motor tics include hitting oneself, jumping, touching oneself or others, and echopraxia (repeating the movements of others). Simple vocal tics are inarticulate noises, such as throat clearing, grunts, coughs, barks, high-pitched noises, and word accentuation. Complex vocal tics range from single words to sentences. Coprolalia (involuntary use of socially unacceptable expressions) is dramatic but not typical, occurring in about 20 percent of tic patients. Sensory tics are recurrent feelings of heaviness, emptiness, tickling, cold, heat, or other sensations in the skin, bones, muscles, or joints.

Tics may be suppressed for only brief periods. The symptoms change in type and severity over time. Psychosocial factors are probably not significant in the development of tic disorders.

Tics are distinguished from compulsions in that tics are involuntary and compulsions have a volitional component, although the urge to enact the compulsive behavior may be experienced as overwhelming. Simple motor tics lack the premovement electrical potential found in voluntary movements.

Family history studies suggest a link among simple tics, Tourette's disorder, and obsessive-compulsive disorder, but the only established comorbid condition is attention-deficit/hyperactivity disorder. A history of tremor and other involuntary movements should be obtained.

INTERVIEWING AND PSYCHOTHERAPEUTIC GUIDELINES

Patients with tic disorders are neither psychotic nor retarded. Pediatricians and other primary care physicians should empathize with the difficulties patients encounter as a result of the condition and be careful not to patronize or laugh at them.

EVALUATION AND MANAGEMENT

A complete psychiatric evaluation should be obtained, with attention in the differential diagnosis to such conditions as schizophrenia with bizarre movements, medication-induced abnormal movements, and comorbid conditions (for example, attention-deficit/hyperactivity disorder). The patient should be evaluated for depressive symptoms, including suicidal ideation and immature behavior, which occasionally necessitate hospitalization.

In addition, a neurological examination should be conducted to rule out neurological disorders of which tics are characteristic (Table 5.7–2).

Behavioral techniques, particularly habit reversal treatments, are effective treatments for chronic motor or vocal tic disorder and transient tic disorder. Psychotherapy or a support group may help the patient cope with social stigmatization and other problems.

DRUG TREATMENT

The mainstay of treatment for tics has been high-potency antipsychotics. Haloperidol (Haldol) decreases 70 to 90 percent of tics in 80 percent of patients. Pimozide (Orap) and clonazepam (Klonopin) have been effective in some cases. Treatment is initiated with 0.25 to 0.5 mg of haloperidol at bedtime, increasing the dosage slowly to minimize the likelihood of neuroleptic-induced dystonia.

In cases of comorbid attention-deficit/hyperactivity disorder, some clinicians recommend an initial trial with a tricyclic antidepressant, such as desipramine (Norpramin) or nortriptyline (Pamelor), before initiating a stimulant trial. Serotonergic agents (for example, clomipramine [Anafranil] or fluoxetine [Prozac]), have been reported to be of use, especially for the treatment of comorbid obsessive-compulsive disorder.

For a more detailed discussion of this topic, see G L Hanna: Tic Disorders, Chap 41, p 2325, in CTP/VI.

TABLE 5.7–2
DIAGNOSIS OF TIC DISORDERS

Disease or Syndrome	Age at Onset	Associated Features	Course	Predominant Type of Movement
Hallervorden-Spatz	Childhood-adolescence	May be associated with optic atrophy, club feet, retinitis pigmentosa, dysarthria, dementia, ataxia, emotional lability, spasticity, autosomal recessive inheritance	Progressive to death in 5 to 20 years	Choreic, athetoid, myoclonic
Dystonia musculorum deformans	Childhood-adolescence	Autosomal recessive inheritance commonly, primarily among Ashkenazi Jews; a more benign autosomal dominant form also occurs	Variable course, often progressive but with rare remissions	Dystonia
Sydenham's chorea	Childhood, usually 5–15 years	More common in females, usually associated with rheumatic fever (carditis elevated ASLO titers)	Usually self-limited	Choreiform
Huntington's disease	Usually 30–50 years, but childhood forms are known	Autosomal dominant inheritance, dementia, caudate atrophy on CT scan	Progressive to death in 10 to 15 years after onset	Choreiform
Wilson's disease (hepatolenticular degeneration)	Usually 10–25 years	Kayser-Fleischer rings, liver dysfunction, inborn error of copper metabolism; autosomal recessive inheritance	Progressive to death without chelating therapy	Wing-beating tremor, dystonia
Hyperreflexias (including latah, myriachit, jumper disease of Maine)	Generally in childhood (dominant inheritance)	Familial; may have generalized rigidity and autosomal inheritance	Nonprogressive	Excessive startle response; may have echolalia, coprolalia, and forced obedience
Myoclonic disorders	Any age	Numerous causes, some familial, usually no vocalizations	Variable, depending on cause	Myoclonus
Myoclonic dystonia	5–47 years	Nonfamilial, no vocalizations	Nonprogressive	Torsion dystonia with myoclonic jerks
Paroxysmal myoclonic dystonia with vocalization	Childhood	Attention, hyperactive, and learning disorders; movements interfere with ongoing activity	Nonprogressive	Bursts of regular, repetitive clonic (less tonic) movements and vocalizations
Tardive Tourette's disorder syndromes	Variable (after antipsychotic medication use)	Reported to be precipitated by discontinuation or reduction of medication	May terminate after increase or decrease of dosage	Orofacial dyskinesias, choreoathetosis, tics, vocalization
Neuroacanthocytosis	Third or fourth decade	Acanthocytosis, muscle wasting, parkinsonism, autosomal recessive inheritance	Variable	Orofacial dyskinesia and limb chorea, tics, vocalization

Condition	Onset	Clinical features	Course	Tics
Encephalitis lethargica	Variable	Shouting fits, bizarre behavior, psychosis, Parkinson's disease	Variable	Simple and complex motor and vocal tics, coprolalia, echolalia, echopraxia, palilalia
Gasoline inhalation	Variable	Abnormal EEG; symmetrical theta and theta bursts frontocentrally	Variable	Simple motor and vocal tics
Postangiographic complications	Variable	Emotional lability, amnestic syndrome	Variable	Simple motor and complex vocal tics, palilalia
Postinfectious	Variable	EEG: occasional asymmetrical theta bursts before movements, elevated ASLO titers	Variable	Simple motor and vocal tics, echopraxia
Posttraumatic	Variable	Asymmetrical tic distribution	Variable	Complex motor tics
Carbon monoxide poisoning	Variable	Inappropriate sexual behavior	Variable	Simple and complex motor and vocal tics, coprolalia, echolalia, palilalia
XYY genetic disorder	Infancy	Aggressive behavior	Static	Simple motor and vocal tics
XXY and 9$_p$ mosaicism	Infancy	Multiple physical anomalies, mental retardation	Static	Simple motor and vocal tics
Duchenne's muscular dystrophy (X-linked recessive)	Childhood	Mild mental retardation	Progressive	Motor and vocal tics
Fragile X syndrome	Childhood	Mental retardation, facial dysmorphism, seizures, autistic features	Static	Simple motor and vocal tics, coprolalia
Developmental and perinatal disorders	Infancy, childhood	Seizures, EEG and CT abnormalities, psychosis, aggressivity, hyperactivity, Ganser's syndrome, compulsivity, torticollis	Variable	Motor and vocal tics, echolalia

Adapted from A K Shapiro, E Shapiro, J G Young, T E Feinberg: *Gilles de la Tourette Syndrome*, ed 2. Raven, New York, 1987. Used with permission.

6

Delirium, Dementia, Amnestic and Other Cognitive Disorders

6.1 Amnesia

Amnesia, an impairment in memory, can be a sign or a symptom of a variety of disorders, including medical conditions, such as brain tumors and central nervous system (CNS) infections, substance-related disorders, and so-called functional disorders, such as posttraumatic stress disorder and dissociative disorders. Amnesia can follow a head trauma, a seizure, or a migraine headache. It may be a side effect of such substances as alcohol, sedative-hypnotics, and hallucinogens. In primary care practice, a decrease has been seen in the frequency of amnesia related to chronic alcohol abuse and an increase in the frequency of amnesia related to head trauma.

CLINICAL FEATURES AND DIAGNOSIS

The disorder usually begins abruptly, and the patients are usually aware that they have lost their memories. Some patients are upset about the memory loss, but others appear to be unconcerned or indifferent. Amnestic patients are usually alert before and after the amnesia occurs. A few patients, however, report a slight clouding of consciousness during the period immediately surrounding the amnestic period. Depression is a common predisposing factor and a coexisting finding on the mental status examination.

The amnesia may take one of several forms: (1) *localized amnesia,* the most common type, characterized by a loss of memory for the events of a short period of time (a few hours to a few days); (2) *generalized amnesia,* the loss of memory for a whole lifetime of experience; (3) *selective* (also known as *systematized*) *amnesia,* failure to recall some but not all events during a short period of time; and (4) *continuous amnesia,* characterized by forgetting each successive event as it occurs, although the patient is clearly alert and aware of what is happening in the environment at the time.

Amnesia may have a primary or secondary gain. The woman who is amnestic for the birth of a dead baby achieves primary gain by protecting herself from painful emotions. Secondary gain would accrue to a soldier who develops sudden amnesia and is removed from combat.

The differential diagnostic considerations for amnesia are listed in Table 6.1-1. Neurological signs are common in organic disorders. Is there a history of seizures or a recent electroconvulsive therapy session with postictal amnesia? Does the patient have CNS neoplasms or infections? Brain lesions (in the brainstem, the hippocampus, the third ventricle, the hypothalamic-diencephalon system, and the cortex), subarachnoid hemorrhages, and diffuse cerebral disease can present with

TABLE 6.1-1
DIFFERENTIAL DIAGNOSTIC CONSIDERATIONS IN DISSOCIATIVE AMNESIA

Dementia
Delirium
Anoxic amnesia
Cerebral infections (e.g., herpes simplex affecting temporal lobes)
Cerebral neoplasms (especially limbic and frontal)
Substance-induced (e.g., ethanol, sedative-hypnotics, anticholinergics, steroids, lithium carbonate,
β-adrenergic antagonists, pentazocine, phencyclidine, hypoglycemic agents, marijuana,
hallucinogens, methyldopa) disorders
Electroconvulsive therapy (or other strong electric shock)
Epilepsy
Metabolic disorders (e.g., uremia, hypoglycemia, hypertensive encephalopathy, porphyria)
Postconcussion (posttraumatic) amnesia
Sleep-related amnesia (e.g., sleepwalking disorder)
Transient global amnesia
Wernicke-Korsakoff syndrome
Postoperative amnesia
Other dissociative disorders
Posttraumatic stress disorder
Acute stress disorder
Somatoform disorders (somatization disorder, conversion disorder)
Malingering (especially when associated with criminal activity)

amnesia. Does the patient have a history of head trauma? Are there metabolic problems, such as hypoglycemia, porphyria, anoxia, and hypertensive encephalopathy? Is there evidence of infection (for example, herpes encephalitis)? A careful neurological examination is necessary, and a computed tomography (CT) scan or magnetic resonance imaging (MRI) is often needed.

Another condition, called transient global amnesia, occurs in middle-aged or older (over 50 years old) patients who present with an abrupt onset, bewilderment, and an inability to form new memories. A profound loss of immediate or short-term memory occurs that usually lasts several hours to a few days. The onset may occur during sexual intercourse, intense emotion, or physical exertion. The amnesia for the period affected may be lasting. The prominent symptoms include anxiety and repeated questioning of others about what happened during the amnestic period. The patient shows no loss of consciousness or of higher cognitive functions and no associated seizures. Transient global amnesia is most often caused by transient ischemic attacks (TIAs) that affect limbic midline brain structures, and it can also be associated with migraine headaches, seizures, and intoxication with sedative-hypnotic drugs. About 25 percent of affected patients have recurrent episodes. No treatment is required.

INTERVIEWING AND PSYCHOTHERAPEUTIC GUIDELINES

Amnestic patients may be confused or frightened; therefore, a calm, reassuring approach is needed. Do not pressure the patient into providing lost memories. Obtain a collateral history.

EVALUATION AND MANAGEMENT

1. The most important task is to thoroughly evaluate the patient for possibly treatable medical conditions.
2. If dissociative amnesia is diagnosed, try to help the patient recover the lost memories to prevent the creation of an amnestic nucleus that may facilitate future amnestic episodes.
3. In dissociative disorders, treatment may also include hypnosis or drug-assisted interviews. In dissociative amnesia, treatment with hypnosis or sedative-hypnotics (for example, intravenous thiopental [Pentothal] or amobarbital [Amytal]) to reduce amnestic barriers can be helpful.

DRUG TREATMENT

Drug treatment depends on the specific disorder underlying the amnesia. For instance, amnestic disorder due to temporal lobe epilepsy is most effectively addressed by treatment with anticonvulsants. The psychogenic and dissociative amnesias may be treated with benzodiazepines. Medical disorders underlying amnesias must be treated specifically. The symptoms of dissociative amnesia usually terminate abruptly, and recovery is generally complete with few recurrences.

For a more detailed discussion of this topic, see L R Squire, R D McKee: Biology of Memory, Sec 3.5, p 317; E D Caine, H Grossman, J M Lyness: Delirium, Dementia, and Amnestic and Other Cognitive Disorders and Mental Disorders Due to a General Medical Condition, Chap 12, p 705; M A Schuckit: Alcohol-Related Disorders, Sec 13.2, p 775; J C Nemiah: Dissociative Disorders, Chap 20, p 1281, in CTP/VI.

6.2 Aphasia (Impaired Language Comprehension and Expression)

Aphasia is an acquired disorder of language (comprehension, word choice, expression, syntax); it is caused by a brain dysfunction.

CLINICAL FEATURES AND DIAGNOSIS

Aphasia can be a symptom of lesions in the frontal, parietal, or temporal lobes that have occurred in the dominant hemisphere. Aphasia is most often caused by a discrete lesion. The primary care physician should always refer a patient with aphasia for a complete neurological evaluation. Often, the lesions involve Wernicke's area (used in the comprehension of speech), Broca's area (used in the motor production of speech), or the arcuate fasciculus (connecting Broca's and Wernicke's

TABLE 6.2-1
APHASIAS

Type	Fluency	Comprehension	Repetition	Naming
Broca's	No*	Yes†	No	No
Wernicke's	Yes	No	No	No
Conduction	Yes	Yes	No	No
Motor transcortical	No	Yes	Yes	No
Sensory transcortical	Yes	No	Yes	No
Mixed transcortical	No	No	Yes	No
Global	No	No	No	No
Anomic	Yes	Yes	Yes	No
Thalamic	Yes	Variable	Yes	No

*No = Impaired.
†Yes = Relatively spared.

TABLE 6.2-2
ASSESSMENT OF THE APHASIC PATIENT

Spontaneous speech
Nonfluent aphasia: Lesion anterior to central sulcus (e.g., Broca's aphasia); <50 words/min; considerable effort required to initiate speech; 1- or 2-word phrases
Fluent aphasia: Lesion posterior to central sulcus (e.g., Wernicke's aphasia); 100 to 200 words/min; easy initiation of speech; uses incorrect words and grammar; makes little sense
Word-finding difficulty
Circumlocutory phrase (e.g., what you use to tell time for clock)
Nonspecific words (e.g., thing)
Incorrect words (paraphasia)
  Literal paraphasia (e.g., pone for phone)
  Verbal paraphasia (e.g., spoon for knife)
  Jargon (googooga joob for egg)

From Speech and language disorders. F T Sherman, S M Meisells, E Margolis, and L S Libow: in The Core of Geriatric Medicine, L S Libow, F T Sherman; CV Mosby, St. Louis, 1981. Used with permission.

areas) (Table 6.2-1). The typical aphasic patient is elderly and has a cardiovascular or cerebrovascular disease.

It is important to distinguish aphasia from the confused disorganized speech sometimes presented by psychiatric patients. In addition, patients with dementia may present with poverty of speech. Dementia is usually caused by diffuse processes, rather than by discrete lesions.

Aphasias are categorized as fluent and nonfluent. *Fluent aphasia* is characterized by a normal amount and rate of speech and correctly structured sentences. However, the words or phrases are used incorrectly, making the patient's speech unintelligible (Table 6.2-2). Incorrect words may be substituted in a correct sentence structure. A patient with *nonfluent aphasia* has largely intact comprehension but an impaired ability to name objects or repeat words. Characteristically, the patient has a minimal amount of slow speech.

Both fluent and nonfluent aphasias must be differentiated from functional psychosis. Nonfluent aphasia may be confused with withdrawn, isolated behavior or elective mutism. Fluent aphasia may be confused with a thought disorder related to schizophrenia or mania. Fluent aphasia is often misdiagnosed as dementia, since the patient appears to have diffuse cognitive impairment on structured cognitive tests.

INTERVIEWING AND PSYCHOTHERAPEUTIC GUIDELINES

Be patient when evaluating aphasic patients. Empathize with patients who are frustrated by the aphasia, and concentrate on the systematic evaluation of language functions. A collateral history may be needed if communication with the patient is difficult.

EVALUATION AND MANAGEMENT

1. Test various language functions. Can the patient understand simple commands, such as "Close your eyes," either spoken or written (comprehension)? Can the patient name common simple objects, such as a pen and a watch (naming)? Can the patient repeat simple short phrases, such as "John opened the door" (repeating)?
2. Order a complete neurological examination and computed tomographic (CT) or magnetic resonance imaging (MRI) scan of the patient's head. Look for paresis of the right arm and the right side of the face in nonfluent aphasia. Nonfluent aphasias are commonly caused by lesions of the middle cerebral artery, which also can damage the motor cortex. Fluent aphasias are less typically associated with obvious motor deficits. A lumbar puncture and an electroencephalogram (EEG) may be indicated if the diagnosis is uncertain.
3. Order screening tests for medical conditions, including a complete blood count (CBC), thyroid function tests, Venereal Disease Research Laboratory (VDRL) tests, urinalysis, urine toxicology screen, tests for B_{12} and folate, and other tests as indicated (for example, human immunodeficiency virus [HIV]).

DRUG TREATMENT

Agitation is common in aphasic patients as they try to communicate, and an anxiolytic—such as lorazepam (Ativan) 1 to 2 mg by mouth or intramuscularly (IM), estazolam (ProSom) 0.5 to 1 mg by mouth, alprazolam (Xanax) 0.5 to 1 mg by mouth, or oxazepam (Serax) 10 to 30 mg by mouth—may be useful.

For a more detailed discussion of this topic, see E D Caine, H Grossman, J M Lyness: Delirium, Dementia, and Amnestic and Other Cognitive Disorders and Mental Disorders Due to a General Medical Condition, Chap 12, p 705; D P Cantwell, L Baker: Mixed Receptive-Expressive Language Disorder, Sec 36.4b, p 2264, in CTP/VI.

6.3 Blackouts

Blackouts are episodes of amnesia associated with intoxication, most commonly with alcohol, during which the patient is awake.

CLINICAL FEATURES AND DIAGNOSIS

Blackouts usually last several hours, but they may persist for days. Drugs such as sedative-hypnotics, including benzodiazepines and barbiturates, produce blackouts less often than alcohol. Brain damage is a risk. During a blackout, an intoxicated person can carry out complex behaviors, such as driving and carrying on a conversation. Sometimes, complex fugue states appear, during which long-distance travel may occur. Blackouts indicate alcohol abuse, are suggestive of alcohol dependence, and are familiar experiences for many alcohol-dependent patients. In some cases, subsequent intoxication brings back the lost memory.

INTERVIEWING AND PSYCHOTHERAPEUTIC GUIDELINES

It is extremely important that the primary care physician conduct collateral interviews with relatives, friends, or those accompanying the patient. Try to confirm alcohol use and patterns of drinking. Reassure the patient that alcohol is the most likely cause and that the condition is reversible and treatable.

EVALUATION AND MANAGEMENT

1. Prevent potential dangers (for example, driving and assaults).
2. Observe the patient for possible alcohol overdose.
3. Check for intoxication or overdose with other drugs by taking a history and conducting urine or blood toxicology screens.
4. Evaluate the patient for other possible medical problems, including head injury and nutritional deficiencies.
5. Provide supportive treatment in a nonstimulating environment.
6. Refer the patient to an alcohol dependence and rehabilitation program.

DRUG TREATMENT

Drugs should be avoided with this disorder. However, give thiamine 100 mg intramuscularly and then by mouth three times a day to treat possible superimposed alcohol-induced persisting amnestic disorder (Korsakoff's syndrome) or Wernicke's encephalopathy.

For a more detailed discussion of this topic, see M A Schuckit: Alcohol-Related Disorders, Sec 13.2, p 775, in CTP/VI.

6.4 Catatonia (Rigid Muscle Tone)

Catatonia is a condition characterized by alteration in muscle tone—for example, fixed posture or immobility, stupor, or rigidity. *Catalepsy* is a general term for a condition in which an immobile or awkward position is maintained for a prolonged period of time. A specific type of catalepsy is *waxy flexibility* (flexibilitas cerea), in which a patient's body part can be moved and, when released, remains in that position, as if the patient were made of wax.

CLINICAL FEATURES AND DIAGNOSIS

Symptoms associated with catatonia include mutism, echolalia, stupor, negativism, excitement, and repetitive motor behavior, as well as catalepsy. Catatonia is a syndrome that can be produced by organic disorders (for example, metabolic conditions and central nervous system [CNS] lesions), mood disorders, schizophrenia (for example, catatonic type), drug toxicity, and severe anxiety states (for example, posttraumatic stress disorder, dissociative disorders, and conversion disorder).

Lethal catatonia is a rare syndrome that occurs in patients receiving long-term treatment with antipsychotic medication. It is characterized by a prodrome of increasing mental and physical agitation that lasts for weeks to months. Lethal catatonia may culminate in stupor, coma, or death. It can resemble neuroleptic malignant syndrome. The two syndromes are compared in Table 6.4-1.

INTERVIEWING AND PSYCHOTHERAPEUTIC GUIDELINES

Catatonic patients may be awake and aware, despite their appearance. Clinicians should identify themselves and explain their actions. Patients may remember events, especially conversations, that occur during their catatonic episodes.

EVALUATION AND MANAGEMENT

The primary case physician should (1) perform a mental status examination if possible, (2) check the patient's vital signs, (3) complete a medical workup to rule out organicity, and (4) obtain a history of drug abuse and medications.

In the absence of a known organic condition, hypnosis should be considered for the relief of the catalepsy and related symptoms.

If the symptoms persist in spite of hypnosis or parenteral benzodiazepines, the patient should be referred for a full neurological workup, including brain scans with computed tomography (CT) or magnetic resonance imaging (MRI).

Treatments are specific to the underlying diagnosis.

DRUG TREATMENT

If the patient has a recent history of antipsychotic exposure, consider giving anticholinergic drugs—for example, benztropine (Cogentin) 2 mg by mouth or intramuscularly (IM)—to treat such extrapyramidal side effects as dystonia. However, if the patient has an underlying organic disorder, the anticholinergic drug could exacerbate the condition. Also consider the possibility of neuroleptic malignant syndrome (Table 6.4-1).

Benzodiazepines—for example, lorazepam (Ativan) 1 to 2 mg IM or intravenously (IV)—may reduce the patient's anxiety, permit cooperation with the interview, or relieve the symptoms altogether.

TABLE 6.4–1
CLINICAL DIFFERENCES BETWEEN LETHAL CATATONIA AND NEUROLEPTIC MALIGNANT SYNDROME

Stage	Lethal Catatonia	Neuroleptic Malignant Syndrome
	Prodrome lasting 2 weeks–2 months, consisting of behavioral and personality changes or frank schizophrenic symptoms Possible acute onset with no prodrome	Period of prior antipsychotic drug exposure can be hours to months Develops rapidly over a few hours to days No prodromal phase has been described
Initial symptoms	Excitement, intense anxiety, and restlessness lasting a few days Possible self-destructive or assaultive behavior Hallucinatory experiences and delusional thinking usually present Possible fever, tachycardia, and acrocyanosis Sudden death may occur	Tremors and dyskinesias are early signs Muscle hypertonicity described as lead pipe or plastic rigidity Severe excitement and intense anxiety are not major features Autonomic instability with tachycardia, labile hypertension, and possible diaphoresis Fever may not be present initially Acrocyanosis has not been described May occur in nonpsychotic patients treated with antipsychotics No deaths reported during early phase
Full syndrome	Continued increasing excitement with wild agitation and violent, destructive behavior, lasting 3–15 days, and possible choreiform movements Mutism, ridigity, or stupor may alternate with excitement Refusal of food and fluids Increasing and fluctuating fever, rapid and weak pulse, profuse, clammy perspiration, hypotension	Appearance of most major symptoms (severe muscle rigidity, persistent autonomic instability, fever) usually occurs after 2–9 days Possible agitation, confusion, and clouding of consciousness
Final stage	Cocheida, convulsions, delirium, coma, exhaustion Death may occur	Severe complications, e.g., rhabdomyolysis with elevated creatine phosphokinase, myoglobinuria, renal failure, and intravascular thrombosis with pulmonary embolism and respiratory failure Possible 20–30% mortality rate with full syndrome
Treatment	Antipsychotic drugs and other treatments to reduce severe psychotic symptoms	Immediate cessation of all dopamine-blocking antipsychotic drugs Dopamine agonists (to reduce central hypodopaminergic state), calcium channel blockers (to reduce muscle rigidity), beta-adrenergic blockers (to reduce tachycardia), other supportive measures as needed Consider using electroconvusive therapy (ECT)

Table adapted from E Castillo, R T Rubin, E Holsboer-Trachsler: Clinical differentiation between lethal catatonia and neuroleptic malignant syndrome. Am J Psychiatry *146:* 326, 1989. Used with permission.

For a more detailed discussion of this topic, see E D Caine, F Grossman, J M Lyness: Delirium, Dementia, and Other Cognitive Disorders and Mental Disorders Due to a General Medical Condition, Chap 12 p 705; A A Lipton, R Cancro: Schizophrenia: Clinical Features, Sec 14.7, p 968, in CTP/VI.

6.5 Confusion

Confusion is a disturbance in the clarity and the coherence of thinking. Confused patients may be brought by relatives to the primary care physician's office, or patients may sometimes become confused during an interview. Confusion is often considered a cardinal (although nonspecific) sign of organic disorders, but confusion can also occur in schizophrenia and psychotic mood disorders.

CLINICAL FEATURES AND DIAGNOSIS

Cognitive impairment is the major sign of confusion. Focus on cognition. Test the patient's orientation; concentration and attention; naming; reading; writing; verbal repetition; copying; and short-term, intermediate-term, and long-term memory. The primary care physician may also consider administering the Mini-Mental State Examination (MMSE), a screening examination for a wide range of cognitive functions (Table 6.5-1).

TABLE 6.5-1
MINI-MENTAL STATE EXAMINATION (MMSE) QUESTIONNAIRE

Orientation (score 1 if correct)
  Name this hospital or building.
  What city are you in now?
  What year is it?
  What month is it?
  What is the date today?
  What state are you in?
  What county is this?
  What floor of the building are you on?
  What day of the week is it?
  What season of the year is it?
Registration
  Name three objects, and have the patient repeat them. Score number
  repeated by the patient. Name the three objects several more times if needed
  for the patient to repeat correctly (record trials _____).
Attention and calculation
  Subtract 7 from 100 in serial fashion to 65. Maximum score = 5
Recall
  Do you recall the three objects named before?
Language tests
  Confrontation naming: watch, pen = 2
  Repetition: "No ifs, ands, or buts" = 1
  Comprehension: Pick up the paper in your right hand, fold it in half, and set
  it on the floor = 3
  Read and perform the command "Close your eyes" = 1
  Write any sentence (subject, object, verb) = 1
Construction
  Copy the design below = 1

Total MMSE questionnaire score (maximum = 30)

Table adapted from M F Folstein, S Folstein, P R McHugh: Mini-mental state: A practical method for grading the cognitive state of patients for the clinician. J Psychiatr Res *12*: 189, 1975. Used with permission.

Although abnormal results on the MMSE do not provide information about organicity or cause, they do provide a reliable screening of cognitive functions that can be followed over time. Psychotic patients may have abnormal MMSE results because of poor cooperation or cognitive deficits.

Table 6.5-2 lists several causes of acute confusional states requiring urgent attention.

INTERVIEWING AND PSYCHOTHERAPEUTIC GUIDELINES

The primary concern in interviewing a confused patient is the possible presence of organic disorders. Immediately assess the patient's condition; orient and reassure the patient. If the patient's behavior seems impulsive or unpredictable, providing enough staff members to ensure environmental control may help establish limits and prevent violent acts. Identify the rate of onset of the confusion and any physical or psychological stressors.

EVALUATION AND MANAGEMENT

1. Check the patient's vital and neurological signs. Abnormal findings suggest possible organic conditions. Is the patient epileptic? Is evidence of a cerebrovascular disease or a head injury present? Are risk factors for a cardiovascular disease, such as hypertension or heart disease, present?
2. Consider the patient's age. Is the patient elderly and likely to have an organic disorder? Is the patient a young person who may be abusing drugs?
3. Obtain the patient's past history of confused episodes and the rate of onset of the current episode.
4. Perform a full mental status examination. Fluctuations in consciousness suggest delirium. Psychotic symptoms and blunted affect suggest schizophrenia. Prominent amnesia and global cognitive impairment suggest dementia. Prominent mood symptoms with psychosis suggest a mood disorder.
5. What medications is the patient currently taking? Include prescribed, over-the-counter, and street drugs. Could any be causing toxic side effects? Could delirium be caused by medications (for example, anticholinergic drugs, antipsychotics, or other psychotropic drugs)?
6. Obtain the patient's medical history. Are systemic diseases, liver disease, cancer, neurological disorders (especially epilepsy), or other diseases increasing the possibility of an organic disorder?
7. Obtain a medical workup, including a physical examination with neurological examination, complete blood count (CBC), chemistry profile, thyroid function tests, urinalysis, urine drug screen, blood concentrations of drugs being taken, Venereal Disease Research Laboratory (VDRL) test, and electrocardiogram (ECG). If an organic disorder is suspected, a computed tomography (CT) or a magnetic resonance imaging (MRI) scan of the head and an electroencephalogram (EEG) are indicated. Other tests, such as a lumbar puncture, may be

TABLE 6.5–2
SOME CLUES TO CAUSES OF ACUTE CONFUSIONAL STATES DEMANDING URGENT ATTENTION

Metabolic disorders
1. Hypoglycemia: history of diabetes or alcoholism; reduced level of consciousness, shaky, sweaty, perhaps combative
2. Hyperglycemia: history of diabetes; complaints of increased thirst, urination, or flulike symptoms
3. Hyponatremia: underlying illness like lung cancer, recent stroke, chronic pulmonary infections, heart failure, cirrhosis, diuretic use
4. Hypernatremia: dehydration from inadequate fluid intake or excessive fluid loss without replacement
5. Hypercalcemia: underlying disorder such as cancer metastatic to bone, sarcoidosis, lung and renal cell cancer, multiple myeloma, and/or prolonged immobilization
6. Hypoxia: inadequate oxygen supplied to the brain because of poor pulmonary or cardiac function or carbon monoxide poisoning
7. Hypercarbia: history of chronic lung disease characterized by carbon dioxide retention; may use oxygen at home
8. Hepatic encephalopathy: history of chronic liver disease or alcoholism; probably jaundiced; ascites
9. Uremia: history of kidney disease, enlarged prostate, recent inability to pass urine
10. Thiamine deficiency (Wernicke's encephalopathy); variable degrees of ophthalmoplegia, ataxia, and mental disturbance; history of nutritional deficiency secondary to alcoholism, particularly of thiamine; since remaining thiamine in the body is rapidly used when the patient is given intravenous glucose, any patient with alcoholism should immediately receive intramuscular thiamine before glucose infusion to prevent precipitating this encephalopathy; untreated, the disorder rapidly progresses to a permanent memory disorder (Korsakoff's syndrome) and, in some advanced cases, death
11. Hypothyroidism: history of progressive fatigue, constipation, sensitivity to cold, weight gain, coarsening of hair and skin, mental slowing; examination shows abnormally low temperature and enlarged heart and slow pulse; may be precipitated by the effects of lithium on thyroid function
12. Hyperthyroidism: patient may be either hyperactive or apathetic; history may reveal rapid weight loss, diarrhea, heat intolerance, and emotional instability; examination shows goiter, silky fine hair, warm moist skin, proptosis and wide-eyed stare, fine tremor, rapid or irregular pulse; in elderly patients muscle weakness and heart failure may be most apparent
Systemic illness
1. Decreased cardiac output from various causes, such as congestive heart failure, arrhythmia, pulmonary embolus, and myocardial infarction; acute myocardial infarction presents with confusion as the major symptom in 13% of elderly patients; aged patients do not complain of typical pain; often they complain of indigestion; vital signs may be abnormal, and patient may look ill (ashen coloring, weak, nauseated, sweaty) and be confused
2. Pneumonia: recent history of a cold, becoming bedridden and aspirating; fever may not be apparent, but tachycardia or hypotension are evident on vital signs
3. Urinary tract infection: especially in patients with indwelling urinary catheters, prostatic hypertrophy, diabetes, neurogenic bladder
4. Anemia: especially with acute blood loss (injury, intestinal bleeding), chronic illness, occult gastrointestinal malignancy
5. Acute surgical emergencies: infarction of the bowel, appendicitis, and volvulus are common and often present only with confusion and no other complaints
6. Hypertension: sustained or rapid increase in blood pressure may cause encephalopathy; often has history of elevated blood pressure; may occur in patient on MAO inhibitor antidepressants who has eaten food containing tyramine
7. Vasculitides: e.g., systemic lupus erythematosus; confusion arises from cerebral involvement or treatment with steroids
8. Any febrile illness and infection can cause confusion in the aged
Central nervous system disorders
1. Subdural or epidural hematoma: may or may not have history of head trauma; fluctuating mental status often present; may have no focal neurological signs
2. Seizure: unwitnessed seizure may be suggested if patient was found on floor with evidence of incontinence or vomiting; history of seizure disorder or alcoholism
3. Stroke: history of transient ischemic attacks or strokes; may have no signs except confusion
4. Infection: meningitis (bacterial, fungal, or tuberculous), viral encephalitis
5. Tumor, primary or metastatic: with a growing mass, raised intracranial pressure may cause local compression of vital structures of herniation of the brain; in the elderly, brain atrophy allows for greater space inside the skull so that symptoms may not appear until the mass is quite large
6. Normal pressure hydrocephalus: presents with triad of gait disturbance, incontinence, dementia; surgery may be curative

Continued

TABLE 6.5–2—*continued*

Drugs and medication
  1. Almost all drugs are capable of causing confusion in the elderly; the most commonly implicated drugs include those with strong anticholinergic effects (antidepressants, antipsychotics, and antiparkinsonian drugs, and many over-the-counter preparations), sedative-hypnotics (barbiturates, benzodiazepines), cardiac medications (digoxin, propranolol, lidocaine, quinidine), antihypertensives, anticonvulsants, cimetidene, nonnarcotic and narcotic analgesics, and corticosteroids
  2. Alcohol: intoxication and withdrawal syndromes occur as in young patients, but poor health in the elderly may put geriatric patients at greater risk
  3. Drug abuse: far less common in elderly persons, but chronic intoxication with bromides, minor tranquilizers (especially meprobamate, barbiturates) occurs

Table from S L Minden: Elderly psychiatric emergency patients. In *Emergency Psychiatry*, E L Bassuk, A W Birk, editors, p 360. Plenum, New York, 1984. Used with permission.

ordered. An HIV infection may be heralded by confusion, so HIV testing may be indicated.

DRUG TREATMENT

Avoid medicating the patient until a definitive diagnosis is made. If severe agitation or potential violence is seen and tranquilization is necessary, a high-potency antipsychotic—for example, haloperidol (Haldol) 2 to 5 mg by mouth or intramuscularly (IM) or fluphenazine (Prolixin) 2 to 5 mg by mouth or IM—may be used, since benzodiazepines may worsen the confusion in organic patients.

For a more detailed discussion of this topic, see E D Caine, H Grossman, J M Lyness: Delirium, Dementia, and Amnestic and Other Cognitive Disorders and Mental Disorders Due to a General Medical Condition, Chap 12, p 705, in CTP/VI.

6.6 Delirium

Delirium is an acute organic mental syndrome involving global cognitive impairment. It is frequently missed or misdiagnosed. The primary care physician's prompt recognition and treatment of this syndrome is essential to avoid attendant morbidity and mortality.

CLINICAL FEATURES AND DIAGNOSIS

The onset of delirium is relatively rapid; the course is usually brief and rapidly fluctuating. The symptoms of delirium are listed in Table 6.6-1. The diagnostic criteria for delirium due to a general medical condition are given in Table 6.6-2.

Delirium is considered a sign of acute brain dysfunction and is, therefore, a medical emergency. The immediate goals are to make a definitive diagnosis of the cause and to reverse the cause before further deterioration, permanent damage, or physical injury occurs. Delirium is common in the medically ill, inpatients on medical and surgical services, postburn patients, and patients in intensive care units.

TABLE 6.6-1
SYMPTOMS OF DELIRIUM IN APPROXIMATE ORDER OF SPECIFICITY

1. Instability of all mental status findings over time
2. Nonauditory hallucinations
3. Misperceptions and illusions
4. Impaired attention span
5. Disorientation
6. Impaired level of consciousness
7. Auditory hallucinations
8. Other cognitive impairment
9. Delusional ideation
10. Affective symptoms

Table from O Thienhaus: Delirium and dementia. In *Manual of Clinical Emergency Psychiatry*, J R Hillard, editor, p 164. American Psychiatric Press, Washington, 1990. Used with permission.

TABLE 6.6-2
DIAGNOSTIC CRITERIA FOR DELIRIUM DUE TO A GENERAL MEDICAL CONDITION

A. Disturbance of consciousness (i.e., reduced clarity of awareness of the environment) with reduced ability to focus, sustain, or shift attention.
B. A change in cognition (such as memory deficit, disorientation, language disturbance) or the development of a perceptual disturbance that is not better accounted for by a preexisting, established, or evolving dementia.
C. The disturbance develops over a short period of time (usually hours to days) and tends to fluctuate during the course of the day.
D. There is evidence from the history, physical examination, or laboratory findings that the disturbance is caused by the direct physiological consequences of a general medical condition.

Coding note: If delirium is superimposed on a preexisting dementia of the Alzheimer's type or vascular dementia, indicate the delirium by coding the appropriate subtype of the dementia, e.g., dementia of the Alzheimer's type, with late onset, with delirium.

Coding note: Include the name of the general medical condition on Axis I, e.g., delirium due to hepatic encephalopathy; also code the general medical condition on Axis III.

Table from DSM-IV, *Diagnostic and Statistical Manual of Mental Disorders*, ed 4. Copyright American Psychiatric Association, Washington, 1994, Used with permission.

The very young and the elderly are most vulnerable. Brain damage, dementia, and a prior history of delirium are also risk factors.

INTERVIEWING AND PSYCHOTHERAPEUTIC GUIDELINES

Delirious patients may present a wide range of psychomotor activity, ranging from agitation with delirium tremens to apathy because of sensory deprivation. Try to use stimuli that balance the level of psychomotor activity—for example, minimally stimulate an agitated patient. The patient's behavior may change suddenly. Keep questions brief, since the patient's attention may be limited. Assess the patient's memory, orientation, and level of consciousness. Orient patients with repeated simple statements regarding their situation (for example, "You are in the hospital. Today is . . ."). Clinicians should give simple, repetitious explanations of who they are and what they are doing. A family member or any familiar face may help calm an agitated patient. The patient's mental status may change considerably within a period of hours. Physical restraints may be needed. Obtaining a history from collateral informants is important in establishing a diagnosis; for example, a relative may reveal that the patient is an insulin-dependent diabetic who has not been eating.

TABLE 6.6–3
PHYSICAL EXAMINATION OF THE DELIRIOUS PATIENT

Parameter	Finding	Clinical Implications
Pulse	Bradycardia	Hypothyroidism
		Stokes-Adams syndrome
		Increased intracranial pressure
	Tachycardia	Hyperthyroidism
		Infection
		Heart failure
Temperature	Fever	Sepsis
		Thyroid storm
		Vasculitis
Blood pressure	Hypotension	Shock
		Hypothyroidism
		Addison's disease
	Hypertension	Encephalopathy
		Intracranial mass
Respiration	Tachypnea	Diabetes
		Pneumonia
		Cardiac failure
		Fever
		Acidosis (metabolic)
	Shallow	Drug or alcohol intoxication
Carotid vessels	Bruits or decreased pulse	Transient cerebral ischemia
Scalp and face	Evidence of trauma	
Neck	Evidence of nuchal rigidity	Meningitis
		Subarachnoid hemorrhage
Eyes	Papilledema	Tumor
		Hypertensive encephalopathy
	Pupillary dilatation	Anxiety
		Autonomic overactivity (e.g., delirium tremens)
Mouth	Tongue or cheek lacerations	Evidence of generalized tonic-clonic seizures
Thyroid	Enlarged	Hyperthyroidism
Heart	Arrhythmia	Inadequate cardiac output, possibility of emboli
	Cardiomegaly	Heart failure
		Hypertensive disease
Lungs	Congestion	Primary pulmonary failure
		Pulmonary edema
		Pneumonia
Breath	Alcohol	
	Ketones	Diabetes
Liver	Enlargement	Cirrhosis
		Liver failure
Nervous System		
Reflexes-muscle stretch	Asymmetry with Babinski's signs	Mass lesion
		Cardiovascular disease
		Preexisting dementia
	Snout	Frontal mass
		Bilateral posterior cerebral artery occlusion
Abducent nerve (sixth cranial nerve)	Weakness in lateral gaze	Increased intracranial pressure
Limb strength	Asymmetrical	Mass lesion
		Cardiovascular disease
Autonomic	Hyperactivity	Anxiety
		Delirium

Table from R L Strub, F W Black: *Neurobehavioral Disorders: A Clinical Approach.* Davis, Philadelphia, 1981. Used with permission.

EVALUATION AND MANAGEMENT

1. Identify any possible causes from the patient's history; if any are identified, try to reverse them immediately. If untreated, delirium can lead to death. List all the patient's drugs—prescribed, over-the-counter, and drugs of abuse—especially anticholinergic drugs, antidepressants, antipsychotics, sedative-hypnotics, psychostimulants, hallucinogens, and alcohol.
2. If the patient is agitated, physical restraint may be necessary, especially in medical and surgical inpatients. Restraint may be preferable to medication if a definitive diagnosis has not been made.
3. Check the patient's vital signs, and perform a complete physical examination. Fever suggests an infection; hypertension and tachycardia suggest withdrawal from alcohol or sedative-hypnotics. Examine the patient for focal neurological signs suggesting an acute central nervous system (CNS) event. Signs of cardiopulmonary instability require prompt treatment (Table 6.6-3).
4. On the mental status examination, document the areas of cognitive impairment and the level of psychomotor activity. Test the patient's language functions. Administer the remainder of the Mini-Mental State Examination (MMSE) as the patient's cooperation permits.
5. Order laboratory tests, including a complete blood count (CBC) with differential, erythrocyte sedimentation rate (ESR), complete blood chemistries, liver and renal function tests, thyroid function tests, urinalysis, urine toxicology screen, electrocardiogram (ECG), chest X-ray, computed tomography (CT) scan of the head, and a lumbar puncture if indicated.
6. Correct any metabolic, nutritional, electrolyte, or fluid abnormalities.
7. Obtain a neurological consultation.
8. Start the treatment when a definitive diagnosis has been made. Delirium may be due to multiple causes; therefore, even after one possible cause has been identified, continue to make a full evaluation (Table 6.6-4).

DRUG TREATMENT

The primary goal is to treat the underlying condition. High-potency antipsychotics are usually the first-choice treatment for psychosis. They have little anticholinergic effects and are less likely than are low-potency antipsychotics to lower the seizure threshold. Haloperidol (Haldol) 2 to 10 mg intramuscularly (IM) may be repeated after one hour if the first dose is ineffective. Antipsychotics are less likely than benzodiazepines to worsen the patient's cognitive function. However, patients in alcohol or sedative-hypnotic withdrawal are best treated with a benzodiazepine.

Benzodiazepines—for example, lorazepam (Ativan) 1 to 2 mg by mouth, IM, or slow intravenous (IV) administration and repeated after one hour as needed—may also be used for agitation if antipsychotics are contraindicated. If several doses of an antipsychotic are ineffective, lorazepam may be added.

TABLE 6.6–4
CAUSES OF DELIRIUM

Intracranial causes
  Epilepsy and postictal states
  Brain trauma (especially concussion)
  Infections
    Meningitis
    Encephalitis
  Neoplasms
  Vascular disorders
Extracranial causes
  Drugs (ingestion or withdrawal) and poisons
    Anticholinergic agents
    Anticonvulsants
    Antihypertensive agents
    Antiparkinsonian agents
    Antipsychotic drugs
    Cardiac glycosides
    Cimetidine
    Clonidine
    Disulfiram
    Insulin
    Opiates
    Phencyclidine
    Phenytoin
    Ranitidine
    Salicylates
    Sedatives (including alcohol) and hypnotics
    Steroids
  Poisons
    Carbon monoxide
    Heavy metals and other industrial poisons

Endocrine dysfunction (hypofunction or hyperfunction)
  Pituitary
  Pancreas
  Adrenal
  Parathyroid
  Thyroid
Diseases of nonendocrine organs
  Liver
    Hepatic encephalopathy
  Kidney and urinary tract
    Uremic encephalopathy
  Lung
    Carbon dioxide narcosis
    Hypoxia
  Cardiovascular system
    Cardiac failure
    Arrhythmias
    Hypotension
Deficiency diseases
  Thiamine, nicotinic acid, B_{12}, or folic acid deficiencies
Systemic infections with fever and sepsis
Electrolyte imbalance of any cause
Postoperative states
Trauma (head or general body)

Table adapted from Charles E. Wells, MD.

For a more detailed discussion of this topic, see E D Caine, H Grossman, J M Lyness: Delirium, Dementia, And Amnestic and Other Cognitive Disorders and Mental Disorders Due to a General Medical Condition, Chap 12, p 705, in CTP/VI.

6.7 Dementia

Dementia is a loss of cognitive and intellectual functions that is sufficiently severe to interfere with the patient's social or occupational functioning and is a decline from a previously higher level of functioning. Dementia is primarily a syndrome of the elderly, who will make up an increasingly larger percentage of the primary care physician's patient load as the United States population continues to age.

CLINICAL FEATURES AND DIAGNOSIS

The essential deficit is a loss of memory, both short-term and long-term. Abstract thinking and judgment are also frequently impaired, often with other signs of high cortical involvement as well as a marked change in personality (Table 6.7-1).

TABLE 6.7-1
DIAGNOSTIC CRITERIA FOR DEMENTIA

A. The development of multiple cognitive deficits manifested by both
  1. Memory impairment (impaired ability to learn new information or to recall previously learned information.
  2. One (or more) of the following disturbances:
    a. Aphasia (language disturbance)
    b. Apraxia (impaired ability to carry out motor activities despite intact motor function)
    c. Agnosia (failure to recognize or identify objects despite intact sensory function)
    d. Disturbance in executive functioning (i.e., planning, organizing, sequencing, abstracting)
B. The cognitive deficits in criteria A1 and A2 each cause significant impairment in social or occupational functioning and represent a significant decline from a previous level of functioning.
C. There is evidence from the history, physical examination, or laboratory fincings that the disturbance is the direct physiological consequence of one of the general medical conditions listed below.
D. The deficits do not occur exclusively during the course of a delirium.

Table from DSM-IV, *Diagnostic and Statistical Manual of Mental Disorders*, ed 4. Copyright American Psychiatric Association, Washington, 1994. Used with permission.

TABLE 6.7-2
CLINICAL DIFFERENTIATION OF DELIRIUM AND DEMENTIA*

	Delirium	Dementia
History	Acute disease	Chronic disease
Onset	Rapid	Insidious (usually)
Duration	Days–weeks	Months–years
Course	Fluctuating	Chronically progressive
Level of consciousness	Fluctuating	Normal
Orientation	Impaired, at least periodically	Intact initially
Affect	Anxious, irritable	Labile but not usually anxious
Thinking	Often disordered	Decreased amount
Memory	Recent memory is markedly impaired	Both recent and remote are impaired
Perception	Hallucinations common (especially visual)	Hallucinations less common (except sundowning)
Psychomotor	Retarded, agitated, or mixed	Normal
Sleep	Disrupted sleep-wake cycle	Less disruption of sleep-wake cycle
Attention and awareness	Prominently impaired	Less impaired
Reversibility	Often reversible	Majority not reversible

* *Note:* Demented patients are more susceptible to delirium, and delirium superimposed on dementia is common.

Dementia must be differentiated from normal aging, delirium, and depression. In *normal aging* the patient may have some loss of cognitive function, but it is not progressive and does not cause impairments in social and occupational functioning. The differential diagnosis between dementia and delirium is summarized in Table 6.7-2. The differential diagnosis between dementia and depression (pseudodementia) is summarized in Table 6.7-3. Demented patients often have a superimposed delirium or depression.

Dementia, although possible at any age after which an intelligence quotient (I.Q.) can be determined, is primarily a syndrome of the elderly. Increasing age is the major risk factor for dementia. The primary short-term objectives in treating demented patients are identifying and reversing any reversible dementias, managing behavioral emergencies, and treating any other medical and psychiatric conditions.

The most common cause of dementia is Alzheimer's disease, followed by vascular dementia. Mixed forms are also common. Acquired immune deficiency syndrome (AIDS) is a common cause in young patients. Other causes are listed in Table 6.7-4.

TABLE 6.7–3
DEMENTIA VERSUS DEPRESSION

Feature	Dementia	Pseudodementia
Age	Usually elderly	Nonspecific
Onset	Vague	Days to weeks
Course	Slow, worse at night	Rapid, even through day
History	Systemic illness or drugs	Mood disorder
Awareness	Unawareness, unconcerned	Aware, distressed
Organic signs	Often present	Absent
Cognition*	Prominent Impairment	Personally changes
Mental status examination	Consistent, spatty deficits	Variable deficits in different modalities
	Approximates, confabulates, perseverates	Apathetic, "I don't know"
	Emphasizes trivial accomplishments	Emphasizes failures
	Shalow or labile mood	Depressed
Behavior	Appropriate to degree of cognitive impairment	Incongruent with degree of cognitive impairment
Cooperation	Cooperative but frustrated	Uncooperative with little effort
CT and EEG	Abnormal	Normal

* Benzodiazepines and barbiturates worsen cognitive impairments in the demented patient, whereas they help the depressed patient to relax.

TABLE 6.7–4
Causes of Dementia

Tumor	Physiological
Primary cerebral[a]	Epilepsy[a]
Trauma	Normal pressure hydrocephalus[a]
Hematomas[a]	Metabolic
Posttraumatic dementia[a]	Vitamin deficiencies[a]
Infection (chronic)	Chronic metabolic disturbances[a]
Metastatic[a]	Chronic anoxic states[a]
Syphilis	Chronic endocrinopathies[a]
Creutzfeldt–Jacob disease[b]	Degenerative dementias
AIDS dementia complex[c]	Alzheimer's disease[b]
Cardiac/vascular	Pick's disease (dementias of frontal lobe type)[b]
Single Infarction[a]	Parkinson's disease[a]
Multiple infarction[b]	Progressive supranuclear palsy[c]
Large infarction	Idiopathic cerebral ferrocalcinosis (Fahr's disease)[c]
Lacunar infarction	Wilson's disease[a]
Strewanger's disease (subcortical arteriosclerotic encephalopathies)	Demyelinating
Hemodynamic type[a]	Multiple sclerosis[c]
Congenital/hereditary	Drugs and toxins
Huntington's disease[c]	Alcohol[a]
Metachromatic leukodystrophy[c]	Heavy metals[a]
Primary psychiatric	Carbon monoxide poisoning[a]
Pseudodementia[c]	Medications[a]
	Irradiation[a]

[a] Variable or missed pattern.
[b] Predominantly cortical pattern.
[c] Predominantly subcortical pattern.

Table from E D Caine, H Grossman, J M Lyness. Delirium, dementia, and amnestic and other cognitive disorders and mental disorders due to a general medical condition. In *Comprehensive Textbook of Psychiatry*, ed 6, H I Kaplan, B J Sadock, editors, p 734. Williams & Wilkins, Baltimore, 1995, p 734.

Patients with dementia are typically brought to the primary care physician's office by their family or caretakers who complain of the patient's wandering, confusion, inappropriate behavior (for example, touching others in a sexually inappropriate way, walking out of the house partially clad), aggression, depression, anxiety, or delusionally driven behavior (for example, accusations of theft). Patients with a known diagnosis of dementia are frequently brought in because of a sudden change in their behavior.

INTERVIEWING AND PSYCHOTHERAPEUTIC GUIDELINES

If patients are disoriented or confused, try to orient them and help them relax. In evaluating the patient's mental status, focus on cognitive functions and administer the Mini-Mental State Examination (MMSE). If the patient seems to be irritated or embarrassed by questions that reveal impaired cognition, change the subject, and return to examining the patient's cognition later. Try to determine the course of the impairment, whether it had a rapid onset or a slow onset, and whether there were physical or psychological precipitants to the present episode.

Note the patient's affect, especially whether the patient is depressed or anxious. What is the patient's attitude toward the impairment? Does it bother the patient, or is the patient unconcerned? Determining the patient's attitude helps identify possible pseudodementia. Patients with dementia often minimize or deny their cognitive deficits; those with pseudodementia often have exaggerated complaints of memory loss (Table 6.7-3).

EVALUATION AND MANAGEMENT

1. Obtain a full physical and neurological examination. The medical workup should include a complete blood count (CBC) with differential white blood count, liver function tests, the blood urea nitrogen (BUN) and creatinine test, thyroid function tests, a Venereal Disease Research Laboratory (VDRL) test, B_{12} and folate levels, a urinalysis, a urine toxicology screen, an electrocardiogram (ECG), a chest X-ray, and a computed tomography (CT) or magnetic resonance imaging (MRI) scan of the head. A lumbar puncture may also be indicated.
2. Interview collaborative sources, such as the family, for the patient's history.
3. The elderly take many more medications than do the young. Identify all the prescribed and over-the-counter drugs the patient takes. The patient may also take alcohol and drugs of abuse. Any drugs that could possibly cause dementia should be systematically discontinued if that is medically possible. Common candidates for discontinuation include antihypertensives, anticonvulsants, antipsychotics, sedative-hypnotics, steroids, antiarrhythmics, anticholinergics, methyldopa, and antidepressants.
4. Perform a mental status examination, including a detailed cognitive examination, and assess depressive or psychotic symptoms.
5. Identify and treat the patient's medical problems; correct any nutritional and metabolic deficiencies. Preventive measures (changes in diet, exercise, and control of diabetes and hypertension) are especially important in vascular dementia. Assess any behavioral changes in a known dementia patient. Evaluate the patient for superimposed delirium, a brain injury (for example, a cerebral infarct or a subdural hematoma secondary to a fall), or an environmental change (for exam-

ple, the recent replacement of a long-time home attendant or some other change in caretaking).
6. Decide whether admission to a hospital or a nursing home is needed. Unless the patient has an acute medical or behavioral emergency, try to avoid hospital admission, since disposition problems (for example, finding a nursing home bed) may produce a long, medically unnecessary hospitalization.
7. Counsel the patient's family regarding the prognosis; the possible need for placement in a nursing home, home care, or legal guardianship; the possible behaviors to expect from the patient; and the syndromes that may develop in the caretakers (for example, burnout, depression, and anxiety). When appropriate, refer the family to the Alzheimer's Disease and Related Disorders Association (ADRDA). The family can obtain information about local groups by writing to ADRDA, 70 East Lake Street, Chicago, IL 60601.

DRUG TREATMENT

Use low dosages of all psychotropic medications in the elderly. Adhere to the maxim, "start low, go slow."

Although antipsychotics such as haloperidol (Haldol) 0.5 to 5 mg a day are the primary psychotropic drugs for behavioral control in demented patients, the elderly clear many drugs more slowly than do young patients because of decreased hepatic and renal function. The primary problems with antipsychotics in the elderly are the acute side effects, including dystonia, parkinsonism, anticholinergic side effects, and hypotension. High-potency antipsychotic agents, such as haloperidol, are preferable to low-potency agents, such as chlorpromazine (Thorazine), whose strong anticholinergic effects can further impair the patient's cognition.

Tacrine (Cognex) (initially 40 mg a day, up to a maximum 160 mg a day in divided doses) has been approved as a treatment for Alzheimer's disease. Well-controlled trials have shown a clinically significant improvement in 20 to 25 percent of patients who take it. However, physicians should be aware of possible adverse effects, especially changes in serum aminotransferase concentrations. In patients with liver dysfunction, tacrine should be used with caution. Serum aminotransferase concentrations should be closely monitored in all patients.

Some clinicians recommend short-acting benzodiazepines for insomnia or anxiety in the elderly, but the risks of cognitive impairment and dependence must be considered. The use of conjugated benzodiazepines—oxazepam (Serax) 7.5 to 15 mg by mouth, lorazepam (Ativan) 0.5 to 1 mg by mouth, temazepam (Restoril) 7.5 to 15 mg by mouth—is recommended because the elimination half-life of those drugs is not increased in the elderly by their impaired liver function.

Antidepressants, lithium, and anticonvulsants may be used, but they should be started at low dosages, increased slowly, and monitored with frequent blood concentrations. Monoamine oxidase inhibitors (MAOIs) may be useful for depression associated with dementia.

Antihistamines may be used in low dosages for anxiety or insomnia, but they may cause anticholinergic side effects to which the demented are especially sensitive.

For a more detailed discussion of this topic, see E D Caine, H Grossman, J M Lyness: Delirium, Dementia, and Amnestic and Other Cognitive Disorders and Mental Disorders Due to a General Medical Condition, Chap 12, p 705, in CTP/VI.

6.8 Disorientation

Disorientation is impaired awareness of time, place, or person. This symptom is often considered a hallmark of organic disorders that produce global cognitive impairment, particularly delirium and dementia.

CLINICAL FEATURES AND DIAGNOSIS

The primary objective for the primary care physician is to determine whether an acute organic disorder is present and, if so, to reverse it. In general, assume that delirium is present, and proceed accordingly. Patients with psychiatric disorders who are severely psychotic may also be disoriented.

INTERVIEWING AND PSYCHOTHERAPEUTIC GUIDELINES

In testing the patient's orientation, do not give any information that reveals the correct answer. Test the patient's orientation in detail, and try to quantify the degree of disorientation. Ask for the patient's name and age. Testing for orientation to time initially includes questions about the day, date, month, and year. If the patient is not oriented to those facts, inquire about the season and whether it is day or night. Similarly, if the patient is not oriented to place (for example, does not know the name of the hospital), inquire whether the patient knows the function of the building ("Is this a police station? A train station?"). If the patient does not know the name or the function of the building, ask for the name of the town, the county, the state, and the country.

If a patient is disoriented, screen for other signs of cognitive impairment. Administer the Mini-Mental State Examination (MMSE) as a broad screening test.

EVALUATION AND MANAGEMENT

1. Obtain the patient's vital signs. If the signs are abnormal, suspect a central nervous system (CNS) infection, delirium from alcohol or sedative-hypnotic withdrawal, or delirium from other causes.
2. Ask about medications. Both psychotropic and medical drugs can cause delirium, of which disorientation may be a sign. Steroids, anticholinergic drugs, anticonvulsants, antiparkinsonian agents, antipsychotics, benzodiazepines, antihypertensives, cardiac glycosides, cimetidine (Tagamet), and disulfiram (Antabuse) should be considered as possible causes of the cognitive impairment.

3. Consider drugs of abuse. Intoxication or withdrawal from alcohol or sedative-hypnotics and intoxication with hallucinogens or psychostimulants may disorient the patient.
4. Examine the patient for medical and neurological conditions. Consider such medical conditions as thyroid disease, cardiac failure, nutritional deficiencies, cancer, hepatic failure, renal failure, sepsis, and electrolyte imbalance. Consider such neurological conditions as head trauma, epilepsy, meningitis, encephalitis, CNS neoplasms, and vascular disorders.
5. Ask for the patient's history and the course of the disorientation. Is it a new condition? If so, the search for a reversible cause must be aggressive.
6. Consider the age of the patient. An adolescent is likely to be abusing street drugs, but an elderly person is likely to be demented or delirious from prescription drugs.
7. Perform a medical workup. The full workup consists of a detailed physical examination and laboratory tests, including a complete blood count with differential white cell count; a chemistry profile, including electrolytes, liver function tests, and blood urea nitrogen; thyroid function tests; tests for B_{12} and folate; Venereal Disease Research Laboratory (VDRL) test; a urinalysis; a urine toxicology screen; an electrocardiogram (ECG); and a chest X-ray. A computed tomographic (CT) scan of the head, an electroencephalogram (EEG), and a lumbar puncture may also be indicated. Neurological and medical consultations may be needed.

DRUG TREATMENT

Although medications should be avoided, pending the results of a definitive workup, severe agitation or uncooperativeness may require medication. High-potency antipsychotics—for example, haloperidol (Haldol), fluphenazine (Prolixin), thiothixene (Navane), and trifluoperazine (Stelazine), all given at 2 to 5 mg by mouth or intramuscularly (IM)—are the drugs of choice over benzodiazepines; antipsychotics are less likely than benzodiazepines to worsen the patient's cognition. However, benzodiazepines are indicated if withdrawal from alcohol or sedative-hypnotics is a possible diagnosis.

For a more detailed discussion of this topic, see E D Caine, H Grossman, J M Lyness: Delirium, Dementia, and Amnestic and Other Cognitive Disorders and Mental Disorders Due to a General Medical Condition, Chap 12, p 705, in CTP/VI.

6.9 Wernicke's Encephalopathy

Wernicke's encephalopathy is characterized by ophthalmoplegia, weakness, a staggering gait, and confusion in the long-term alcoholic person. The diagnosis is critical, since the acute encephalopathy is treatable with thiamine and usually resolves in a matter of days; if untreated, the condition progresses to Korsakoff's syndrome. Other signs of thiamine deficiency may also be present, such as cardiovascular disease.

CLINICAL FEATURES AND DIAGNOSIS

The hallmark of Wernicke's encephalopathy is confusion, so a reliable history is difficult to obtain. In addition, the patient may not be currently drinking, making the association with alcohol difficult to establish. The confusion is marked by apathy, slowed responses, and disorientation, despite gross awareness, lack of drowsiness, and superficially appropriate behavior.

The patient's apathy may impress the primary care physician as a lack of effort. A thorough examination, however, reveals that the patient cannot retain new information, despite repeated efforts.

The ocular symptoms are related to sixth cranial nerve palsy and include internal strabismus, dysconjugate gaze, and nystagmus. A staggering gait is present even in the absence of acute intoxication.

INTERVIEWING AND PSYCHOTHERAPEUTIC GUIDELINES

The patient's apathetic demeanor and superficial cooperation may foster an unfortunate lack of concern or even antipathy in the physician. A disposition made too rapidly because of bias will frustrate an accurate diagnosis, with catastrophic results. A structured approach to the diagnosis of organic mental syndromes is always suggested. An appropriate and reliable screening tool is the Mini-Mental State Examination (MMSE). Do not ignore disturbances of consciousness, as they are associated with a high rate of serious occult medical illness and subsequent mortality.

EVALUATION AND MANAGEMENT

1. A neurological examination is necessary to establish the diagnosis.
2. The onset may be sudden or gradual, and it is unrelated to the presence of alcohol, so the patient may present in any stage of intoxication or withdrawal.
3. A thiamine level may confirm the diagnosis, but treatment should proceed without awaiting the results.
4. The short-term treatment is the correction of the nutritional deficiency. Early Wernicke's encephalopathy is largely reversible with timely treatment. The remainder of the patient's care is directed at alcohol detoxification and rehabilitation. Admission to a medical service is usually indicated.
5. Observe the patient closely to prevent self-harm secondary to confusion.

DRUG TREATMENT

Alcohol-dependent patients should be given thiamine 100 mg parenterally and subsequently placed on daily supplements of thiamine 100 mg, folic acid 1 mg, and multivitamins. Elevated vital signs, tremor, and vomiting are consistent with concurrent alcohol withdrawal and can be treated with diazepam (Valium) 5 mg intravenously (IV) or lorazepam (Ativan) 2 mg intramuscularly (IM) or IV repeated at 30-minute intervals until the withdrawal symptoms are controlled. The total benzodiazepine dose during the first 24 hours may then be tapered by 20 percent a day.

For a more detailed discussion of this topic, see M A Schuckit: Alcohol-Related Disorders, Sec 13.2, p 775, in CTP/VI.

6.10 Korsakoff's Syndrome

Korsakoff's syndrome (also called alcohol-induced persisting amnestic disorder) is an amnestic syndrome caused by thiamine (vitamin B_1) deficiency related to long-standing severe alcohol dependence and general nutritional deficiency. It often follows an acute episode of Wernicke's encephalopathy (confusion, ataxia, nystagmus, ophthalmoplegia), which is also due to thiamine deficiency. Wernicke's encephalopathy, the acute stage of the syndrome, usually has an abrupt onset; Korsakoff's syndrome has a slow onset and a chronic course. Once Korsakoff's syndrome emerges, the prognosis is poor; only 20 percent of patients make a substantial recovery. Thus, it is important that the primary care physician treat any manifestation of Wernicke's encephalopathy immediately.

CLINICAL FEATURES AND DIAGNOSIS

In Korsakoff's syndrome the patient has an irreversible short-term memory impairment in the presence of a clear sensorium. The syndrome is associated with confabulation (the filling in of memory deficits with false information). Since the disorder usually occurs in persons who have been drinking heavily for many years, it rarely occurs before the age of 35. Postmortem brain biopsies often reveal bilateral structural lesions in the mamillary bodies.

INTERVIEWING AND PSYCHOTHERAPEUTIC GUIDELINES

The patients are generally alert and cooperative but completely disoriented, not knowing the place, the time, or in some cases even their own identities. The physician must be calm, supportive, and empathic, as the patients can be severely confused and vulnerable.

EVALUATION AND MANAGEMENT

1. Prompt diagnosis and treatment by the primary care physician is crucial.
2. Thiamine treatment improves the ocular symptoms, the ataxia, and the confusional symptoms within days.

3. The administration of carbohydrates (including intravenous [IV] dextrose) before thiamine replacement has been reported to worsen the patient's symptoms. Therefore, give thiamine first to all alcoholic and nutritionally deficient patients before starting any other treatment.
4. An adequate diet should be instituted.

DRUG TREATMENT

Treatment includes immediate thiamine supplementation—100 mg given by mouth two to three times daily; the treatment should be continued for 3 to 12 months.

No specific drug treatment is indicated other than thiamine. If severe agitation or confusion makes the patient unmanageable, a short-acting benzodiazepine—for example, lorazepam (Ativan) 0.5 to 1 mg by mouth or intramuscularly (IM)—or a high-potency antipsychotic—for example, haloperidol (Haldol) or fluphenazine (Prolixin), both given at 1 to 2 mg by mouth or IM—may be used.

For a more detailed discussion of this topic, see E D Caine, H Grossman, J M Lyness: Delirium, Dementia, and Amnestic and Other Cognitive Disorders and Mental Disorders Due to a General Medical Condition, Chap 12, p 705; M A Schuckit: Alcohol-Related Disorders, Sec 13.2, p 775, in CTP/VI.

6.11 Sundowner Syndrome

Sundowner syndrome is seen in the elderly, usually at night. It is characterized by drowsiness, confusion, disorientation, transient psychotic symptoms, ataxia, and falling. It occurs in the aged as a result of being overly sedated with medications and in demented patients who react adversely to even a small dose of a psychoactive drug. The primary care physician should exercise great caution in prescribing sedatives to the elderly. If their use is necessary, they should be prescribed in the smallest dose possible. The patient and the patient's relatives or caretakers should be cautioned about the possibility of sundowning.

CLINICAL FEATURES AND DIAGNOSIS

Sundowner syndrome is a variant of delirium and may present dramatically with delusions and hallucinations. Depression, anxiety, and irritability can be the presenting symptoms. Some patients are demanding and uncooperative and attempt to leave the hospital against medical advice. Sundowner syndrome may be secondary to the sensory deprivation that occurs when elderly, cognitively impaired patients are placed in a new environment, such as a hospital.

INTERVIEWING AND PSYCHOTHERAPEUTIC GUIDELINES

The key to interviewing any disorganized patient, whatever the cause, is to gently but firmly impose a high degree of structure. The first questions may be abstract, but, as soon as the patient fails to respond appropriately, substitute concrete questions. Rambling, pointless responses may be interrupted after a brief unstructured speech sample has been obtained.

Ask the patient about delusions, hallucinations, and suicidal and aggressive ideas, even if the answers are fragmentary and inconsistent.

Document cognitive deficits using the Mini-Mental State Examination (MMSE).

The patients' irritability and poor responses should not provoke the physician to discontinue an examination in frustration.

EVALUATION AND MANAGEMENT

1. Management focuses on establishing and treating the underlying condition.
2. Restraints may be necessary. A waist or camisole restraint may suffice to prevent wandering. Two-point or three-point restraints (legs together constituting one point) may be necessary if the patient is agitated or aggressive. Patients attempting to leave should be restrained and held for the consultant. Emergency treatment should proceed while awaiting the consultation.
3. Parenteral medication may be preferable to the prolonged use of restraints and may be administered under the emergency exception to the doctrine of informed consent. In fact, patients with sundowner syndrome are incapable of informed consent, and the physician who allows such patients to leave or fails to render appropriate treatment because of their refusal may be liable for any damages that result.
4. The use of clocks, calendars, radios, and televisions and the presence of family or friends at the bedside may be useful in treating sundowner syndrome secondary to sensory deprivation.

DRUG TREATMENT

For agitation, lorazepam (Ativan) may be given in 1 to 2 mg doses by mouth or intramuscularly (IM). Low-dose antipsychotics—for example, haloperidol (Haldol) 0.5 mg—at bedtime may be of use in treating sundowner syndrome in elderly demented patients. However, if the syndrome is the result of medication excess, use only supportive or restraining methods.

For a more detailed discussion of this topic, see E D Caine, H Grossman, J M Lyness: Delirium, Dementia, and Amnestic and Other Cognitive Disorders and Mental Disorders Due to a General Medical Condition, Chap 12, p 705; M A Schuckit: Alcohol-Related Disorders, Sec 13.2, p 775, in CTP/VI.

6.12 Syncope (Fainting)

Syncope is the brief loss of consciousness, usually lasting no longer than 15 seconds, caused by decreased perfusion, generally in the carotid arteries and occasionally in the vertebral-basilar system. The most common causes of syncope are vasovagal dysfunction, orthostatic hypotension, cardiac arrhythmia, and, much less often, vertebral-basilar artery insufficiency. The most commonly associated psychiatric disorder is blood-injection-injury phobia, in which fainting is common on exposure to a phobic stimulus because of a vasovagal mechanism. Many psychotropic medications have orthostatic hypotension as a side effect.

CLINICAL FEATURES AND DIAGNOSIS

The primary care physician should begin the assessment of syncope with a medication history, and continue with the patient's postural vital signs, auscultation of the heart and the neck, a thorough neurological examination, and an electrocardiogram (Table 6.12-1). Do not ascribe alterations in the patient's mental state to a psychiatric condition until possible medical causes, some of which are life-threatening or disabling, have been thoroughly considered.

The psychiatric causes of syncope have historically included hysteria and, recently, anxiety disorders. Fainting was at one time a culturally accepted response to stress among women and was described as hysterical. It is still the kind of dramatic attention-seeking behavior that, although now not common, suggests the diagnosis of histrionic personality disorder.

Exposure to blood, the threat of injury, or the news of illness can provoke a vasovagal episode, resulting in syncope. That type of phobic response is unusual. More commonly, specific phobia results in autonomic arousal, resembling panic. If the patient can avoid phobic stimuli, the condition results in little distress. Occasionally, blood-injection-injury phobia causes delayed medical attention. Because of avoidance, few phobics are seen in clinical settings, but they are common in the community. Although most specific phobias are fears of animals and have their onset in childhood, blood-injection-injury phobias typically begin in adolescence. Unlike panic disorder, the phobia may be causatively related. Patients are invariably aware that their fears are excessive or unreasonable.

INTERVIEWING AND PSYCHOTHERAPEUTIC GUIDELINES

The loss of consciousness for any reason is a frightening experience for the patient and should be taken seriously. Try to determine the cause; for example, patients with blood-injection-injury phobia may report prior episodes.

If the patient appears to be genuinely unconcerned, that unconcern may be *la belle indifférence* and may point to a conversion disorder.

It is important to determine whether or not the symptom is deliberately produced, as in factitious disorder. Detailed questioning about the context of the episode may uncover evidence of a strong affect associated with conflicts that relate to a recent real or imagined event involving significant others.

EVALUATION AND MANAGEMENT

1. If organic causes have been eliminated, no specific management is required for psychogenic syncope.

TABLE 6.12–1
CLINICAL APPROACH TO SYNCOPE

Evaluation and Assessment	Clinical Syndrome	Second-Order Evaluation
History		
Provocation		
Upright position	Postural hypotension	
Recumbent position	Hysteria, hyperventilation hypoglycemia, arrhythmia	
Exercise	Aortic stenosis, IHSS,[1] arrhythmia	
Emotional stress	Vasodepressor, hyperventilation	
Food intake	Fasting or reactive hypoglycemia	Blood sugar
Drugs and toxin exposure	Iatrogenic or abuse	
Duration		
Prolonged	Aortic stenosis, IHSS	
Seconds	Hypoglycemia, hysteria, cerebrovascular disease, arrhythmia	
Premonitory symptoms		
None	Arrhythmia, postural hypotension	
Palpitations	Arrhythmia	
Vagal	Vasodepressor	
Dyspnea, light-headedness, numbness	Hyperventilation	
Neurological symptoms	Cerebrovascular disease	EEG, CT, MRI, lumbar puncture
Physical examination		
Orthostatic hypotension		
Tachycardia	Volume loss	Tests for volume loss, adrenal insufficiency
Normal heart rate	Autonomic postural hypotension	Tests for integrity of autonomic and voluntary nervous systems (tabes, diabetes, β-blockers, or other drug-related cause)
Carotid pulse, cardiac murmur	Left ventricular outflow obstruction, localized vascular disease	Echocardiogram, ECG, carotid duplex, catheterization
Carotid sinus massage	Carotid sinus hypersensitivity	
Voluntary hyperventilation	Hyperventilation	
Electrocardiogram		
Heart block, bilateral bundle branch block		
Sinus bradycardia, block, arrest	Bradycardia	Prolonged monitoring, resting or ambulatory; stress test, pacing and His bundle electrophysiologic studies
Supraventricular tachycardia, WPW[2]	Tachycardia	
PVC[3] or ventricular tachycardia	Tachycardia	

Adapted from R J Noble: The patient with syncope. JAMA *237:* 1375, 1977. Used with permission. Table from L Goldfrank, N A Lewin, M A Howland, R S Weisman: Diets. In *Goldfrank's Toxicologic Emergencies,* L Goldfrank, N E Flomenbaum, N A Lewin, R S Weisman, M A Howland, editors, p 297. Appleton Lange, Norwalk, Conn, 1990.
[1] IHSS = ideopathic hypertrophic subaortic stenosis
[2] WPW = Wolff-Parkinson-White syndrome
[3] PVCs = premature ventricular contractions

2. Patients with blood-injection-injury phobia do not respond to simple reassurance, since the patients are already aware that their fears are unrealistic.
3. If the patient is unable to avoid the stimulus on a regular basis, a variety of behavioral techniques involving systematic exposure to the phobic stimulus may be useful.

DRUG TREATMENT

If orthostatic hypotension is the result of adrenergic side effects of medication, the dosage may require adjustment. Encourage oral hydration. Some patients respond to fludrocortisone (Florinef) 0.025 to 0.05 mg twice a day. High-potency antipsychotics may be used instead of low-potency drugs.

If a phobic patient must be regularly exposed to a phobic situation, a β-blocker, such as atenolol (Tenormin) 50 to 100 mg as needed, may be sufficient.

Benzodiazepines may be useful for a short time if the patient is overwhelmed, but regular use must be weighed against the risks of benzodiazepine dependence.

For a more detailed discussion of this topic, see A J Fyer, S Mannuzza, J D Coplan: Panic Disorders and Agoraphobia, Sec 17.1, p 1191; D H Barlow, M R Liebowitz: Specific Phobia and Social Phobia, Sec 17.2, p 1204, in CTP/VI.

7

Mental Disorders Associated with a General Medical Condition

7.1 Acquired Immune Deficiency Syndrome (AIDS)

Acquired immune deficiency syndrome (AIDS) results from infection by the human immunodeficiency virus (HIV), which is associated with a broad array of other medical conditions and neuropsychiatric syndromes. Primary care physicians will be treating increasing numbers of HIV infected persons, and should therefore be familiar with HIV-associated psychiatric conditions. Clinically, neuropsychiatric complications (for example, HIV encephalopathy) occur in at least 50 percent of HIV-infected patients and may be the first signs of the disease in about 10 percent of patients. Classic psychiatric syndromes (for example, anxiety disorders, depressive disorders, and psychotic disorders) are commonly associated with HIV-related disorders.

Primary care physicians should be familiar with the Centers for Disease Control (CDC) guidelines for the prevention of HIV transmission (Table 7.1-1), and prepared to discuss safe-sex practices with their patients (Table 7.1-2). Possible indications for HIV testing are included in Table 7.1-3. Patients belonging to high-risk groups are also listed there.

CLINICAL FEATURES AND DIAGNOSIS

A diagnosis of AIDS is made in an HIV-positive patient with findings of decreased cell-mediated immunity and subsequent opportunistic infections (such as *Pneumo-*

TABLE 7.1-1
CDC GUIDELINES FOR THE PREVENTION OF HIV TRANSMISSION FROM INFECTED TO UNINFECTED PERSONS

Infected persons should be counseled to prevent the further transmission of HIV by

1. Informing prospective sex partners of their infection with HIV, so they can take appropriate precautions. Abstention from sexual activity with another person is one option that would eliminate any risk of sexually transmitted HIV infection.
2. Protecting a partner during any sexual activity by taking appropriate precautions to prevent that person's coming into contact with the infected person's blood, semen, urine, feces, saliva, cervical secretions, or vaginal secretions. Although the efficacy of using condoms to prevent infections with HIV is still under study, the consistent use of condoms should reduce the transmission of HIV by preventing exposure to semen and infected lymphocytes.
3. Informing previous sex partners and any persons with whom needles were shared of their potential exposure to HIV and encouraging them to seek counseling and testing.
4. For IV drug abusers, enrolling or continuing in programs to eliminate the abuse of IV substances. Needles, other apparatus, and drugs must never be shared.
5. Never sharing toothbrushes, razors, or other items that could become contaminated with blood.
6. Refraining from donating blood, plasma, body organs, other tissue, or semen.
7. Avoiding pregnancy until more is known about the risks of transmitting HIV from the mother to the fetus or newborn.
8. Cleaning and disinfecting surfaces on which blood or other body fluids have spilled, in accordance with previous recommendations.
9. Informing physicians, dentists, and other appropriate health professionals of antibody status when seeking medical care, so that the patient can be appropriately evaluated.

Table from MMWR *35*:182, 1986. Used with permission.

TABLE 7.1-2
SAFE-SEX GUIDELINES

Remember: Any activity that allows for the exchange of body fluids of one person through the mouth, anus, vagina, bloodstream, cuts, or sores of another person is considered unsafe at this time.

Safe-Sex Practices
Massage, hugging, body-to-body rubbing
Dry social kissing
Masturbation
Acting out sexual fantasies (that do not include any unsafe-sex practices)
Using vibrators or other instruments (provided they are not shared)

Low-Risk Sex Practices
These activities are not considered completely safe:
French (wet) kissing (without mouth sores)
Mutual masturbation
Vaginal and anal intercourse while using a condom
Oral sex, male (fellatio), while using a condom
Oral sex, female (cunnilingus), while using a barrier
External contact with semen or urine, provided there are no breaks in the skin

Unsafe-Sex Practices
Vaginal or anal intercourse without a condom
Semen, urine, or feces in the mouth or the vagina
Unprotected oral sex (fellatio or cunnilingus)
Blood contact of any kind
Sharing sex instruments or needles

Table from B Moffatt, J Splegal, S Parrish, M Helquist: *AIDS: A Self-Care Manual*, p. 125. IBS Press, Santa Monica, CA, 1987. Used with permission.

TABLE 7.1-3
POSSIBLE INDICATIONS FOR HUMAN IMMUNODEFICIENCY VIRUS (HIV) TESTING

1. Patients who belong to a high-risk group: (1) men who have had sex with another man since 1977; (2) intravenous drug abusers since 1977; (3) hemophiliacs and other patients who have received since 1977 blood or blood product transfusions not screened for HIV; (4) sexual partners of people from any of those groups; (5) sexual partners of people with known HIV exposure—people with cuts, wounds, sores, or needlesticks whose lesions have had direct contact with HIV-infected blood.
2. Patients who request testing. Not all patients admit to the presence of risk factors (e.g., because of shame, fear).
3. Patients with symptoms of AIDS.
4. Women belonging to a high-risk group who are planning pregnancy or who are pregnant.
5. Blood, semen, or organ donors.
6. Patients with dementia in a high-risk group.

Table adapted from R B Rosse, A A Giese, S I Deutsch, J M Morihisa: *Laboratory and Diagnostic Testing in Psychiatry*, p 54. American Psychiatric Press. Washington, 1989. Used with permission.

cystis carinii pneumonia) or neoplasms (such as Kaposi's sarcoma). In addition, the expanded AIDS surveillance case definition includes all HIV-infected persons (1) who have less than 200 T lymphocytes (also called CD4+ lymphocytes) per μL or (2) who have a T lymphocyte percent of total lymphocytes less than 14 or (3) who have received a diagnosis of pulmonary tuberculosis, invasive cervical cancer, or recurrent pneumonia. If a screening test is positive for HIV antibodies, it is confirmed by a Western blot analysis test. HIV often infects the central nervous system (CNS) directly.

Making a diagnosis of infection with HIV by blood tests is important because (1) the treatment of asymptomatic HIV-infected patients with zidovudine (Retrovir), previously called azidothymidine (AZT), and other medications is useful and (2) behavior can be changed to avoid spreading HIV (for example, by safe sex and by not sharing needles). HIV screening is indicated in any person in a high-risk group.

Psychiatric conditions that often develop as a consequence of having AIDS include delirium, dementia, depression, personality change, frank neurological signs, anxiety disorders, adjustment disorders, and, less commonly, psychosis or mania. HIV-infected patients can present with organic disorders resulting from direct CNS infection with HIV or an opportunistic CNS infection such as toxoplasmosis, cryptococcosis, cytomegalovirus, and herpes. CNS metastases of Kaposi's sarcoma and primary CNS lymphoma are common.

A full dementia syndrome in AIDS is also common. AIDS dementia may present with memory loss and other cognitive dysfunctions, psychomotor retardation, social withdrawal, and apathy. Neurological signs, motor deficits, and seizures (including temporal lobe seizures) can occur. AIDS dementia is believed to be due to a chronic, progressive encephalitis from HIV infection. The medical workup of an AIDS patient usually includes specific blood tests, a computed tomography (CT) or magnetic resonance imaging (MRI) scan, a lumbar puncture, and cultures of the blood and the cerebrospinal fluid (CSF).

INTERVIEWING AND PSYCHOTHERAPEUTIC GUIDELINES

Ask all patients whether they have been tested for HIV. Any patient in a high-risk group should be counseled about possible HIV testing and about changing behavior to reduce risk. Major psychological implications surround the HIV test. Extensive pretest and posttest counseling and a written informed consent are required (Tables 7.1-4 and 7.1-5).

EVALUATION AND MANAGEMENT

1. When treating a known or suspected HIV-positive patient, protect others from possible exposure. Staff members should be immediately instructed to practice

TABLE 7.1-4
PRETEST HIV COUNSELING

1. Discuss meaning of a positive result and clarify distortions (e.g., the test detects exposure to the AIDS virus; it is not a test for AIDS).
2. Discuss the meaning of a negative result (e.g., seroconversion requires time, recent high-risk behavior may require follow-up testing).
3. Be available to discuss the patient's fears and concerns (unrealistic fears may require appropriate psychological intervention).
4. Discuss why the test is necessary. (Not all patients will admit to high-risk behaviors.)
5. Explore the patient's potential reactions to a positive result (e.g., "I'll kill myself if I'm positive"). Take appropriate necessary steps to intervene in a potentially catastrophic reaction.
6. Explore past reactions to severe stresses.
7. Discuss the confidentiality issues relevant to the testing situation (e.g., is it an anonymous or nonanonymous setting?). Inform the patient of other possible testing options where the counseling and testing can be done completely anonymously (e.g., where the result is not made a permanent part of a hospital chart). Discuss who has access to the test results.
8. Discuss with the patient how being seropositive can potentially affect social status (e.g., health and life insurance coverage, employment, housing).
9. Explore high-risk behaviors and recommend risk-reducing interventions.
10. Document discussions in chart.
11. Allow the patient time to ask questions.

Table from R B Rosse, A A Giese, S I Deutsch, J M Morihisa: *Laboratory and Diagnostic Testing in Psychiatry*, p 55. American Psychiatric Press, Washington, 1989. Used with permission.

TABLE 7.1–5
PROTEST HIV COUNSELING

1. Interpretation of test result: Clarify distortion (e.g., "a negative test still means you could contract the virus at a future time; it does not mean you are immune from AIDS"). Ask questions about the patient's understanding and emotional reaction to the test result.
2. Recommendations for prevention of transmission (careful discussion of high-risk behaviors and guideline for prevention of transmission).
3. Recommendations on the follow-up of sexual partners and needle contacts.
4. If test result is positive, recommendations against donating blood, sperm, or organs and against sharing razors, toothbrushes, and anything else that may have blood on it.
5. Referral for appropriate psychological support: HIV-positive patients often need access to a mental health team (assess need for inpatient versus outpatient care; consider individual or group supportive therapy). Common themes include the shock of the diagnosis, the fear of death, social consequences, grief over potential losses, and dashed hopes for good news. Also look for depression, hopelessness, anger, frustration, guilt, and obsessional themes. Activate supports available to patient (e.g., family, friends, community services).

Table from R B Rosse, A A Giese, S I Deutsch, J M Morihisa: *Laboratory and Diagnostic Testing in Psychiatric*, p. 58. American Psychiatric Press, Washington, 1989. Used with permission.

universal precautions, especially when invasive procedures, a physical examination, or blood tests are indicated. AIDS patients require a thorough physical examination and medical evaluation for signs of opportunistic infection. An infectious-disease consultation is often helpful.

2. Carefully evaluate the patient's cognition, which is often impaired in HIV-positive patients who have no other manifestations of AIDS. Subtle signs, such as impaired concentration and diminished memory, may be the sole initial findings.
3. Mild adjustment disorders, anxiety disorders, and depression can generally be treated with brief supportive psychotherapy. The general approach is similar to that used with cancer patients. Group therapy is sometimes helpful for the patient and for family members. Working through guilt feelings about high-risk behavior is often important. Talking about safe sexual practices and the cessation of intravenous (IV) drug use should be a priority.
4. Many ethical issues arise in treating AIDS patients: HIV testing, experimental treatments, the duty to warn sexual partners and family members, the effects on health insurance, and the potential loss of employment. Although few standardized guidelines exist for handling those ethical questions, they should be addressed directly and worked through.

DRUG TREATMENT

Psychotropic medications should be avoided if possible; if they are necessary, use only low dosages, since AIDS patients are very susceptible to side effects. AIDS patients may have personality disorders or substance-related disorders that antedate AIDS. Mood, anxiety, and psychotic disorders that are not responsive to psychotherapy can be treated with medication, although high dosages should be avoided. While antidepressants with strong anticholinergic effects may cause a worsening of cognitive deficits, some depressed AIDS patients may respond well to low dosages of amphetamines. Severe behavioral problems, such as agitation and assaultiveness, that do not respond to psychotherapeutic interventions can be treated with medication. Generally, benzodiazepines should be avoided because of the possibility of worsening any cognitive impairment, and high-potency antipsy-

TABLE 7.1–6
DRUGS FOR HIV INFECTION

Class/Generic Name	Trade Name	Typical Daily Dosage (mg/day)
Nucleoside analogs		
Didanosine	Videx	400
Lamivudine	Epivir	300
Stavudine	Zerit	80
Zalcitabine	Hivid	2.25
Zidovudine	Retrovir	600
Protease inhibitors		
Indinavir	Crixivan	2,400
Ritonavir	Norvir	1,200
Saquinavir	Invirase	1,800

chotics—such as haloperidol (Haldol) in doses of 0.5 to 2 mg by mouth or intramuscularly (IM)—should be given.

The Food and Drug Administration (FDA) has recently approved several new drugs for the treatment of HIV infection, and single-drug therapy is no longer the treatment of choice. The nucleosides and the protease inhibitors are the two classes of drugs used to treat HIV infection (Table 7.1-6). Some studies indicate that triple-drug therapy with two nucleosides and one protease inhibitor is the most potent antiretroviral treatment available. Double-drug treatment with two nucleosides or one nucleoside and one protease inhibitor may also be effective. Many other drugs not approved by the FDA are used by AIDS patients; therefore, a careful medication history is imperative.

For a more detailed discussion of this topic, see W G Van Gorp, J L Cummings: Neuropsychiatric Aspects of Infectious Disorders, Sec 2.7, p 235; I Grant, J Hampton Atkinson Jr: Psychiatric Aspects of Acquired Immune Deficiency Syndrome, Sec 29.2, p 1644; C H Hinkin, W G Van Gorp, P Satz: Neuropsychological and Neuropsychiatric Aspects of HIV Infection in Adults, Sec 29.2a, p 1669 in CTP/VI.

7.2 Cardiac Arrhythmia

Cardiac arrhythmia is a disorder characterized by irregular heartbeats, which the patient usually describes to the primary care physician as a pounding heartbeat or a fluttering sensation. The disorder may occur as a symptom of anxiety or panic, as a side effect of cocaine or other psychostimulant drug, or as a toxic effect of psychotropic drugs, such as tricyclic antidepressants and antipsychotics. Cardiac arrhythmia may also be a sign of cardiac disease.

CLINICAL FEATURES AND DIAGNOSIS

Arrhythmia can be brought on by anxiety. Death as a result of overwhelming shock may be due to cardiac arrhythmia. Anxiety-related arrhythmia may be worsened by withdrawal from alcohol or sedative-hypnotics. Tachycardia is common in anxiety, but arrhythmia is uncommon and typically occurs only during the acute episode of anxiety.

INTERVIEWING AND PSYCHOTHERAPEUTIC GUIDELINES

Provide a nonstimulating environment and reassure the patient, who is likely to be anxious. Explain all medical procedures concisely and clearly, and tell the patient that all efforts are being made to make an accurate diagnosis and to initiate appropriate treatment.

EVALUATION AND MANAGEMENT

1. Obtain a full medical and psychiatric history from any patient with complaints that may indicate arrhythmia, such as dizziness, syncope, blackouts, light-headedness, and palpitations.
2. Obtain an electrocardiogram (ECG), thyroid function tests, toxicology screen, and other tests as indicated.
3. Determine if the patient has a history of substance abuse. Cocaine-induced and other stimulant-induced arrhythmias are potentially life-threatening. Tachycardia can be treated with β-blockers. Benzodiazepines are also helpful in relieving anxiety and reducing agitation, which may decrease the risk of arrhythmia. If arrhythmia persists, admission to an intensive care unit may be required.
4. Determine if the patient is taking psychotropic agents that may be arrhythmogenic. Tricyclic antidepressants at therapeutic blood concentrations have a quinidinelike antiarrhythmic effect. However, at toxic blood concentrations they are arrhythmogenic. Cardiac side effects that are more common than arrhythmia include conduction delays, tachycardia, and nonspecific ST changes. Patients taking tricyclic antidepressants who have arrhythmia should have the medication withheld until a blood concentration can be obtained; the antidepressant should be resumed only after a cardiology consultation.
5. Arrhythmia induced by prescription medications mandates a discontinuation of those medications.

DRUG TREATMENT

Severe associated anxiety can be treated with a short-acting benzodiazepine—for example, estazolam (ProSom) 0.5 to 1 mg by mouth, lorazepam (Ativan) 1 to 2 mg by mouth, or oxazepam (Serax) 10 to 30 mg by mouth, all given every four to six hours—until the underlying problem is resolved. Associated diagnoses of substance abuse, anxiety disorders, and other disorders should be treated as needed.

For more a more detailed discussion of this topic, see J H Jaffe: Cocaine-Related Disorders, Sec 13.6, p 817; Anxiety Disorders, Chap 17, pp 1191–1249; W Katon, M D Sullivan, M R Clark: Cardiovascular Disorders, Sec 26.4, p 1491, in CTP/VI.

7.3 Cataplexy (Sudden Loss of Muscle Tone)

Cataplexy is the sudden, temporary loss of voluntary muscle tone in response to emotional stimulation. Cataplexy is a symptom of narcolepsy, although it can also occur in other neurological disorders.

CLINICAL FEATURES AND DIAGNOSIS

Typically, the patient's history includes uncontrollable daytime sleep attacks (from which the patient awakens refreshed), hypnagogic hallucinations (which occur while the patient is falling asleep), sleep paralysis (in which the patient feels unable to move while falling asleep), and restless sleep with vivid, terrifying dreams. Cataplectic attacks are typically brought on by laughter or elation, although other emotions may also trigger an attack. The patient is usually awake during the cataplectic attack and is aware of the surroundings, even though temporarily paralyzed. A sleep laboratory evaluation reveals that the electroencephalogram (EEG) during a cataplectic attack is that of rapid eye movement (REM) sleep, a sleep stage associated with decreased muscle tone (hence the paralysis). A polysomnogram reveals REM periods shortly after the onset of sleep (rather than the usual delay of at least 70 minutes) and an abnormal sleep architecture. Primary narcolepsy runs in families and is, at least in part, genetically based. Other causes of narcolepsy include brain tumors, encephalitis, head injury, and cerebrovascular diseases.

Cataplexy can be differentiated from petit mal seizures in that the patient is awake during the attack and also by the characteristic precipitation of cataplexy by emotional stimuli. Hypoglycemia, multiple sclerosis, and myasthenia gravis must be considered as part of the differential diagnosis.

INTERVIEWING AND PSYCHOTHERAPEUTIC GUIDELINES

The primary care physician should reassure the patient that treatment is available to ameliorate some of the symptoms. The patient should understand that while a thorough medical workup is necessary to rule out rare causes of the disorder, the condition is most likely a sleep disorder.

EVALUATION AND MANAGEMENT

1. Obtain a complete neurological examination and medical screening tests, including thyroid tests.
2. Refer the patient for an EEG, polysomnography, and daytime multiple sleep latency tests.
3. Advise the patient to avoid emotionally provocative stimuli to prevent cataplectic attacks.

DRUG TREATMENT

Narcolepsy is usually treated with sympathomimetics, such as amphetamines and methylphenidate (Ritalin), but those drugs usually do not help with the cataplectic attacks.

Tricyclic antidepressants, such as imipramine (Tofranil) and clomipramine (Anafranil), are often helpful. Monoamine oxidase inhibitors (MAOIs), such as phenelzine (Nardil), may also be useful if tricyclics are ineffective.

For a more detailed discussion of this topic, see J C Gillin, R K Zoltoski, R J Salin-Pascual: Basic Science of Sleep, Sec 1.9, p 80; J Yager, M J Gitlin: Clinical Manifestations of Psychiatric Disorders, Chap 10, p 637; R L Williams, I Karacan, C A Moore, M Hirshkowitz: Sleep Disorders, Chap 23, p 1373 in CTP/VI.

7.4 Coma

Coma is a severe state of impaired consciousness that indicates depression of the central nervous system (CNS); the patient is unresponsive to the environment or to internal needs, shows no purposeful spontaneous movement, and shows no evidence of thinking.

CLINICAL FEATURES AND DIAGNOSIS

Coma is a neurological emergency that is often an end stage mental status; it indicates severe brain dysfunction. It can be distinguished from deep sleep in that the comatose patient cannot be awakened by any stimulus, and the patient's eyes do not open (Table 7.4-1).

Coma can be caused by a wide range of conditions. An acute onset suggests cerebrovascular disease, head trauma, toxic conditions, overdose, or heatstroke. A gradual onset suggests CNS infection, intracranial mass, or systemic disease.

INTERVIEWING AND PSYCHOTHERAPEUTIC GUIDELINES

The patient's history should be obtained from the person accompanying the patient. Some comatose patients are aware of their surroundings and remember events occurring during the coma. Patients with akinetic mutism and catatonia may erupt into explosive outbursts and should be approached with caution.

EVALUATION AND MANAGEMENT

1. Refer the patient for a complete neurological examination.
2. Differentiate organic coma from psychogenic unresponsiveness or other comalike states (Table 7.4-2). Normal muscle tone and reflexes, a normal electroencephalogram (EEG), forcible closing of the eyes, eyes kept open but interrupted by

TABLE 7.4-1
LEVELS OF CONSCIOUSNESS

Alert wakefulness—The patient responds immediately, fully, and appropriately to visual, auditory, or tactile stimulation.
Lethargy—The patient appears drowsy and inactive; responses are delayed or incomplete.
Obtundation—The patient seems indifferent and maintains wakefulness but little more.
Stupor—The patient can be aroused only by vigorous and continuous external stimulation.
Coma—The patient's responses to stimulation are either completely lost (deep coma) or reduced to only rudimentary reflex motor responses (moderately deep coma).

Table from F Plum, M Posner. *Diagnosis of Stupor and Coma,* p 2. Davis, Philadelphia, 1966. Used with permission.

TABLE 7.4–2
COMA STATES

Condition	Features
Akinetic mutism	Absence of muscle activity, lack of movement, mutism; alert-appearing eye movements; periods of sleep and decreased wakefulness in the isthargic form; midbrain lesion often pressed
Catatonic stupor	Perseveration, rigidity, waxy flexibility, mutism, negativism, tachycardia, low-grade fever, diaphoresis, mydriasis, tachypnea, choreiform movements, violent outbursts; possible multiple causes, including organicity, schizophrenia, and mood disorders
Coma vigil	Apparently asleep and ready to be aroused; similar to akinetic mutism
Locked-in syndrome	Total body paralysis secondary to brainstem damage, with preservation of eye movements and mentation; mute but alert with intact hemispheric function; communication by blinking
Persistent vegetative state	Rare random or absent motor responses; evidence of meaningful contact with the environment; blood pressure and respiratory control maintained, eye movements present, sleep-wake cycles present; usually caused by severe brain damage
Psychogenic coma	No signs of neurological disease or dysfunction or changes in respiratory function, pupils, or eye movements; sometimes apparently aware of surroundings; urinary or fecal incontinence, insensitivity to pain, and no swallowing of secretions or fluids placed in the mouth

TABLE 7.4–3
GLASGOW COMA SCALE*

Eye opening	
None	1
To pain	2
To speech	3
Spontaneous	4
Motor Response	
No response	1
Extension	2
Abnormal flexion	3
Withdrawal	4
Localizes pain	5
Obeys commands	6
Verbal Response	
No response	1
Incomprehensible	2
Inappropriate	3
Confused	4
Oriented	5

Glasgow Coma Scale Score = Eye Opening + Motor Response + Verbal Response

Table adapted from B Jennett, G Teasdale: *Management of Head Injuries.* Davis, Philadelphia, 1981.
*The higher the point score, the better the prognosis.

quick blinks, normally reactive pupils, and random or no eye movements in response to head turning (doll's-eye maneuver)—all suggest a psychogenic origin. Bárány's caloric test (putting 10 cc of ice water into the external ear and observing for the quick component of nystagmus) can be performed. The presence of the quick component of nystagmus during the caloric test suggests a state of alertness. In an organically comatose patient, the quick component is absent, and the eyes slowly deviate to the side of the cooled ear. Those tests are also useful in identifying a malingering patient who is attempting to simulate coma.
3. Determine the level of coma, using the Glasgow Coma Scale (Table 7.4-3). Document any efforts to ward off painful stimuli. Document the specific stimuli

used and the response, so that the tests may be repeated serially by other examiners to measure the patient's progress.

4. Obtain a full medical workup, including complete blood count (CBC) with differential, complete blood chemistries, Venereal Disease Research Laboratory (VDRL) test, thyroid profile, urine and blood toxicology screens, urinalysis, chest X-ray, computed tomography (CT) or magnetic resonance imaging (MRI) scan of the head, an EEG, a lumbar puncture, and other diagnostic tests as indicated.

5. Give supportive care and treat as the workup results indicate.

DRUG TREATMENT

Medications are indicated only according to the definitive diagnosis. In general, CNS-depressant drugs should be avoided.

For a more detailed discussion of this topic, see A A Lipton, R Cancro: Schizophrenia: Clinical Features, Sec 14.7, p 968; E D Caine, H Grossman, J M Lyness: Delirium, Dementia, and Amnestic and Other Cognitive Disorders and Mental Disorders Due to a General Medical Condition, Chap 12, p 705; B J Fauman: Other Psychiatric Emergencies, Sec 30.2, p 1752, in CTP/VI.

7.5 Dysarthria

Dysarthria is an impairment of speech articulation usually caused by neurological involvement of the motor systems controlling speech. It can occur independently of neurological disorders affecting language expression or reception.

CLINICAL FEATURES AND DIAGNOSIS

Dysarthria can be caused by conditions affecting the lower motor neurons, cerebellum, extrapyramidal system, or brainstem. Intoxication with alcohol or sedative-hypnotics is a common cause of transient dysarthria through cerebellar involvement. Anticonvulsants can also cause dysarthria. Less commonly, dysarthria is a hysterical sign without any identifiable neurological basis. In children, dysarthria may be a sign of phonological disorder or a pervasive developmental disorder.

INTERVIEWING AND PSYCHOTHERAPEUTIC GUIDELINES

Ask the patient to speak slowly. If communication is still difficult, see if the patient can communicate by writing, although motor involvement may make this means of communication ineffective.

EVALUATION AND MANAGEMENT

1. Ask what medications or drugs the patient has taken. Look for obvious intoxication with alcohol or sedative-hypnotics. Urine and blood screens for drugs and blood drug levels may be helpful.

2. Look for associated neurological signs. The presence of other neurological signs and subtle differences in the quality of the dysarthria may indicate an involvement of specific neurological sites. Unless the dysarthria can be easily explained (for example, by alcohol or sedative-hypnotic intoxication), a full neurological evaluation is indicated.
3. Dysarthria, unless it is a sign of an acute central nervous system (CNS) event, is seldom an emergency. The patient can usually be referred for outpatient neurological or psychiatric evaluation.
4. If no definitive treatment is indicated after a neurological workup, refer the patient for speech therapy.

DRUG TREATMENT

No specific medications are indicated.

For a more detailed discussion of this topic, see M A Schuckit: Alcohol-Related Disorders, Sec 13.2, p 775; J H Jaffe: Amphetamine (Or Amphetaminelike)-Related Disorders, Sec 13.3, p 791; D A Ciraulo, D J Greenblatt: Sedative-, Hypnotic-, or Anxiolytic-Related Disorders, Sec 13.11, p 872; E D Caine, H Grossman, J M Lyness: Delirium, Dementia, and Amnestic and Other Cognitive Disorders and Mental Disorders Due to a General Medical Condition, Chap 12, p 705, in CTP/VI.

7.6 Epilepsy

Epilepsy is characterized by recurrent seizures caused by central nervous system (CNS) disease or dysfunction. The symptoms of a seizure can range from the tonic-clonic movements of a grand mal seizure to such subtle symptoms as akinesia, abnormal sensations and perceptions, disturbed behavior, automatisms, and impaired consciousness.

Epilepsy is the most common chronic neurological condition; it affects 1 percent of the population. Comorbidity with psychiatric conditions is common; 30 to 50 percent of epileptic patients have a diagnosable mental disorder, and 7 to 10 percent have psychotic symptoms. Epilepsy is three to seven times more common in psychotic patients than in the general population.

Recurrent seizures are usually treated by a neurologist. Primary care physicians may be involved for many reasons, including the diagnosis of epilepsy when the symptoms are behavioral, perceptual, or affective; the differentiation of true seizures from pseudoseizures; the treatment of depression, personality changes, and psychotic symptoms; and the management of postictal and interictal behavioral problems.

CLINICAL FEATURES AND DIAGNOSIS

The definitive diagnosis of epilepsy relies on an electroencephalogram (EEG), although normal findings on an EEG do not exclude the diagnosis of epilepsy.

TABLE 7.6-1
INTERNATIONAL CLASSIFICATION OF EPILEPTIC SEIZURES

I. Partial seizures (seizures beginning locally)
    A. Partial seizures with elementary symptoms (generally without impairment of consciousness)
        1. With motor symptoms
        2. With sensory symptoms
        3. With automatic symptoms
        4. Compound forms
    B. Partial seizures with complex symptoms (generally with impairment of consciousness;
        temporal lobe or psychomotor seizures)
        1. With impairment of consciousness only
        2. With cognitive symptoms
        3. With affective symptoms
        4. With psychosensory symptoms
        5. With psychosensory symptoms (automatisms)
        6. Compound forms
    C. Partial seizures secondary generalized
II. Generalized seizures (bilaterally symmetrical and without local onset)
    A. Absences (petit mal)
    B. Myoclonus
    C. Infantile spasms
    D. Clonic seizures
    E. Tonic seizures
    F. Tonic-clonic seizures (grand mal)
    G. Atonic seizures
    H. Akinetic seizures
III. Unilateral seizures
IV. Unclassified seizures (because of incomplete data)

Table adapted from H Gastaut: Clinical and electroencephalographical classification of epileptic seizures. Epilepsia *11:* 102, 1970.

Seizures can be broadly divided into generalized and focal (partial). Table 7.6-1 lists a classification of seizure types.

Generalized Seizures

In generalized seizures the EEG paroxysms are bilaterally symmetrical, synchronous, and present in all leads. Generalized seizures almost always involve altered or lost consciousness. The most common types are generalized convulsive seizures (grand mal or tonic-clonic) and petit mal seizures. Generalized convulsive seizures produce clinical convulsions and postictal confusion. They are characterized by bilaterally synchronous polyspike and slow-wave bursts on the EEG. Petit mal seizures usually begin between ages 5 and 10 years. These seizures are abrupt, brief (seconds), and frequent episodes of loss of consciousness (absences) associated with automatisms, akinetic episodes, and myoclonic jerks. They are characterized by a 3-cycles-per-second spike-and-slow-wave pattern on the EEG.

Partial (Focal) Seizures

The type of seizure most likely seen by the primary care physician is the partial (focal) seizure, which can mimic several psychiatric disorders.

Partial seizures show localized spike discharges on the EEG and are divided according to whether they show simple symptoms or complex symptoms. They may spread and develop into secondarily generalized seizures.

Partial Simple Seizures. Partial simple seizures are usually motor seizures and involve clonic movements or the loss of muscle tone on the side of the body contralateral to the focus of the seizure discharge. Sensory symptoms—such as abdominal pain, pain localized elsewhere, paroxysmal autonomic discharges, and hallucinations (visual, auditory, olfactory, and gustatory)—are other presentations.

Partial Complex Seizures. Temporal lobe epilepsy is a partial complex seizure with a focus in the temporal lobe. It may confuse the diagnostician because patients often present with behavior problems. The patient may be brought to the primary care physician's office with a history of sudden, irrational, agitated, and possibly violent behavior. On examination, the patient appears to be sleepy and confused, with no memory for the events in question. The history may be divided into preictal, ictal, postictal, and interictal symptoms.

Preictal events, including auras, may or may not occur or may occur irregularly. They include autonomic sensations (for example, stomach fullness, hunger, nausea, and blushing), cognitive events (for example, déjà vu, *jamais vu*, hallucinations, and forced thinking), affective states (for example, fear, depression, and elation), and automatisms (for example, lip smacking and chewing).

The ictal event is characterized by a three-to-five-minute loss of consciousness and by disorganized, disinhibited behavior. Violence is rare; since the patient is unconscious, any aggressive behavior is random, undirected, and disorganized. Patients may experience dissociative phenomena, including changes in personality characteristics, handedness, and speech. Prolonged dissociation secondary to complex partial status epilepticus may resemble catatonia.

After the seizure, the patient may experience a variable period of postictal confusion and, possibly, bizarre or agitated behavior. The postictal confusion passes, but amnesia for the ictal period remains, and the patient's memory is cloudy for events in the preictal and postictal periods.

INTERVIEWING AND PSYCHOTHERAPEUTIC GUIDELINES

In general, if epilepsy is a diagnostic consideration, assume first that the symptoms are related to an organic condition, rather than a psychiatric disorder. That approach leads to the full exploration of possible organic causes. All patients with seizure disorders should be asked about the frequency and the duration of the seizures; the events before, during, and after a seizure (is there an aura? loss of consciousness? postictal amnesia or fatigue?); the relation of the seizures to drug or alcohol use; and their treatment history. Do not overlook the many psychosocial factors that may affect patients. Work to identify the possible definitive organic causes, but also emphasize adaptation strategies for coping with any impairment. How have the symptoms affected the patient's occupational, familial, sexual, and social functioning? Is the patient able to drive? Does driving affect the patient's ability to work? Might any personality changes benefit from psychotherapeutic interventions? What were the patient's premorbid psychological substrates and traits that may make adaptation easy or difficult?

Cognitive assessment is crucial, as delirium is associated with high mortality. Any recurrent abrupt and spontaneous onset and remission of a psychiatric disturbance should increase the suspicion of epilepsy. Obtaining the patient's history from the family is usually critical because of the patient's amnesia during the ictal period. A patient who does appear to be conscious and responsive during a seizure and who remembers events during the seizure is probably experiencing pseudoseizures or attempting to produce factitious symptoms.

EVALUATION AND MANAGEMENT

1. The mainstay of management during the ictal event is restraint to prevent injury. Episodes are generally brief, and patients are usually in the postictal period by the time they reach an emergency room or the primary care physician's office.
2. The patients' sensoria may be clouded, and their activities should be restricted until normal cognition is restored. At that point, if no family member has been reached, the patient is usually able to clarify the situation. No further short-term care is necessary unless seizures recur or psychosis is present.
3. If psychosis is present, evaluation and treatment proceed as for other psychoses, except for the medication used.
4. A full medical workup and a neurological evaluation are needed.
5. A thorough search for the cause is mandatory. The causes to rule out include anoxia, head trauma, cerebrovascular diseases, infections, intracranial bleeding, drug abuse and withdrawal, alcohol withdrawal, electrolyte imbalances, hypoglycemia, hyperglycemia, and CNS tremor. Start with a detailed clinical history, focusing on headache, head injury, childhood seizures, and febrile seizures. Order a complete neurological examination, EEG, computed tomography (CT) or magnetic resonance imaging (MRI) scan, and a full battery of blood tests and urine drug screens.
6. Epilepsy should be managed by a neurologist with appropriate anticonvulsant medication.

Depression

Depression is common in epilepsy. Among epileptic patients, those with partial complex seizures have the highest suicide rate. Treatment may include psychotherapy and antidepressants, such as serotonin-specific reuptake inhibitors, tricyclics, or monoamine oxidase inhibitors. Electroconvulsive therapy is another option that itself has anticonvulsant effects.

Personality Changes

Personality changes are common, but their cause is controversial and may be related to the stress of coping with epilepsy, to anticonvulsant medications, or to a primary organic condition. Personality changes are more related to the duration of epilepsy than to the frequency of seizures.

Psychosis

Psychosis of a schizophreniform type may develop in patients who have long-standing temporal lobe epilepsy. Usually, the psychosis is preceded by personality changes. Responses to treatment are unpredictable. Treatment may include antipsychotics and anticonvulsants; however, low-potency antipsychotics are likely to lower the seizure threshold and should be avoided.

Impaired Cognition

Impaired cognition is not common, although some patients clearly show a progressive deterioration in cognition. The possible causes include anticonvulsant drugs, a CNS lesion (often the same one causing the seizures), and repeated prolonged seizures. Consider whether the patient can be treated with a lower dosage of an anticonvulsant or a different anticonvulsant.

Status Epilepticus

In status epilepticus, a potentially fatal condition, seizures follow one another with no intervening periods of consciousness. Partial continuous epilepsy is a rare type of sensory or motor seizure that may last for days to weeks. These conditions are considered neurological emergencies.

Pseudoseizures

In a pseudoseizure the patient has some conscious control over mimicking the symptoms of a seizure. Some cases of pseudoseizures are obvious; for difficult cases, the distinctions in Table 7.6-2 may help.

Violence

Violence rarely occurs during a seizure, but it may be a problem in some epileptic patients as an interictal or postictal phenomenon, particularly in patients with

TABLE 7.6–2
CLINICAL FEATURES DISTINGUISHING SEIZURES AND PSEUDOSEIZURES*

Feature	Organic Seizure	Pseudoseizure
Aura	Common stereotyped	Rare
Timing	Nocturnal common	Only when awake
Incontinence	Common	Rare
Cyanosis	Common	Rare
Postictal confusion	Yes	No
Body movement	Tonic-clonic	Nonstereotyped and asynchronous
Self-injury	Common	Rare
EEG	May be abnormal	Normal
Affected by suggestion	No	Yes
Secondary gain	No	Yes

*Some patients with organic seizure disorders may also have pseudoseizures.

TABLE 7.6–3
DRUGS OF CHOICE FOR VARIOUS TYPES OF SEIZURES

Generalized tonic-clonic (grand mal) seizures: Phenobarbital Phenytoin (Dilantin) Carbamazepine (Tegretol)	Myoclonic, atonic, akinetic, and atypical absence seizures: Clonazepam (Klonopin) Diazepam (Valium)
Absence (petit mal) seizures: Ethosuximide (Zarontin) Valproic acid (Depakene)	Infantile spasms: Adrenocorticotropic hormone Corticosteroids
Simple partial (focal) seizures: Phenobarbital Phenytoin (Dilantin)	Status epilepticus: Diazepam (Valium) Phenobarbital Amobarbital (Amytal) Phenytoin (Dilantin) Paraldehyde Anesthetic agent
Complex partial (temporal lobe) seizures: Phenytoin (Dilantin) Carbamazepine (Tegretol)	

temporal lobe epilepsy. Carbamazepine (Tegretol), other anticonvulsants, antipsychotics, or β-adrenergic receptor antagonists may help.

DRUG TREATMENT

In general, use a single anticonvulsant drug and increase the dosage until it is effective or not tolerated. Table 7.6-3 lists the drugs of choice for various types of seizures. Polypharmacotherapy should be avoided because of drug interactions and the compounding of side effects.

For a more detailed discussion of this topic, see E D Caine, H Grossman, J M Lyness: Delirium, Dementia, and Amnestic and Other Cognitive Disorders and Mental Disorders Due to a General Medical Condition, Chap 12, p 705; J C Nemiah: Dissociative Disorders, Chap 20, p 1281; B J Fauman: Psychiatric Emergencies, Sec 30.2, p 1752, in CTP/VI.

7.7 Headache

Headache is a clinical complaint experienced by more than 75 percent of the population each year; 10 to 20 percent of the population go to physicians with headache as their primary complaint. Headaches have a wide range of causes, ranging from mild stress to life-threatening intracranial disease. Many psychiatric disorders, including anxiety and depressive disorders, frequently have headaches as a prominent symptom.

CLINICAL FEATURES AND DIAGNOSIS

The differential diagnosis of headache includes chronic syndromes, such as migraine, tension, cluster, and postconcussional headaches (Table 7.7-1). Trigeminal neuralgia (tic douloureux), other neuralgias, and temporomandibular joint syndrome are other causes of pain in the head area. Headaches, both acute and chronic, may

TABLE 7.7–1
DIFFERENTIATING FEATURES OF COMMON TYPES OF HEADACHE

| | Muscle Contraction (Tension) Headache | Vascular Headaches | |
		Migraine	Cluster Headache
Sex	Male = female	Female > male	Male > female
Age of onset	Not specific	Puberty to menopause	20 to 50 years
Family history	Not specific	Often familial	Not familial
Quality of pain	Pressure, tightness, bandlike, or not specific	Throbbing	Excruciating, boring, piercing, burning
Location of pain	Bilateral, occipital > frontal	Unilateral, often temporal	Unilateral orbital or adjacent head or face or both
Time of onset	Afternoon or evening more than morning	Early morning, often on weekends	Soon after onset of sleep, and daytime
Mode of onset	Gradual	Abrupt or gradual, often prodromata	Abrupt
Duration	Hours, days, or weeks; often continuous	Hours, 1 to 2 days	20 minutes to 2 hours
Frequency	Not specific; chronic daily headache	Not specific	Cluster, such as one or more a day for 2 to 10 weeks
Precipitating aggravating factors	Emotional stress or not apparent	Emotional stress, menstruation, vasodilators; alcohol, certain foods; change in weather	Alcohol, lying down, REM sleep
Ameliorating factors	Nonspecific: relaxation, alcohol; Rx: analgesics, tricyclics	Rest, compression of scalp arteries; pregnancy; Rx: ergotamine, propranolol	Activity: Rx: oxygen, ergotamine, methysergide, lithium, steroids
Associated symptoms or signs	None or not specific symptoms—tenderness of scalp or neck muscles	Prodromata: scintillating scotomata, hemianopsia, other brain signs

During attack: nausea, vomiting, photophobia, irritability; tender scalp | Ipsilateral redness and tearing of eye, stuffiness and discharge of nostril, ptosis and myosis |
| Personality traits | Competitive, sensitive, conscientious > perfectionistic | Perfectionistic, neat, efficient, restrained, ambitious > compulsive | Not specific > perfectionist |

Table from S Solomon, J C Masdeu: Neuropsychiatry and behavioral neurology. In *Comprehensive Textbook of Psychiatry*, ed 5, H I Kaplan, B J Sadock, editors, p 217. Williams & Wilkins, Baltimore, 1989. Used with permission.

also herald serious intracranial pathology, including subdural and subarachnoid hemorrhage, tumors, pseudotumor cerebri, meningitis, temporal arteritis, and uncontrolled hypertension.

Unless a headache is mild, transitory, and clearly in response to an identified stress, it warrants a workup. The patient's description of the headache does not usually lead to a definitive diagnosis. Laboratory tests and brain imaging are all part of the workup, which typically includes computed tomography (CT) or magnetic resonance imaging (MRI) of the brain, even though the results of the majority of brain-imaging studies are negative.

Migraine

Migraine is often (but not always) preceded by an aura, including visual abnormalities (scotoma, scintillating scotomata, tubular vision) and autonomic dysfunction.

The headache is described by the patient as throbbing, unilateral, and often periorbital. It is precipitated by bright light, alcohol, certain foods (for example, chocolate), changes in sleep or eating habits, and medications (for example, oral contraceptives), and it may be associated with hypersensitivity to noise or light. The headache can occur when a person is asleep or awake. Migraine is thought to be related to cerebral vasoconstriction.

Tension Headache

Tension headache (muscle contraction headache) is caused by the contraction of muscles of the head and the neck. The onset is late in the day. The headache is exacerbated by fatigue, stress (as in migraines), and emotional factors. Combined migraine and tension headaches are common. In combined cases, the focus is on first treating the migraine.

Cluster Headaches

Several headaches daily that persist for days to weeks are known as cluster headaches. Each lasts several hours. The headache is typically periorbital and nonthrobbing but with sharp pain. It may be associated with local symptoms, such as Horner's syndrome, tearing, and nasal congestion. The headache is precipitated by alcohol and may occur during sleep.

INTERVIEWING AND PSYCHOTHERAPEUTIC GUIDELINES

Although headaches are often affected by psychological factors, the primary care physician should approach the patient with the assumption that the headache is due to an organic condition until proved otherwise. However, the majority of headaches do not have an identifiable organic cause. Headaches often respond to medication and psychotherapeutic interventions.

EVALUATION AND MANAGEMENT

1. The patient's history should include the headache's location, duration, quality (sharp, throbbing, tight), timing, rate of onset, frequency, and precipitating and ameliorating factors. Find out whether the headaches occur during sleep and whether associated symptoms and signs, such as hallucinations and gastrointestinal disturbances, are present. A family history of migraine headache is often found in migraine sufferers.
2. Document the pattern of the headaches in a written record of all the headaches, their circumstances, possible precipitants, and what relieved them.
3. Over-the-counter medications—such as acetaminophen, aspirin, nonsteroidal anti-inflammatory drugs, caffeine, and phenacetin—may have been taken. Prescription medications—such as barbiturates, opioids, benzodiazepines, anticholinergics, tricyclic antidepressants, β-blockers, ergot alkaloids, lithium (Eskalith), and steroids—may have been taken. The evaluation should include inquiring about which medications have helped and those still being taken that may produce side effects.
4. A thorough physical and neurological examination is mandatory. Intracranial masses may be stretching or irritating the meninges. Nuchal rigidity is a sign of meningeal irritation and may be caused by hemorrhage or infection. Headaches caused by a brain tumor progress in intensity and duration as the tumor grows but are usually constant in location. Such headaches may be worsened by coughing or changing positions.
5. Biofeedback may be useful in tension headache. Oxygen inhalation is useful in cluster headaches.
6. Although psychotherapy is not a definitive treatment of headache, psychological stressors can often exacerbate headaches, and the relief of stress may improve the symptoms. Chronic headache syndromes can lead to disability and depression and should be dealt with by using a rehabilitation model that emphasizes functioning.

DRUG TREATMENT

Medications are given either abortively (to be taken after the headache has started) or prophylactically.

Begin treatment with common analgesics, such as aspirin, acetaminophen, and nonsteroidal anti-inflammatory drugs.

If those drugs are ineffective, treat migraines with ergot alkaloids, tension headaches with benzodiazepines, and cluster headaches with steroids and lithium. Sumatriptan (Imitrex) is also used to treat migraines.

β-Blockers and methysergide (Sansert) have been used for the prophylaxis of migraine. Tricyclic antidepressants—for example, low to moderate doses of amitriptyline (Elavil)—are effective in the prophylaxis of both migraine and tension headache.

Trigeminal neuralgia is treated with carbamazepine (Tegretol), and temporal arteritis is treated with steroids.

For a more detailed discussion of this topic, see E J Singer: Neuropsychiatric Aspects of Headache, Sec 2.9, p 251, in CTP/VI.

7.8 Head Trauma

The most common causes of *head trauma* are motor vehicle accidents, gunshot wounds, or occupational accidents. Head trauma can produce a wide range of psychiatric syndromes, including depression, mania, psychosis, personality change, and (rarely) dementia.

CLINICAL FEATURES AND DIAGNOSIS

Postconcussional disorder (Table 7.8-1) appears within hours to days of a mild head injury. It is characterized by dizziness, anxiety, lability, headache, and personality change. The symptoms may be exacerbated by alcohol, exercise, or exposure to heat or sunlight. Those factors may help differentiate the syndrome from emotional responses to the trauma. The duration of disorientation is an approximate guide to the prognosis. Posttraumatic amnesia is often retrograde and usually does not extend beyond one week. In severe trauma cases, computed tomography (CT) or magnetic resonance imaging (MRI) may show a contrecoup lesion, with atrophy in the frontal

TABLE 7.8–1
RESEARCH CRITERIA FOR POSTCONCUSSIONAL DISORDER

A. A history of head trauma that has caused significant cerebral concussion.

 Note: The manifestations of concussion include loss of consciousness, posttraumatic amnesia, and, less commonly, posttraumatic onset of seizures. The specific method of defining this criterion needs to be established by further research.

B. Evidence from neuropsychological testing or quantified cognitive assessment of difficulty in attention (concentrating, shifting focus of attention, performing simultaneous cognitive tasks) or memory (learning or recalling information).

C. Three (or more) of the following occur shortly after the trauma and last at least 3 months:
 (1) becoming fatigued easily
 (2) disordered sleep
 (3) headache
 (4) vertigo or dizziness
 (5) irritability or aggression on little or no provocation
 (6) anxiety, depression, or affective lability
 (7) changes in personality (e.g., social or sexual inappropriateness)
 (8) apathy or lack of spontaneity

D. The symptoms in criteria B and C have their onset following head trauma or else represent a substantial worsening or preexisting symptoms.

E. The disturbance causes significant impairment in social or occupational functioning and represents a significant decline from a previous level of functioning. In school-age children, the impairment may be manifested by a significant worsening in school or academic performance dating from the trauma.

F. The symptoms do not meet criteria for dementia due to head trauma and are not better accounted for by another mental disorder (e.g., amnestic disorder due to head trauma, personality change due to head trauma).

Table from DSM-IV, *Diagnostic and Statistical Manual of Mental Disorders,* ed 4. Copyright American Psychiatric Association, Washington, 1994. Used with permission.

TABLE 7.8–2
HEAD INJURY CLASSIFICATION

Head Injury	Glasgow Coma Score	Acute Clinical Features
Mild	13 to 15*	Headache, fatigue, dizziness
Moderate	9 to 12*	Impaired consciousness, no coma
Severe	3 to 8	Coma: no eye opening, inability to obey commands, no understandable speech

*Initial and lowest score.

and occipital poles and widespread edema from an anteroposterior injury. Head injury classification is summarized in Table 7.8-2.

INTERVIEWING AND PSYCHOTHERAPEUTIC GUIDELINES

The primary care physician should obtain as much information as possible from anyone who witnessed the trauma. The patient may be able to provide bits of information, but they may be unreliable.

EVALUATION AND MANAGEMENT

1. In the mental status examination, focus on cognition. In the physical and neurological examinations, check for signs of intracranial hemorrhage (for example, focal neurological signs, nuchal rigidity, headache, sudden mental status change, delirium), which warrant an immediate CT or MRI of the head.
2. Factors affecting the prognosis include the presence of epilepsy, litigation, the patient's premorbid personality and coping mechanisms, the emotional repercussions of the injury, and the severity and the location of the brain damage.
3. With time, an organic personality syndrome may develop (Table 7.8-3).

DRUG TREATMENT

Drug treatment depends on the specific syndromes present. Head trauma patients may be vulnerable to the side effects of psychotropic drugs, including amnesia from benzodiazepines, and to extrapyramidal side effects, including tardive dyskinesia caused by antipsychotics. Medication may also mask more severe pathology, such as impending subdural hematoma; therefore, it is rarely used.

For a more detailed discussion of this topic, see D X Capruso, H S Levin: Neuropsychiatric Aspects of Head Trauma, Sec 2.4, p 207; E D Caine, H Grossman, J M Lyness: Delirium, Dementia, and Amnestic and Other Cognitive Disorders and Mental Disorders Due to a General Medical Condition, Chap 12, p 705, in CTP/VI.

7.9 Hemodialysis

Hemodialysis is a complex treatment process that can cause many maladaptive behaviors. Most hemodialysis patients are coping with a chronic, debilitating, life-

TABLE 7.8–3
DIAGNOSTIC CRITERIA FOR PERSONALITY CHANGE DUE TO A GENERAL MEDICAL CONDITION

A. A persistent personality disturbance that represents a change from the individual's previous characteristic personality pattern. (In children, the disturbance involves a marked deviation from normal development or a significant change in the child's usual behavior patterns lasting at least 1 year).

B. There is evidence from the history, physical examination, or laboratory findings that the disturbance is the direct physiological consequence of a general medical condition.

C. The disturbance is not better accounted for by another mental disorder (including other mental disorders due to a general medical condition).

D. The disturbance does not occur exclusively during the course of a delirium and does not meet criteria for a dementia.

E. The disturbance causes clinically significant distress or impairment in social, occupational, or other important areas of functioning.

Specify type:
  Labile type: if the predominant feature is affective lability
  Disinhibited type: if the predominant feature is poor impulse control as evidenced by sexual indiscretions, etc.
  Aggressive type: if the predominant feature is aggressive behavior
  Apathetic type: if the predominant feature is marked apathy and indifference
  Paranoid type: if the predominant feature is suspiciousness or paranoid ideation
  Other type: if the predominant feature is not one of the above, e.g., personality change associated with seizure disorder
  Combined type: if more than one feature predominates in the clinical picture
  Unspecified type

  Coding note: Include the name of the general medical condition on Axis I, e.g., personality change due to temporal lobe epilepsy; also code the general medical condition on Axis III

Table from *DSM-IV, Diagnostic and Statistical Manual of Mental Disorders,* ed 4. Copyright American Psychiatric Association, Washington, 1994. Used with permission.

long disease; its treatment requires tedious attachment to a machine for up to six hours three or more times each week. Hemodialysis patients spend a major portion of their lives coping with the consequences of renal failure, and the process of dialysis itself severely disrupts their daily lives, depriving them of their autonomy. Although primary care physicians may be consulted for acute situations, they must evaluate the patient in terms of chronic symptoms and long-term plans.

CLINICAL FEATURES AND DIAGNOSIS

Depression is common in hemodialysis patients, and suicide is 300 times more common in hemodialysis patients than in otherwise comparable normal controls. The behavioral problems that can arise include acting out, noncompliance with the prescribed diet, missing dialysis sessions, anger toward staff members, regression, infantilization, bargaining, and pleading. The premorbid personalities of the patients are important determinants of how they will handle the process of hemodialysis.

INTERVIEWING AND PSYCHOTHERAPEUTIC GUIDELINES

Hemodialysis patients are confronted by disturbances of body image, by depression, and by fears of death. The primary care physician should counsel patients before hemodialysis begins, and directly address the issues of denial and unrealistic expectations. Discuss the benefits of alternative treatment plans, such as home dialysis and renal transplants. Evaluate the family and how the hemodialysis will change the roles of the family members. How will dialysis affect the patient's financial situation and ability to work? During dialysis, make periodic evaluations of the patient's adaptation to the process.

EVALUATION AND MANAGEMENT

1. Hemodialysis patients are subject to frequent and rapid shifts in fluids, electrolytes, and nutrients. Those changes can produce vitamin deficiencies, electrolyte imbalances, and osmotic disequilibrium in the brain.
2. Some patients complain of headache during dialysis, probably because the rapid changes in osmolality cause edema and increased water in the brain. In severe cases, nausea, muscle cramps, short-term mental status changes, delirium, and seizures can occur.
3. Long-term hemodialysis (several years) can lead to dialysis dementia, which is accompanied by dyspraxia, myoclonus, asterixis, grimacing, and seizures. Organic mental syndromes may also result from hypercalcemia, anemia, nitrogen retention, and cerebral infections.
4. Subdural hematomas can be caused by the anticoagulants that are administered to keep the arteriovenous shunt open.
5. Patients should strive to achieve an adaptive acceptance of the situation. The new hemodialysis patient may start with a feeling of euphoria, which then progresses to a stage of depression before progressing to acceptance. A steady, supportive family and treatment team are important in facilitating the process. Group therapy with other dialysis patients is often helpful.

DRUG TREATMENT

Any medications used must have their dosages adjusted according to their effects on the patient's renal function and should be prescribed in consultation with a nephrologist. Antidepressants are often indicated. Blood concentrations of drugs should be measured after each dialysis treatment.

For a more detailed discussion of this topic, see S C Schulz: Schizophrenia: Somatic Treatment, Sec 14.8, p 987; A Roy: Suicide, Sec 30.1, p 1739; B J Sadock, H I Kaplan: Other Biological Therapies, Sec 32.30, p 2144, in CTP/VI.

7.10 Hypothermia

Hypothermia is a medical emergency that is usually caused by prolonged exposure to cold temperatures.

CLINICAL FEATURES AND DIAGNOSIS

The behavioral symptoms include confusion, lethargy, combativeness, low body temperature and shivering, and a paradoxical feeling of warmth. The typical patient

with hypothermia has been exposed for a prolonged period to cold external temperature after the heavy use of alcohol or other central nervous system (CNS) depressants.
Medically ill patients may have hypothermia even without prolonged exposure to
the cold.

The presence of hypoglycemia or hypothyroidism predisposes the patient to
hypothermia. Antipsychotic medications can decrease the central thermoregulation,
causing patients to be susceptible to hypothermia when exposed to the cold. Other
medical conditions that increase the patient's susceptibility to the cold include
pituitary insufficiency, Addison's disease, cerebrovascular disease, Wernicke's
encephalopathy, myocardial infarction, cirrhosis, and pancreatitis. The most common clinical feature is alcohol intoxication.

INTERVIEWING AND PSYCHOTHERAPEUTIC GUIDELINES

Focus on the medical emergency and its potential sequelae. Inquire about the
duration of exposure to the cold, the medications taken (especially antipsychotics),
and the use of alcohol and drugs of abuse. If the patient is confused or delirious, focus
on maintaining a safe, controlled environment and initiating immediate emergency
medical treatment.

EVALUATION AND MANAGEMENT

1. Monitor the patient's temperature frequently, and institute cardiac monitoring.
   Order blood tests (including a complete blood count), thyroid function tests,
   blood urea nitrogen (BUN) and creatinine tests, electrolytes, liver function tests,
   amylase tests, blood alcohol level, and other screening tests for possible medical problems.
2. Warm the patient. Mild hypothermia can be treated by wrapping the patient in
   blankets in a warm room, but moderate hypothermia may require warm baths.
   In severely hypothermic patients, external warming can cause vasodilation that
   diverts blood from the viscera and can lead to rewarming shock. Patients with
   severe hypothermia require core warming with hemodialysis or peritoneal dialysis with warmed blood or dialysate.
3. Do not give the patient alcohol, which causes vasodilation and increases heat
   loss in spite of producing a subjective feeling of warmth.
4. If frostbite is present, warm the affected area gradually (starting with water at
   50°F) after raising the patient's core temperature.

DRUG TREATMENT

Provide intravenous (IV) fluids, and carefully monitor the patient's pH and
potassium. Treat acidosis with IV bicarbonate, and treat hypokalemia to reduce the
risk of cardiac arrhythmias. No specific drugs are used for this condition.

For a more detailed discussion of this topic, see M A Schuckit: Alcohol-Related Disorders, Sec 13.2, p 775; E D Caine, H Grossman, J M Lyness: Delirium, Dementia, and Amnestic and Other Cognitive Disorders and Mental Disorders Due to a General Medical Condition, Chap 12, p 705, in CTP/VI.

7.11 Mitral Valve Prolapse

Mitral valve prolapse is a bulging of the mitral valve into the left atrial chamber during left ventricular systole. This condition is considered to be an associated feature of panic disorder. Although some cardiologists consider it the cause of panic disorder, in some patients the mitral valve prolapse is caused by hemodynamic factors associated with panic attacks. In those patients, when the panic disorder is treated, the mitral valve prolapse also resolves.

CLINICAL FEATURES AND DIAGNOSIS

Mitral valve prolapse produces a midsystolic click and a systolic murmur (systolic click-murmur syndrome). It is more common in females than in males, especially between the ages of 14 and 30 years; as many as 10 percent of females in this age group present with asymptomatic mitral valve prolapse. The patients are often tall and thin and may also have connective tissue diseases, such as Marfan's syndrome. Mitral valve prolapse is usually a benign finding, but it may be associated with mitral regurgitation that is significant enough to cause ventricular hypertrophy.

The symptoms of mitral valve prolapse are similar to those of panic disorder and include chest pain, palpitations, tachycardia, dyspnea, extrasystoles, weakness, fatigue, dizziness, syncope, and anxiety. Perhaps up to one half of all patients who have panic disorder have mitral valve prolapse. The symptoms are thought to be related to arrhythmias.

The diagnosis is confirmed by echocardiography. An electrocardiogram (ECG) typically shows biphasic or inverted T waves in leads II, III, and aVF.

INTERVIEWING AND PSYCHOTHERAPEUTIC GUIDELINES

The patient's history alone is unlikely to provide enough information to distinguish between mitral valve prolapse and panic disorder. In fact, many patients have both conditions. Consider mitral valve prolapse in the differential diagnosis of paniclike symptoms, and proceed with an appropriate medical workup, even though the patient may be young and generally healthy. Anxiety is usually prominent. Be calm and reassuring. The disorder need not interfere with any of the patient's activities of daily living. Anxiety superimposed on a cardiac condition can increase the possibility of arrhythmias and angina.

EVALUATION AND MANAGEMENT

1. Refer the patient to a cardiologist. An electrocardiogram and an echocardiogram are noninvasive parts of the workup.

2. Order thyroid function tests—triiodothyronine (T_3), thyroxine (T_4), T_3 resin uptake (T_3RU), and thyroid stimulating hormone (TSH). Thyrotoxicosis can produce symptoms identical to those of mitral valve prolapse.
3. Obtain the patient's vital signs and order screening tests—complete blood count (CBC), a chemistry profile, and liver and renal function tests—before initiating any drug treatments.
4. Behavioral treatment, such as in vivo exposure, is effective in panic disorder.

DRUG TREATMENT

β-Blockers—for example, propranolol (Inderal)—are helpful in mitral valve prolapse but are usually not completely effective in panic disorder. Many mitral valve prolapse patients also fulfill the diagnostic criteria for panic disorder. Panic disorder can be treated with benzodiazepines (for example, alprazolam [Xanax] and clonazepam [Klonopin]), tricyclic antidepressants (for example, imipramine [Tofranil]), monoamine oxidase inhibitors (MAOIs) (for example, phenelzine [Nardil]), and serotonergic agents.

For a more detailed discussion of this topic, see A J Fyer, S Mannuzza, J D Coplan: Panic Disorders and Agoraphobia, Sec 17.1, p 1191; W Katon, M D Sullivan, M R Clark: Cardiovascular Disorders, Sec 26.4, p 1491, in CTP/VI.

7.12 Parkinsonism

Parkinsonism is an extrapyramidal syndrome which may be due to Parkinson's disease (idiopathic), may be a side effect of high-potency antipsychotic medication (see Chapter 23), may follow head trauma or exposure to such toxins as N-methyl-4-phenyl-1,2,3,6-tetrahydropyridine (MTPT, an illicit opioid of abuse), or may be due to other neurological conditions.

CLINICAL FEATURES AND DIAGNOSIS

Parkinsonism is characterized by cogwheel rigidity, a flattened affect, drooling, and a shuffling gait. The tremor is greatest at rest and can often be seen in a pill-rolling motion of the hands.

Parkinson's disease occurs in the elderly; antipsychotic-induced parkinsonism (in which the tremor is usually bilateral) usually begins shortly after starting the medication or increasing the dosage; MTPT-induced parkinsonism is associated with a history of intravenous (IV) drug abuse; and parkinsonism caused by head trauma is likely only after a history of repeated trauma, as in boxing.

The primary mechanism in parkinsonism is believed to be a decrease in dopaminergic activity in the nigrostriatal pathway. In Parkinson's disease, MTPT use, and head trauma, the decrease in dopaminergic activity is due to the loss of dopaminergic cells. In antipsychotic-induced parkinsonism, the decrease is due to the blockade of dopaminergic receptors. Treatments of parkinsonism are based either on increasing the stimulation of dopaminergic receptors or decreasing the stimulation of cholinergic receptors. Dopaminergic and cholinergic activity are in a balance; decreasing cholinergic activity is another way to compensate for decreased dopaminergic activity.

INTERVIEWING AND PSYCHOTHERAPEUTIC GUIDELINES

The patient's degree of distress varies according to the specific syndrome causing the parkinsonism. Antipsychotic-induced parkinsonism may be associated with acute dystonia, which can be a frightening experience for the patient. Reassure the patient that an effective treatment is readily available. Patients with Parkinson's disease are commonly depressed and may also be demented.

EVALUATION AND MANAGEMENT

1. Make a definitive diagnosis that accounts for the cause of the parkinsonism.
2. Unless the parkinsonism is obviously antipsychotic-induced, perform a neurological examination, looking for focal neurological findings. Look for stiffness, cogwheeling, decreased arm swing, and other features of parkinsonism. Examine the patient taking an antipsychotic agent for dystonia and neuroleptic malignant syndrome, particularly if the rigidity is severe.
3. Conduct a full psychiatric mental status examination and obtain the patient's history, looking for depression, dementia, and psychosis.
4. Evaluate the patient's present antipsychotic drug regimen (if any) and consider whether (a) the dose is sufficient, (b) the duration of treatment is sufficient, (c) the patient has responded, (d) a change of drug or a change in dosage could be made, and (e) dopaminergic agonists or cholinergic antagonists are indicated.
5. A surgical treatment involving the brain implantation of tissue from the adrenal medulla has helped some patients.

DRUG TREATMENT

Antipsychotic-induced parkinsonism is a common side effect of high-potency antipsychotics—for example, haloperidol (Haldol) and fluphenazine (Prolixin). A dosage reduction may decrease the risk of parkinsonism, but usually the patient requires rapid relief, which can be given with anticholinergic drugs, such as benztropine (Cogentin) 1 to 2 mg by mouth twice a day (Table 7.12-1). Benztropine 1 to 2 mg is also rapidly effective when given intramuscularly (IM) or IV if the patient is in acute distress. The benztropine should then be given on a standing basis.

If the high-potency antipsychotic is ineffective or if its side effects are severe enough to warrant its discontinuation, the drug should be changed to a low-potency antipsychotic, such as chlorpromazine (Thorazine) or thioridazine (Mellaril). Those drugs are not likely to cause extrapyramidal side effects, such as parkinsonism, and they have strong anticholinergic effects. Amantadine (Symmetrel) 100 to 300 mg a day increases dopaminergic activity and is sometimes useful. However, a

TABLE 7.12–1
DRUGS USED TO MANAGE PARKINSONISM

Class/Generic Name	Trade Names	Usual Dosage (mg per day)
Anticholinergics		
Benztropine	Cogentin	1–6
Biperiden	Akineton	2–6
Ethopropazine	Parsidol	50
Orphenadrine	Dispal, Norflex	300
Procyclidine	Kemardrin	6–20
Trihexyphenidyl	Artane	5–15
Antihistamine		
Diphenhydramine	Benadryl	25–100
Dopamine Agonist		
Amantadine	Symadine, Symmetrel	100–300

problem with amantadine is its possible precipitation of psychotic symptoms. It may be a good alternative to anticholinergics for the elderly and for other patients who are particularly susceptible to anticholinergic toxicity. Another alternative is clozapine (Clozaril), which may not cause any extrapyramidal side effects.

Parkinson's disease is usually treated with levodopa (Larodopa), a dopamine precursor. Levodopa is sometimes combined with carbidopa (Sinemet), a dopa decarboxylase inhibitor that further increases brain dopamine levels. Amantadine and deprenyl (a selective inhibitor of monoamine oxidase type B that selectively catabolizes dopamine) have also been used.

Depression in Parkinson's disease should be treated with antidepressants. Electroconvulsive therapy (ECT) can be considered in refractory cases.

For a more detailed discussion of this topic, see W C Wirshing: Neuropsychiatric Aspects of Movement Disorders, Sec 2.5, p 220; E D Caine, H Grossman, J M Lyness: Delirium, Dementia, and Amnestic and Other Cognitive Disorders and Mental Disorders Due to a General Medical Condition, Chap 12, p 705, in CTP/VI.

7.13 Starvation

Starvation involves a series of physiological changes that the body undergoes in the course of reduced food intake. Psychiatric disturbances may lead to inanition, but starvation also produces secondary psychiatric symptoms, including intense preoccupation with food, food hoarding and stealing, binge eating, food dreams, sleep disturbance, loss of sexual interest, reduced concentration, decreased alertness, diminished ambition, and social withdrawal. Depression and a mild organic mental syndrome may result. Physical changes include a loss of fat, reduced muscle mass, reduced thyroid metabolism, cold intolerance, and difficulty in maintaining the core body temperature. Cardiac muscle condition and conduction are affected by cardiac muscle loss, atrial and ventricular premature contractions, ventricular tachycardia, and sudden death. The gastrointestinal effects are bloating, constipation, and abdominal pain. Menstrual irregularities are common, and amenorrhea ultimately develops in the course of starvation. Lanugo, edema, leukopenia, and osteoporosis are frequently found.

CLINICAL FEATURES AND DIAGNOSIS

Starvation may be deliberately self-induced for cultural reasons, as in hunger strikes, or may result from true anorexia, anorexia nervosa, or schizophrenic apathy. True anorexia is the loss of appetite and may occur in depression, grief, and anxiety disorders. The appetite is not affected in anorexia nervosa. Instead, patients with anorexia nervosa have a marked preoccupation with food, cook elaborate meals, eat surreptitiously, and binge eat. In addition, they suffer from a disturbance of body image, with the persistent belief that they are fat, despite all evidence to the contrary.

The elderly are vulnerable to starvation because of preexisting physical debilitation, dementia, social isolation, and poverty.

Schizophrenic persons among the homeless mentally ill may suffer starvation as a result of complete self-neglect. Hematological changes are common in those people partly because of nutritional reasons and partly because of lice infestation. They often deny any evidence of illness or social deterioration. Most will eat if meals are provided, but they do not have the motivation to obtain food. Some are too apathetic or paranoid to take meals that are offered to them.

INTERVIEWING AND PSYCHOTHERAPEUTIC GUIDELINES

Patients with social reasons to starve themselves and those with true anorexia are usually able to provide a reliable history. Patients with anorexia nervosa, however, are resistant. Schizophrenic patients may also be resistant, but the examiner need not focus directly on appetite and weight loss but can question patients indirectly and concretely. How do the patients support themselves? If they have money, how much do they spend on food? What do they like to eat?

EVALUATION AND MANAGEMENT

1. Any patient with significant weight loss or decreased appetite should be evaluated medically to rule out any underlying physical illness (for example, malignancy). Starvation without complicating mental illness responds to feeding and vitamin supplementation.
2. Starving patients may require admission to the hospital to ensure an adequate intake of food. Involuntary hospitalization in such circumstances is controversial in some jurisdictions, as inanition may not be viewed as an imminent danger. However, most physicians agree that involuntary hospitalization is warranted in extreme cases. Once hospitalized, most patients respond to coaxing to eat.
3. In anorexia nervosa, a 20 percent reduction from the patient's ideal weight or significant electrolyte disturbances, particularly hypokalemia, suggest the need for hospital admission. The threat of hospitalization can be used to set limits on further starvation as long as binging and vomiting do not derange the patient's electrolytes. Patients with anorexia nervosa do not respond to simple reasoning and advice.

4. Occasionally, electroconvulsive therapy (ECT) may be indicated for severe depression with inanition.
5. In severe cases, a nasogastric tube can be used.

DRUG TREATMENT

Anorexia in the case of depressed patients and apathy in the case of schizophrenic patients respond to treatment of the underlying condition.

For a more detailed discussion of this topic, see P E Garfinkel: Eating Disorders, Chap 22. p 1361, in CTP/VI.

7.14 Thyrotoxicosis

Thyrotoxicosis results from the sustained elevation of plasma concentrations of free thyroid hormone (T_2). The resulting psychological state is best described as tense dysphoria. Common causes of thyrotoxicosis include Graves' disease, toxic multinodular goiter, thyroiditis, and exogenous iodide.

CLINICAL FEATURES AND DIAGNOSIS

Patients with hyperthyroidism report heat intolerance, excessive sweating, weight loss despite hyperphagia, increased bowel movements, palpitations, fine tremor, and hyperkinesis. Insomnia, irritability, episodic anxiety, affective lability, and rapid tangential speech are typical. Despite motor restlessness and hyperkinesis, energy levels are usually subjectively depressed. Thyrotoxicosis may eventuate in psychosis or delirium. It is more commonly found in women than in men.

Muscle wasting is common, particularly the muscles of the limb girdles. Deep tendon reflexes are hyperactive. Tachycardia, paroxysmal arrhythmias, and cardiomegaly occur with increased contractility, increased cardiac output, and increased pulse pressure mediated by catecholamines. Tachycardia is maintained even during sleep. The skin is moist and velvety smooth, with vasodilation. The hair is fine and thin. Patients with Graves' disease may have pretibial myxedema and vitiligo. Ocular signs include fixed stare, lid lag, infrequent blinking, widened palpebral fissures, and exophthalmos. However, goiter, tachycardia, and exophthalmos may not be present in all cases. Laboratory evaluation reveals undetectable thyroid-stimulating hormone (TSH), blunted thyrotropin-releasing hormone (TRH), and elevated thyroxine (T_4) serum concentrations, triiodothyronine (T_3), and free thyroxin index (T_2I).

Both hyperthyroid and hypothyroid patients can appear depressed, especially hypothyroid patients. Hyperthyroidism may also present as mania or anxiety. Apathetic hyperthyroidism, which occurs predominately in the elderly, is indistinguishable from major depression with melancholia. It may present as dementia.

INTERVIEWING AND PSYCHOTHERAPEUTIC GUIDELINES

Interview techniques depend on the clinical status of the patient. Apathetic depressed patients may need gentle encouragement to answer specific questions. Patients with organic disorders may need frequent reorientation and repetition of questions and information. Anxious patients need reassurance, support, and a calm environment. Manic and psychotic patients need redirection, limit setting, and a nonstimulating environment.

EVALUATION AND MANAGEMENT

1. Consider the diagnosis of hyperthyroidism in all patients with psychotic, mood, anxiety, and organic disorders.
2. Order thyroid function tests (for example, TSH, T_4, T_3) as part of the routine evaluation of such patients.
3. Psychopathology secondary to thyrotoxicosis may remit with the reduction of circulating hormone levels.

DRUG TREATMENT

β-Blockers—for example, propranolol (Inderal) 10 to 40 mg by mouth four times a day—reduce arrhythmias, tremor, and many behavioral symptoms but not muscle wasting. Lithium (Eskalith) has also been used. Agitated patients can be sedated with oxazepam (Serax) 10 to 30 mg by mouth, estazolam (ProSom) 0.5 to 1 mg by mouth, lorazepam (Ativan) 1 to 2 mg by mouth or intramuscularly (IM), or alprazolam (Xanax) 0.25 to 0.5 mg by mouth. Long-term therapy involves the use of propylthiouracil to block synthesis; it inhibits the deiodination of all iodothyronines. Radioactive iodine is effective but may result in permanent hypothyroidism that requires replacement therapy.

For a more detailed discussion of this topic, see E D Caine, H Grossman, J M Lyness: Delirium, Dementia, and Amnestic and Other Cognitive Disorders and Mental Disorders Due to a General Medical Condition, Chap 12, p 705; R T Rubin, B H King: Endocrine and Metabolic Disorders, Sec 26.6, p 1514, in CTP/VI.

7.15 Vitamin B_{12} Deficiency

Anemia combined with neurological symptoms, personality change, or confusion may suggest vitamin B_{12} deficiency. Although megaloblastic anemia is typical in vitamin B_{12} deficiency, mental symptoms may precede the development of anemia. The psychiatric symptoms include irritability, psychomotor agitation or retardation, depression, neurovegetative disturbances, delirium, dementia, and schizophrenialike symptoms. The neurological complaints include paresthesias, weakness, poor coordination, and an unsteady gait. A prompt diagnosis is vital, as the neurological symptoms can be completely reversed with rapid parenteral vitamin therapy.

CLINICAL FEATURES AND DIAGNOSIS

Patients with vitamin B_{12} deficiency are typically in middle to late life with malabsorption secondary to pernicious anemia. Strict vegetarians are also at risk and may have a folate intake inadequate to prevent anemia. Gastrectomy and bacterial and parasitic competition account for some cases.

The onset is insidious. Anemia develops gradually and hence is tolerated, but it may result in pallor, mild splenomegaly, and jaundice. The patient may have a low-grade fever. B_{12} deficiency is one of several deficiencies that cause glossitis. The loss of fine motor skills is related to the loss of vibratory sensation and two-point discrimination. Patchy central nervous system (CNS) degeneration ultimately results.

Psychiatrically, the condition is classified as an organic mental syndrome, whether its major psychiatric manifestation is affective, cognitive, or perceptual. The diagnosis is critical, as the condition is one of the few treatable types of dementia, and it is gradually progressive if untreated. A routine complete blood count (CBC) may reveal the classic megaloblastic anemia. A low B_{12} level confirms the diagnosis.

INTERVIEWING AND PSYCHOTHERAPEUTIC GUIDELINES

Detailed neurological and cognitive examinations are essential. For the cognitive examination use a structured instrument, such as the Mini-Mental State Examination (MMSE). Reassure patients that they will improve with treatment.

EVALUATION AND MANAGEMENT

1. Parenteral vitamin B_{12} rapidly corrects many manifestations of vitamin B_{12} deficiency, including fever, anemia, and glossitis.
2. Establish the underlying cause.
3. A transfusion is generally not required.
4. Advanced cases with neurological deficits do not respond well to vitamin B_{12} replacement. The patient may be left with persistent neurological or psychiatric sequelae and require rehabilitation.

DRUG TREATMENT

Vitamin B_{12} 100 μg daily should be administered parenterally for 10 to 14 days and then given monthly. Any excess vitamin B_{12} is excreted in the urine. If sedation is necessary, lorazepam (Ativan) 1 to 2 mg by mouth or oxazepam (Serax) 10 to 30 mg by mouth may be given safely at frequent intervals in the short term.

For a more detailed discussion of this topic, see L A Papp, J M Gorman: Generalized Anxiety Disorder, Sec 17.5, p 1236, in CTP/VI.

8

Substance-Related Disorders

8.1. Alcohol Abuse and Dependence

The excessive use of alcohol that is harmful to physical and mental health constitutes alcohol dependence and abuse. Alcohol dependence runs in families; children of alcohol-abusing parents are at high risk of developing alcohol abuse whether or not they are raised by their biological parents.

CLINICAL FEATURES AND DIAGNOSIS

The need for the daily use of large amounts of alcohol for adequate functioning, a regular pattern of heavy drinking limited to weekends, and long periods of sobriety interspersed with periods of heavy alcohol intake lasting from minutes to weeks are strongly suggestive of alcohol use disorders. The patterns are often associated with such behaviors as (1) the inability to cut down or stop drinking, (2) repeated efforts to control or reduce excessive drinking by periods of temporary abstinence (going on the wagon) or restricting drinking to certain times of the day, (3) binges (remaining intoxicated throughout the day for at least two days), (4) the occasional consumption of a fifth of spirits (or its equivalent in wine or beer), (5) amnestic periods for events occurring while intoxicated (blackouts), (6) the continuation of drinking despite a serious physical disorder that the person knows is exacerbated by alcohol use, and (7) the drinking of nonbeverage alcohol, such as fuel and commercial products containing alcohol. In addition, people with alcohol dependence and abuse show impaired social or occupational functioning; such dysfunction may include violence while intoxicated, absence from work, loss of job, legal difficulties (for example, arrest for intoxicated behavior and traffic accidents while intoxicated), and arguments or difficulties with family members or friends because of excessive alcohol use.

INTERVIEWING AND PSYCHOTHERAPEUTIC GUIDELINES

The proper evaluation of the alcohol user requires some suspiciousness. In general, most people, when questioned, underreport the amount of alcohol they consume. When obtaining a history of alcohol usage, it might be helpful to ask open-ended questions. For example, ask, "How much alcohol do you drink?" rather than, "Do you drink alcohol?" Other questions that may give important clues include how often the patient drinks in the morning, how often he or she has blackouts (amnesia while intoxicated), and how often friends or relatives have told the patient to cut down on drinking. Always look for subtle signs of alcohol abuse and always inquire about use of other substances. Does the patient seem to be accident prone (head injury, rib fracture, motor vehicle accidents)? Is he or she often in fights? Are there frequent absences from work? Are there social or family problems?

EVALUATION AND MANAGEMENT

Prolonged maintenance of total sobriety is the goal. The patient must first acknowledge the drinking problem—perhaps overcoming severe denial—before he or she will cooperate in seeking treatment. Referral for group therapy may be more acceptable to patients who perceive alcohol dependence as a social problem rather than a personal psychiatric problem.

DRUG TREATMENT

Disulfiram (Antabuse)—125 to 500 mg a day—may be used if the patient desires enforced sobriety. Patients taking disulfiram develop an extremely unpleasant reaction when they ingest even small amounts of alcohol. The reaction, caused by an accumulation of acetaldehyde, includes flushing, headache, throbbing in head and neck, dyspnea, hyperventilation, tachycardia, hypotension, sweating, anxiety, weakness, and confusion. Life-threatening complications, although uncommon, can occur. Disulfiram is useful only temporarily to help establish a long-term pattern of sobriety and to change long-standing alcohol-related coping mechanisms.

Naltrexone (ReVia) decreases alcohol craving—probably by blocking the release of endogenous opioids—and aids in achieving abstinence by preventing relapse and lowering alcohol consumption. A dosage of 50 mg once daily is recommended for most patients.

8.2. Alcohol Dementia

Chronic alcohol dependence is believed to be able to cause a dementia similar to Wernicke's encephalopathy and Korsakoff's syndrome. In the context of ongoing alcohol use, the signs of dementia may be difficult to differentiate from signs of intoxication. Alcohol withdrawal or alcohol withdrawal delirium may further complicate the clinical picture. Alcohol dementia may also be superimposed on either Alzheimer's disease or vascular dementia.

CLINICAL FEATURES AND DIAGNOSIS

Proper diagnosis requires that the patient be free of alcohol for several weeks. If dementia is diagnosed, the goal is to identify the possible reversible causes. Early signs of alcohol dementia may be reversible.

The clinical features are similar to other dementias which are described in Section 6.7.

INTERVIEWING AND PSYCHOTHERAPEUTIC GUIDELINES

Orient the patient as much and as often as possible. A calm, reassuring attitude may help assuage agitation, which is common in alcohol dementia. Obtain the patient's history of alcohol use from relatives and friends. Assess the use of other drugs (for example, cocaine and benzodiazepines). Ask about falls, head injuries, and other traumas. Assess the patient's nutritional status if possible.

EVALUATION AND MANAGEMENT

1. Obtain the patient's vital signs.
2. Do a complete physical examination and workup for medical problems, including a complete blood count (CBC), complete chemistry panel, thyroid function tests, Venereal Disease Research Laboratory (VDRL) tests, and serum B_{12} and folate concentration tests. A computed tomography (CT) scan of the head and an electroencephalogram (EEG) are also indicated. Obtain routine screening tests, such as urinalysis, urine toxicology screen, electrocardiogram (ECG), and chest X-ray.
3. Other tests—such as a lumbar puncture, magnetic resonance imaging (MRI), and neuropsychological testing—may be indicated after detoxification and stabilization.
4. Reassurance is often effective in relieving the depression and anxiety in demented patients. Support and structure are very important.

DRUG TREATMENT

Give thiamine 100 mg intramuscularly (IM) and then 100 mg by mouth three times a day. Give one multivitamin (B_{12} and folate) twice a day.

Treat any medical problems found. If the patient is dehydrated, encourage the ingestion of fluids to maintain adequate hydration. Agitation or insomnia may be treated with either benzodiazepines or antipsychotics. Benzodiazepines—for example, oxazepam (Serax) 10 to 30 mg by mouth or lorazepam (Ativan) 1 to 2 mg by mouth or IM—are suggested for patients with recent alcohol use or dependence, since benzodiazepines are not likely to precipitate withdrawal seizures. Antipsychotics—for example, fluphenazine (Prolixin) or haloperidol (Haldol), both given at 2 to 5 mg by mouth or IM—are preferable in demented patients without recent alcohol use, because antipsychotics are less likely than are benzodiazepines to worsen the patient's cognitive impairment.

For a more detailed discussion of this topic, see M A Schuckit: Alcohol-Related Disorders, Sec 13.2, p 775, in CTP/VI.

8.3. Alcohol Hallucinosis

Alcohol hallucinosis is defined as hallucinations that occur in an alcohol-dependent patient within two days of a decrease or cessation of drinking and that persist after the symptoms of withdrawal have disappeared. The disorder is uncommon and occurs more often in men than in women.

CLINICAL FEATURES AND DIAGNOSIS

The hallucinations are auditory or visual; often they are unpleasant buzzing sounds. The patient may also have delusions and paranoid ideas of reference. The patient shows no evidence of a decreased level of consciousness, and the patient's orientation for person, place, and time is intact. The duration is variable. The symptoms may last from a few hours to a few weeks; 10 percent of all patients have symptoms that persist indefinitely.

The differential diagnosis includes schizophreniform disorder, schizophrenia, mood disorders, and medically caused organic disorders. The possibility of the concomitant abuse of drugs (for example, cocaine and hallucinogens) should always be considered.

INTERVIEWING AND PSYCHOTHERAPEUTIC GUIDELINES

Calmly reassure the patient. Explain the origin of the hallucinations if reality testing is intact. Do not argue about the sources of the hallucinations if the patient has a delusional interpretation of their origin. Provide a quiet, safe environment.

EVALUATION AND MANAGEMENT

1. Obtain the patient's vital signs. Rule out alcohol withdrawal, which can be accompanied by hallucinations.
2. Conduct a full medical and psychiatric evaluation, giving attention to comorbid psychiatric disorders and the physical sequelae of alcohol abuse.
3. Order a urine toxicology screen.
4. Provide a safe environment and be alert for violent outbursts in which the patient reacts to the hallucinations. Dangerous patients may need hospitalization.
5. Refer patients for treatment of alcoholism when appropriate.

DRUG TREATMENT

Administer thiamine 100 mg intramuscularly (IM) and then 100 mg orally three times a day.

Give benzodiazepines, such as lorazepam (Ativan) 1 to 2 mg by mouth or IM every four to six hours as needed. If benzodiazepines are ineffective, consider giving antipsychotics, such as haloperidol (Haldol) 2 to 5 mg by mouth or IM every four to six hours as needed.

For a more detailed discussion of this topic, see M A Schuckit: Alcohol-Related Disorders, Sec 13.2, p 775, in CTP/VI.

8.4. Alcohol Idiosyncratic Intoxication

Alcohol idiosyncratic intoxication (also called pathological intoxication) is maladaptive behavior, usually aggressive (for example, fighting), that is not characteristic of the patient and that occurs after consuming an amount of alcohol that does not cause intoxication in an average person.

CLINICAL FEATURES AND DIAGNOSIS

The onset is rapid, and the duration is usually minutes to hours, terminating in impaired consciousness, disorientation, confusion, and prolonged sleep. Transient hallucinations, illusions, and delusions may be present, as well as rage, agitation, and violence. The patient is often amnestic for the episode. An underlying organic pathology—such as temporal lobe epilepsy, head trauma, or encephalitis—may make the patient susceptible to the effects of alcohol. The disorder is reportedly most common in the elderly, patients taking sedative-hypnotics, patients who feel tired, chronically anxious people, and people with impaired impulse control. The differential diagnosis includes temporal lobe epilepsy and impulse-control disorders.

INTERVIEWING AND PSYCHOTHERAPEUTIC GUIDELINES

The interviewer should be calm and nonthreatening. Security guards should be available as needed. The patient should not be challenged or provoked; if possible, provide an isolated, quiet area for the patient.

EVALUATION AND MANAGEMENT

1. Take immediate steps to protect patients from harming themselves or others. Restraints and sedation may be needed.
2. Conduct a full medical evaluation for underlying organic disorders and medical complications of intoxication.
3. Conduct a psychiatric reevaluation when the patient is sober to evaluate for dangerousness and to determine whether psychiatric disorders are present.
4. Evaluate the patient for polysubstance abuse.

DRUG TREATMENT

Severe agitation or assaultive behavior can usually be controlled with low doses of a benzodiazepine (for example, lorazepam [Ativan] 1 to 2 mg by mouth or intramuscularly [IM]) or a high-potency antipsychotic (for example, haloperidol [Haldol] 2 to 5 mg by mouth or IM). Low-potency antipsychotics, such as chlorpromazine (Thorazine) and thioridazine (Mellaril), should not be used, because they pose an increased risk of postural hypotension and because they lower the seizure threshold. Long-term dosing is not indicated, because of the risk of long-term side effects.

For a more detailed discussion of this topic, see M A Schuckit: Alcohol-Related Disorders, Sec 13.2, p 775, in CTP/VI.

8.5. Alcohol Intoxication, Alcohol Withdrawal, and Alcohol Withdrawal Delirium

Alcohol Intoxication

Alcohol intoxication (simple drunkenness) is defined as maladaptive behavior after the recent consumption of an amount of alcohol adequate to produce intoxication in most people. A blood alcohol concentration of 30 to 60 mg/dL is generally necessary. Legal intoxication is defined as a blood alcohol concentration of 100 mg/dL (Table 8.5–1).

CLINICAL FEATURES AND DIAGNOSIS

The physical signs of alcohol intoxication include dysarthria, incoordination, ataxia, nystagmus, and a flushed face. The condition may be associated with behavioral changes, including giddiness and disinhibition, increased talkativeness, withdrawal, and argumentativeness. The patient's judgment and recent memory are impaired.

Carefully examine the patient for signs of withdrawal, such as tremor. Look for (1) signs of trauma, especially head injury, subdural hematoma, rib fractures, and facial hematoma; (2) direct effects of alcohol such as cirrhosis, hepatitis, pancreatitis, gastritis, gastrointestinal (GI) bleeding, neuropathy, and cardiomyopathy; infections; and (3) signs of exposure to the elements. See Table 8.5–2 for the differential diagnosis of alcohol intoxication.

INTERVIEWING AND PSYCHOTHERAPEUTIC GUIDELINES

Conduct the interview in a quiet, nonstimulating room. Intoxicated patients are often difficult to evaluate and frustrating to interview because their mental status may change rapidly as they become sober. Patients with other mental disorders who are also intoxicated may be suicidal or homicidal while intoxicated but not after they are sober. Carefully evaluate the intoxicated patient; the first goal of treatment is to maintain safety while the patient becomes sober. If the intoxicated patient is agitated or belligerent, security guards should be available. Do not challenge, provoke, or reprimand the patient. Be as nonthreatening as possible.

EVALUATION AND MANAGEMENT

1. The goal is to help the patient through acute intoxication without injury to self or others; when the patient is sober, reevaluate for a definitive treatment.
2. Evaluate the patient for other alcohol-related disorders (especially dependence and withdrawal) and for other mental disorders.
3. Consider hospitalization for detoxification if necessary.

TABLE 8.5–1
STAGES OF ALCOHOL INTOXICATION

Blood Alcohol Level (mg/dL)[1]	Effects on Feeling and Behavior	Time Required for All Alcohol to Leave the Body
0.02–0.03%	Absence of obvious effects; mild alteration of feelings; slight intensification of existing moods; minor impairment of judgment and memory	2 hours
0.03–0.06%	Feeling of warmth, relaxation, mild sedation; exaggeration of emotion and behavior, slight impairment of the fine motor skills; slight increase in reaction time	4 hours
0.08–0.09%	Visual and hearing acuity reduced; slight speech impairment; minor disturbance of balance; increased difficulty in performing motor skills; feeling of elation or depression; desire for more to drink; speaks louder and becomes more argumentative	6 hours
0.11–0.12%	Difficulty in performing many gross motor skills; uncoordinated behavior; definite impairment of mental facilities, i.e., judgment and memory, decreased inhibitions; becomes angered if he cannot have another drink or is told he has had enough	8 hours
0.14–0.15%	Major impairment of all physical and mental functions; irresponsible behavior; general feeling of euphoria; difficulty in standing, walking, talking; distorted perception and judgment; feels confident of driving skills; cannot recognize impairment	10 hours
0.20%	Feels confused or dazed; gross body movements cannot be made without assistance; inability to maintain a steady upright position	12 hours
0.30%	Minimum perception and comprehension; general suspension or diminution of sensibility	
0.40%	Nearly complete anesthesia, absence of perception; state of unconsciousness, coma	
0.50%	Deep coma	
0.60%	Death is possible after complete anesthesia of the respiratory center	

[1] Milligrams per deciliter.
Table From W R Cote, F D Lisnow: Alcohol use and abuse. In *Emergency Psychiatry*, E L Bassuk, A W Birk, editors, p 132. Plenum, New York, 1984. Used with permission.

TABLE 8.5–2
DIFFERENTIAL DIAGNOSIS OF ALCOHOL INTOXICATION

1. Sedative-hypnotic intoxication
2. Hypoglycemia
3. Diabetic ketoacidosis
4. Subdural hematoma; head injury
5. Postictal states
6. Hepatic encephalopathy
7. Encephalitis
8. Other causes of ataxia (e.g., multiple sclerosis, neurodegenerative disorders)

Table adapted from S E Hyman, B E Bierer: Alcohol-related emergencies. In *Manual of Psychiatric Emergencies*, ed 2, S E Hyman, editor, p 247. Little, Brown, Boston, 1988. Used with permission.

4. Intoxicated patients who make statements about suicide or other dangerous acts may have to be admitted to an inpatient psychiatry service.
5. Protect the patient from falls and accidental injury. Also, prevent the patient, if belligerent, from assaulting others.
6. Obtain the patient's vital signs. If they are elevated, treat the patient immediately for alcohol withdrawal. Intoxication and withdrawal present in a patient at the same time suggests a long-standing pattern of heavy alcohol use that has recently decreased, typically because of the unavailability of alcohol. Anxiety, irritability, tremor, and insomnia are other signs of withdrawal.
7. Find out if the patient also abused other drugs.
8. Evaluate the patient's mental status as completely as possible, particularly focusing on current dangerousness. Identify any other mental disorders present. Alcohol is commonly used to self-medicate anxiety, psychotic symptoms, and depression. Suicide is common in alcohol-dependent patients, and alcohol is commonly consumed before suicide attempts. Homicide attempts and other violence are also much more likely when the patient is intoxicated than when sober.
9. Decide whether withdrawal is from either alcohol or sedative-hypnotics, which have cross-tolerance and cross-dependence with alcohol. Withdrawal implies dependence.
10. Provide a safe environment where the patient can become sober. It may be in the emergency room, in the waiting room, in the physician's office, at a shelter, at a sobering-up station, or at home if a family member can be responsible. Ideally, monitoring for signs of withdrawal should be available.

DRUG TREATMENT

High-dose or frequent medication is not indicated, as any sedating medication would most likely interact synergistically with the alcohol already in the patient. Handle agitation with physical restraint and, in extreme circumstances, the careful use of a benzodiazepine—for example, lorazepam (Ativan) 1 to 2 mg by mouth or intramuscularly (IM), oxazepam (Serax) 10 to 30 mg by mouth, or chlordiazepoxide (Librium) 10 to 25 mg by mouth. Always carefully monitor the patient.

Alcohol Withdrawal

Alcohol withdrawal is a syndrome affecting alcohol-dependent patients when they cease or a markedly decrease alcohol consumption. The presence of the disorder usually implies heavy alcohol use for at least several days. Most symptoms are attributable to central nervous system (CNS) hyperirritability.

CLINICAL FEATURES AND DIAGNOSIS

The onset of withdrawal begins several hours (usually six to eight) after a decrease in alcohol intake. The disorder is usually self-limited in otherwise healthy patients. Alcohol withdrawal is easily identified by the patient's history and by the presence of a mild coarse tremor and at least one of the following symptoms: nausea or vomiting, malaise or weakness, tachycardia, hypertension, sweating, anxiety, depressed mood, irritability, restlessness, transient hallucinations, illusions, headache, insomnia (Table 8.5-3).

INTERVIEWING AND PSYCHOTHERAPEUTIC GUIDELINES

Reassurance—coupled with a calm, specific elicitation of the patient's history—is essential.

EVALUATION AND MANAGEMENT

1. Evaluate the patient's hydration and electrolytes. Either dehydration or overhydration may be present. Correct any electrolyte deficiencies, including calcium and magnesium deficiencies. Intravenous (IV) fluids are usually not necessary.
2. Carefully evaluate the patient for concomitant medical problems, especially head trauma, rib fractures, infections, gastrointestinal bleeding, and hepatic disease.
3. Prevent the progression to alcohol withdrawal delirium.
4. Outpatient management is contraindicated if the patient is febrile (over 101°F), has seizures, is unable to retain fluids, shows signs of Wernicke's encephalopathy or Korsakoff's syndrome, or has a serious underlying medical disorder.

TABLE 8.5–3
SIGNS AND SYMPTOMS OF ALCOHOL WITHDRAWAL

Autonomic overactivity
1. Tachycardia
2. Hypertension
3. Diaphoresis
4. Tremor
5. Fever
6. Respiratory alkalosis

Sleep disturbance
1. Sleep latency insomnia
2. Increased rapid eye movement (REM) sleep
3. Decreased deep sleep (stages 3 and 4)

Gastrointestinal
1. Anorexia
2. Nausea and vomiting

Psychological
1. Agitation, anxiety
2. Restlessness
3. Irritability
4. Distractability, poor concentration
5. Impaired memory
6. Impaired judgment
7. Hallucinosis (may be calmly tolerated; often visual, but may affect all sensory modalities)

Generalized tonic-clonic seizures

Table from R D Weiss, S M Mirin: Intoxication and withdrawal syndromes. In *Manual of Psychiatric Emergencies*, ed 2, S E Hyman, editor, p 249. Little, Brown, Boston, 1988. Used with permission.

DRUG TREATMENT

Benzodiazepines (chlordiazepoxide 25 to 100 mg by mouth four times a day is the usual dosage) relieves the withdrawal and can be tapered over several days. Lorazepam 1 to 2 mg is an alternative. Lorazepam may theoretically be preferable in patients with hepatic impairment, since the elimination half-life of lorazepam is more predictable than the elimination half-life of chlordiazepoxide in patients with liver disease.

Administer thiamine 100 mg IM and then 100 mg by mouth three times a day. Thiamine is mandatory, since malabsorption is common in alcohol-dependent patients, and the consequences of thiamine deficiency are serious. Multivitamins, one capsule twice a day, are also mandatory, since the patient may be deficient in vitamin B_{12} and folate.

Monitor the patient's vital signs, and adjust the benzodiazepine dosage accordingly. If signs of withdrawal are present, increase the benzodiazepine dosage. If the patient is sedated and no withdrawal signs are present, taper the benzodiazepine dosage.

If the patient is being treated in a private office, instruct the patient to go to the emergency room if the withdrawal symptoms do not abate or if a seizure occurs. Ensure adequate sleep and seizure prevention with benzodiazepines.

See Table 8.5-4 for the treatment of mild to moderate alcohol withdrawal.

Alcohol Withdrawal Delirium (Delirium Tremens)

Alcohol withdrawal delirium, also called delirium tremens (DTs), is a severe complication of alcohol withdrawal that occurs in about 5 percent of patients

TABLE 8.5-4
TREATMENT OF ALCOHOL WITHDRAWAL

Stage I: Mild to moderate withdrawal
1. Regular diet as tolerated.
2. Encourage physical activity.
3. Assess hydration (i.e., skin turgor, change in normal body weight, urine specific gravity); force fluids as necessary (120 mL orange juice or milk every 30 min × 8 then 120 mL orange juice or milk every hr × 6).
4. Vital signs every 4 hr × 48 hr, then during each shift.
5. PPD intermediate strength.
6. CBC, urinalysis, prothrombin time, fasting glucose, BUN, electrolytes, alk phos., bilirubin, SGOT, CPK, LDH, uric acid, total protein, albumin, globulin, stool for occult blood, VDRL, serum calcium, magnesium, amylase.
7. Chest X-ray, ECG as soon as possible.
8. Urine toxicology screen for other drugs of abuse.
9. Chlordiazepoxide 25–100 mg by mouth on admission, repeat in 1 hr.[1]
10. Chlordiazepoxide 25–100 mg by mouth every 6 hours × 24 hr.[1]
    Day 2: Cut day 1 dose in half.
    Day 3: Cut day 2 dose in half.
    Day 4: Discontinue.
11. Thiamine HCl 100 mg IM stat and 100 mg by mouth three times a day and every night × 10 days.
12. Folic acid 1 to 5 mg IM or by mouth every day.
13. Berocca C of Solu B Forte, 2 cc IM or IV on admission, then daily × 2 days (IM administered in gluteal muscle only).
14. After third dose of Berocca, stress caps twice a day.
15. Vitamin K 5 to 10 mg IV (only if protime 3 sec control).

[1]Diazepam may be substituted for chlordiazepoxide; 1 mg diazepam—2.5 mg chlordiazepoxide. Table adapted from W R Cose, F D Lisnow: Alcohol use and abuse. In *Emergency Psychiatry,* E L Bassuk, A W Birk, editors, p 135. Plenum, New York, 1984. Used with permission.

withdrawing from alcohol. It usually occurs in medically compromised patients with a long history of heavy alcohol dependence who stop drinking or who markedly decrease their intake of alcohol. The condition is potentially life-threatening; the untreated mortality rate is 20 percent. Even with optimal therapy, delirium tremens has a mortality rate of 5 to 10 percent. Death generally occurs as the result of hyperthermia, volume depletion, electrolyte imbalance, infection, or, ultimately, cardiovascular collapse.

CLINICAL FEATURES AND DIAGNOSIS

In 90 percent of patients, the onset of the condition is within one week of a marked decrease in alcohol consumption, most often after 24 to 72 hours of abstinence.

The condition often develops on the third hospital day in a patient who has been admitted for other medical reasons and who is not known to be dependent.

The signs and symptoms include delirium with a severely impaired sensorium, marked autonomic hyperactivity (for example, tachycardia, hypertension, increased respiration, fever, sweating), tremor, seizures (rum fits), vivid hallucinations that are often visual or tactile, and changing levels of psychomotor activity ranging from agitation to lethargy. Nightmares and insomnia are common.

INTERVIEWING AND PSYCHOTHERAPEUTIC GUIDELINES

Use a supportive approach for those patients who are confused, bewildered, and severely anxious. Reassurance and explanations are helpful.

EVALUATION AND MANAGEMENT

1. Vigorous, intensive inpatient treatment is required. The immediate goals of treatment are to prevent exhaustion, reduce central nervous system hyperirritability, and correct life-threatening electrolyte and fluid imbalances.
2. Avoid physical restraints; they may cause injury if the patient fights against them.
3. Evaluate the patient's hydration and electrolytes. Dehydration is common and may warrant intravenous fluids. Electrolyte deficiencies, including those of calcium and magnesium, must be corrected.
4. Carefully evaluate the patient for concomitant medical problems, especially head trauma, rib fractures, infections, gastrointestinal bleeding, and hepatic disease.
5. Observe the patient closely for the development of possible focal neurological signs, which, if present, require a further neurological workup.
6. Institute a high-calorie, high-carbohydrate diet.
7. Always be alert for infections (for example, aspiration pneumonia) and treat them aggressively.

DRUG TREATMENT

Benzodiazepines (chlordiazepoxide 50 mg or lorazepam 2 mg is the usual choice) may be given IM if they cannot be given orally. Repeat as necessary on the basis of elevated vital signs until the withdrawal signs are no longer present. Use the total dosage given in the first day as the standing dosage for the next day. Avoid antipsychotics, as they lower the seizure threshold and lead to dystonias.

Give thiamine 100 mg IM and then 100 mg orally three times a day.

Multivitamins given twice a day are mandatory, since vitamin B_{12} and folate are often deficient.

Monitor the patient's vital signs, and adjust the benzodiazepine dosage accordingly. If signs of withdrawal are present, increase the benzodiazepine dosage. If the patient is sedated and no withdrawal signs are present, taper the benzodiazepine dosage. Ensure adequate sleep with benzodiazepines.

Maintenance with anticonvulsants is usually not indicated for seizures that develop only in the context of alcohol withdrawal.

For a more detailed discussion of this topic, see M A Schuckit: Alcohol-Related Disorders, Sec 13.2, p 775, in CTP/VI.

8.6. Alcohol Overdose (Poisoning)

Alcohol overdose is the ingestion of a quantity of alcohol sufficient to cause severe toxicity, coma, or death.

CLINICAL FEATURES AND DIAGNOSIS

Alcohol overdose typically occurs under two conditions, either as part of a suicide attempt or as an accident (for example, after a challenge at a fraternity party). In accidental overdoses the patient rapidly consumes a large volume of liquor. In suicide attempts, alcohol is usually consumed with other drugs, such as diazepam (Valium). A blood concentration of 0.1 to 0.15 percent alcohol indicates intoxication, a concentration of 0.3 to 0.4 percent alcohol usually induces coma, and higher concentrations cause death. Alcohol is a central nervous system depressant, and death is due to respiratory depression or the aspiration of vomitus.

INTERVIEWING AND PSYCHOTHERAPEUTIC GUIDELINES

Prompt medical attention is essential. If the patient is comatose or too ill to interview, obtain a history from collateral sources.

EVALUATION AND MANAGEMENT

1. A toxicological emergency may require gastric lavage, intubation, and admission to a medical intensive care unit.
2. In patients who overdose as part of a suicide attempt, always consider the possibility of polyoverdose, and obtain a urine toxicology screen.
3. The patient's blood alcohol concentration is helpful information in an overdose situation. (see Table 8.5-1).

DRUG TREATMENT

After drawing blood samples, administer thiamine 100 mg as prophylaxis against Wernicke's encephalopathy.

Administer 50 mL of 50 percent dextrose intravenously (IV) to prevent hypoglycemia.

Administer naloxone (Narcan) because of the possibility of concomitant opioid use.

For a more detailed discussion of this topic, see M A Schuckit: Alcohol-Related Disorders, Sec 13.2, p 775, in CTP/VI.

8.7. Alcohol Seizures

Alcohol seizures (rum fits) occur in the context of alcohol withdrawal. They are associated with alcohol withdrawal delirium (delirium tremens). Left untreated, alcohol withdrawal seizures and delirium result in significant mortality.

CLINICAL FEATURES AND DIAGNOSIS

Seizures almost always occur 24 to 72 hours after the last drink or decrease in drinking and usually precede delirium. Patients who are medically compromised are especially prone to seizures. The seizures are typically generalized tonic-clonic (grand mal) and are self-limited, with an average of one to four. Many patients experience multiple seizures.

INTERVIEWING AND PSYCHOTHERAPEUTIC GUIDELINES

After immediate medical intervention, a collateral history should be obtained. Be alert to postictal confusion and agitation. Reassure the patient and explain that future seizures can be controlled.

EVALUATION AND MANAGEMENT

1. Carefully evaluate for other medical conditions, especially head trauma.
2. Consider withdrawal from other drugs (for example, sedative-hypnotics and anticonvulsants).
3. Evaluate for other possible causes of seizures or delirium. Usually, seizures do not indicate an underlying seizure disorder, and the electroencephalogram (EEG) after withdrawal shows no abnormalities.
4. If the seizures continue for an extended period, if status epilepticus is present, or if the seizures are focal, (rather than generalized), a cause other than alcohol withdrawal must be considered.

TABLE 8.7–1
TREATMENT OF ALCOHOL SEIZURES

1. Diazepam 10 mg IV (stat) given slowly.[1]
2. Diazepam 5 mg IV every 5 min until calm but awake; then
3. Diazepam 5 mg IV or by mouth every 4 hours until delirium clears, then decrease dose by 50% every day until the patient is withdrawn completely.
4. Optional prophylaxis. Phenytoin loading dose 1 gm IV undiluted given slowly over 4 hours (rate no higher than 50 mg/min). ECG monitoring is helpful during IV administration.
5. IV loading followed by phenytoin 100 mg by mouth three times a day through withdrawal period. Maintain blood level between 10 and 20 mg/mL

[1] Chlordiazepoxide 2.5 mg may be substituted for each 1 mg of diazepam.
Table from W R Cote, F D Lisnow: Alcohol use and abuse. In *Emergency Psychiatry*. E L Bassuk, A W Birk, editors, p 135. Plenum, New York, 1984. Used with permission.

DRUG TREATMENT

The treatment is the same as for alcohol withdrawal delirium, but also consider magnesium supplementation and anticonvulsants, in addition to benzodiazepines.

Treat the seizures aggressively with benzodiazepines—for example, chlordiazepoxide (Librium) or diazepam (Valium) (Table 8.7-1).

The prophylactic use of anticonvulsant medications for alcohol withdrawal seizures is controversial. In patients with pure alcohol withdrawal seizures, the use of long-term anticonvulsant medication is not usually recommended.

For a more detailed discussion of this topic, see M A Schuckit: Alcohol-Related Disorders, Sec 13.2, p 775, in CTP/VI.

8.8. Amphetamine (or Amphetaminelike) Intoxication and Withdrawal

Amphetamine or Similarly Acting Sympathomimetic Intoxication

Amphetamine intoxication, a syndrome produced by amphetamine ingestion, is characterized by behavioral effects—including hypervigilance, grandiosity, euphoria, and agitation—combined with physical effects that include hypertension, tachycardia, and dilated pupils.

CLINICAL FEATURES AND DIAGNOSIS

Amphetamines are the prototypical stimulants of a pharmacologically similar class of drugs that includes cocaine; however, cocaine, specifically crack cocaine (a purified form that is smoked), is abused more often. Other drugs in the class include methamphetamine (Desoxyn), dextroamphetamine (Dexedrine), phenmetrazine (Preludin), and methylphenidate (Ritalin). All those drugs have similar pharmacological properties.

The amphetamines can be orally ingested, injected, snorted, or smoked. Cocaine is usually snorted or smoked, but it can also be injected or absorbed through the mucous membranes. Episodes of intoxication may last days or weeks, followed by a withdrawal syndrome when the drug supply is exhausted.

Many amphetamine abusers are first introduced to the drug as a treatment for obesity or depression. Other abusers are those most likely to use the drug to prevent fatigue, such as doctors, students, and truck drivers. Some abusers use the drug solely to get high; those abusers are usually young, tend to abuse other drugs, and often use stimulants intravenously. Significant toxic reactions occur most often in infrequent users who ingest large doses over a short period.

Amphetamines and other sympathomimetic drugs produce both behavioral and physical symptoms. The behavioral and emotional symptoms range from mood elevation and an increased sense of confidence and mental alertness to grandiosity, hypervigilance, fighting, psychomotor agitation, anxiety, and impaired judgment. Social or occupational functioning may be markedly impaired. The physical symptoms include tachycardia, tremulousness, headaches, dizziness, pupillary dilation, hypertension, perspiration, chills, nausea, and vomiting. Chronically intoxicated users exhibit repetitive, stereotyped movements, such as picking at clothes or sheets and taking things apart and putting them back together. With severe intoxication, delirium, a delusional disorder (typically paranoid), and auditory, visual, and tactile hallucinations can be produced. With overdose, seizures and death may occur. Sudden death related to cardiac complications has been reported. Abuse of the drugs frequently leads to dependence. Unprovoked violence may occur, especially when amphetamines are combined with barbiturates.

INTERVIEWING AND PSYCHOTHERAPEUTIC GUIDELINES

Reassure the patient that the symptoms are self-limiting. Approach paranoid patients with caution; explain every action taken, and keep some physical distance from the potentially violent patient.

EVALUATION AND MANAGEMENT

1. The immediate goals are to reduce the central nervous system (CNS) irritability and autonomic hyperactivity, control psychotic symptoms if present, and effect rapid drug excretion.
2. The intoxication is usually self-limited, and treatment is generally supportive. However, agitation, elevated vital signs (especially an elevated temperature), status epilepticus, and potential violence warrant medication.
3. Prevent excessive stimulation by secluding the patient in a quiet, calm environment.
4. Increase the excretion of amphetamine by urinary acidification—for example, ammonium chloride 500 mg by mouth every three to four hours if no signs of liver or kidney failure are seen.
5. Obtain a history of the type and the amount of drug taken.
6. Obtain and monitor the patient's vital signs.
7. Refer the patient for psychotherapy and a drug treatment program if indicated.

DRUG TREATMENT

To treat the patient's behavioral problems, start with a benzodiazepine—for example, oxazepam (Serax) 10 to 30 mg by mouth, estazolam (ProSom) 0.5 to 1 mg by mouth, or lorazepam (Ativan) 1 to 2 mg by mouth or intramuscularly (IM)—and repeat as needed.

Psychotic symptoms are well controlled with antipsychotics. Antipsychotics should be monitored closely, since they lower the seizure threshold and cause hypotension. Also, anticholinergic contaminants in the amphetamines may potentiate the anticholinergic effects of antipsychotics.

β-blockers—for example, propranolol (Inderal) and clonidine (Catapres)—are effective in treating elevated vital signs but are not at all effective in treating the patient's behavioral symptoms.

Amphetamine or Similarly Acting Sympathomimetic Withdrawal

Amphetamine withdrawal is characterized by severe fatigue, insomnia or hypersomnia, agitation, anxiety, drug craving, and depression after the discontinuation of heavy amphetamine abuse.

CLINICAL FEATURES AND DIAGNOSIS

Withdrawal generally begins within three days after heavy users cease or decrease drug use. The signs and symptoms peak in two to four days and include dysphoria, depression, anxiety, irritability, disturbed sleep, fatigue, and apathy. Patients may present with suicidality, which can persist with severe depressive symptoms for months.

INTERVIEWING AND PSYCHOTHERAPEUTIC GUIDELINES

Provide reassurance by explaining the cause of the symptoms and their self-limited nature. Educate and reassure the patient that dysphoria and fatigue are expected withdrawal symptoms that dissipate with time.

EVALUATION AND MANAGEMENT

1. Obtain a history of the quantity, frequency, and duration of drug use, including polysubstance abuse.
2. Evaluate the patient for suicidality carefully and thoroughly, take appropriate steps, including hospitalization if needed, to protect the patient.
3. Evaluate the patient for coexisting depression that may warrant treatment.
4. Refer the patient for psychotherapy and a drug treatment program if needed.

DRUG TREATMENT

Drug treatment may not be necessary when the symptoms are self-limited, mild, or amenable to psychosocial intervention. If anxiety is prominent, consider the short-term use of a benzodiazepine—for example, lorazepam 1 to 2 mg by mouth three times a day. Persistent or severe depressive symptoms may require antidepressant medication. Withdrawal accompanied by psychotic symptoms should be treated with low dosages of a high-potency antipsychotic, such as thiothixene (Navane), trifluoperazine (Stelazine), fluphenazine (Prolixin), or haloperidol (Haldol), all given at 2 to 5 mg by mouth twice a day.

For a more detailed discussion of this topic, see J H Jaffe: Amphetamine (or Amphetaminelike)-Related Disorders, Sec 13.3, p 791, in CTP/VI.

8.9. Anticholinergic Intoxication

Anticholinergic intoxication is a syndrome of specific signs and symptoms, including mydriasis, constipation, elevated temperature, tachycardia, urinary retention, flushing, dry skin, and delirium caused by parasympathetic blockade. Anticholinergic (antimuscarinic) intoxication can be caused by many psychotropic drugs. Most often, the syndrome is produced by anticholinergic drugs that are coadministered with antipsychotic drugs to prevent extrapyramidal side effects, particularly antipsychotic-induced parkinsonism and antipsychotic-induced dystonia. All antipsychotics have some anticholinergic effects, but the effects are most prominent with low-potency antipsychotics, such as chlorpromazine (Thorazine) and thioridazine (Mellaril). Clozapine (Clozaril) also has prominent anticholinergic effects. Some chronically mentally ill patients abuse anticholinergic drugs for their hallucinatory effects.

Other psychotropic drugs can also produce anticholinergic effects. The most commonly implicated are tricyclic antidepressants, such as amitriptyline (Elavil) and imipramine (Tofranil). Other heterocyclic antidepressants, antihistamines, and monoamine oxidase inhibitors can also produce anticholinergic effects. Some over-the-counter hypnotics (for example, Sominex), eye drops, and asthma preparations also have anticholinergic effects, as do some cough preparations. Elderly patients are at a higher risk of anticholinergic delirium than are young adults.

CLINICAL FEATURES AND DIAGNOSIS

The peripheral symptoms include flushing, mydriasis, dry skin, hyperthermia, urinary hesitancy, acute urinary retention, and decreased bowel sounds.

The central symptoms include agitation, hallucinations (often visual), hypotension, tachycardia, fever, seizures, delirium, coma, and eventually death. A medical aphorism describing anticholinergic intoxication is "red as a beet, dry as a bone, mad as a hatter" (Table 8.9-1).

TABLE 8.9–1
ANTICHOLINERGIC SYNDROME MANIFESTATIONS

Systemic manifestations
Tachycardia
Dilated, sluggishly reactive pupils
Blurred vision
Warm dry skin
Dry mucous membranes
Fever
Reduced or absent bowel sounds
Urinary retention

Neuropsychiatric manifestations
Agitation
Motor restlessness
Confusion
Disturbance of recent memory
Dysarthria
Myoclonus
Hallucinations (including visual)
Delirium
Seizures

Table from S E Hyman: Toxic side effects of psychotropic medications and their management. In *Manual of Psychiatric Emergencies*. S E Hyman, editor, ed 2, p 158. Little, Brown, Boston, 1988. Used with permission.

INTERVIEWING AND PSYCHOTHERAPEUTIC GUIDELINES

In mild cases, reassure patients by explaining the cause and the treatability of their symptoms. Delirious patients may alternate between lethargy and agitation. The interview has to accommodate those fluctuations in activity—for example, be minimally stimulating with agitated patients. Questions should be brief, simple, and repeated as needed. Reorient confused patients, and provide explanations of the procedures. Identify all personnel as often as needed. The presence of a family member or a friend may help calm the patient.

EVALUATION AND MANAGEMENT

1. Immediately discontinue all drugs with possible anticholinergic effects.
2. Consider toxicity from other drugs (for example, alcohol and sedative-hypnotics), in addition to the anticholinergic drugs.

DRUG TREATMENT

In severely agitated patients, give oxazepam (Serax) 10 to 30 mg by mouth or lorazepam (Ativan) 1 to 2 mg by mouth or intramuscularly (IM) or by slow intravenous (IV) injection. Repeat every hour as needed. Antipsychotics should be avoided because of their anticholinergic effects.

Physostigmine (Antilirium) inhibits acetylcholinesterase (the enzyme that breaks down acetylcholine) and reverses the syndrome. Give physostigmine 1 to 2 mg IV over a one-to-two-minute period, and repeat in 20 minutes if no response is seen. Physostigmine can also be given IM every 30 to 60 minutes, but IM absorption is unpredictable. Only give physostigmine in settings in which cardiac monitoring and life-support systems are available, since its use may precipitate severe hypotension and bronchial constriction. Physostigmine is usually used either to confirm a diagnosis of anticholinergic intoxication or to reverse the dangerous symptoms of the syndrome (for example, seizures, delirium, hypotension, hallucinations). It is contraindicated in patients with cardiac abnormalities or asthma.

Physostigmine toxicity can be reversed with atropine 0.5 mg IV for every mg of physostigmine given.

For a more detailed discussion of this topic, see T J Crowley: Hallucinogen-Related Disorders, Sec 13.7, p 831; G W Arana, A B Santos: Anticholinergics and Amantadine, Sec. 32.4, p 1919, in CTP/VI.

8.10. Anticonvulsant Intoxication

Anticonvulsant intoxication is a syndrome of signs and symptoms caused by anticonvulsant ingestion. Anticonvulsants are typically prescribed as maintenance drugs for the prophylaxis of epilepsy. Toxicity can develop as a complication. All anticonvulsants are monitored by testing blood concentrations. Phenytoin (Dilantin) does not have linear pharmacokinetics at all blood concentration ranges, so a small increase in dosage may produce a marked increase in blood concentration.

CLINICAL FEATURES AND DIAGNOSIS

Check the patient's anticonvulsant blood concentration and folic acid concentration because many anticonvulsants produce folic acid deficiency. If the patient's folic acid concentration is low, check the vitamin B_{12} concentration, since they tend to fall together.

Look for cognitive deficits. Although controlling the seizures can produce a marked improvement in cognitive functioning, anticonvulsants can produce cognitive impairment. The symptoms include sedation, sluggishness, poor concentration, and memory impairment. They may be present even when the blood concentration is in the therapeutic range. Typical signs of toxicity may not be present when toxicity is manifested by psychotic symptoms.

The short-term toxic effects include nystagmus, ataxia, dysarthria, tremor, hyperreflexia or hyporeflexia, lethargy, nausea, vomiting, slurred speech, hypotension, and coma.

INTERVIEWING AND PSYCHOTHERAPEUTIC GUIDELINES

Obtain a history of the nature of the seizure disorder, including the time of the last seizure (the patient may have postictal confusion and not intoxication). Interview collateral informants. If the patient is confused, be reassuring and direct while asking simple questions in a structured interview. Repeat any instructions or explanations, and reorient the patient throughout the evaluation.

EVALUATION AND MANAGEMENT

1. The usual treatment for anticonvulsant toxicity is a reduction in the dosage and the remeasurement of the patient's blood concentrations when a normal state has been reached, usually in four to seven days.
2. Adjust the dosage, supplement the folic acid and vitamin B_{12} if needed, and arrange for a repeat blood concentration test in one week.
3. Always assess intoxicated patients for intentional overdoses. Take appropriate steps when dealing with suicidal patients. Since some anticonvulsants are not completely protein-bound, hemodialysis may be an alternative, in addition to the usual gastric lavage and charcoal administration.

DRUG TREATMENT

No specific antidotes are available, but reports indicate that valproic acid (Depakene) intoxication can be reversed with naloxone (Narcan). Use naloxone with caution, since it may induce seizures by reversing the anticonvulsant effects of valproic acid.

For a more detailed discussion of this topic, see R M Post: Carbamazepine, Sec 32.11, p 1964; H G Pope Jr, S L McElroy: Valproate, Sec 32.25, p 2112, in CTP/VI.

8.11. Barbiturate and Similarly Acting Sedative, Hypnotic, or Anxiolytic Intoxication and Withdrawal

Barbiturate And Similarly Acting Sedative, Hypnotic, or Anxiolytic Intoxication

Intoxication by barbiturates and similarly acting drugs is a substance use disorder that follows the ingestion of the offending substance.

CLINICAL FEATURES AND DIAGNOSIS

The signs of intoxication include sedation, poor concentration, slurred speech, incoordination, nystagmus, ataxia, disinhibition, and poor judgment (Table 8.11-1). The drugs can also cause an organic amnestic disorder (blackout). All barbiturates, benzodiazepines, other sedative-hypnotics, and alcohol produce intoxication and have cross-tolerance with each other.

Mild intoxication is relatively safe, but an overdose can be dangerous, especially with barbiturates, which have a low therapeutic index (ratio of lethal dose to effective dose) and are often taken in combination with other drugs, typically alcohol. The combination of barbiturates and alcohol produces additive effects that can cause death through respiratory and central nervous system (CNS) depression with subsequent cardiovascular collapse.

TABLE 8.11–1
DIAGNOSTIC CRITERIA FOR SEDATIVE, HYPNOTIC, OR ANXIOLYTIC INTOXICATION

A. Recent use of a sedative, hypnotic, or anxiolytic.
B. Clinically significant maladaptive behavioral or psychological changes (e.g., inappropriate sexual or aggressive behavior, mood lability, impaired judgment, impaired social or occupational functioning) that developed during, or shortly after, sedative, hypnotic, or anxiolytic use.
C. One (or more) of the following signs, developing during, or shortly after, sedative, hypnotic, or anxiolytic use:
    (1) slurred speech
    (2) incoordination
    (3) unsteady gait
    (4) nystagmus
    (5) impairment in attention or memory
    (6) stupor or coma
D. The symptoms are not due to a general medical condition and are not better accounted for by another mental disorder.

Table from DSM-IV, *Diagnostic and Statistical Manual of Mental Disorders*, ed 4. Copyright American Psychiatric Association, Washington, 1994. Used with permission.

Benzodiazepines are much safer than barbiturates, since benzodiazepines have a much higher therapeutic index. Sedative-hypnotics, especially benzodiazepines, are the most frequently prescribed class of psychotropic drug; therefore, they are readily available to patients attempting suicide. In addition, they are a common source of accidental overdose in children.

INTERVIEWING AND PSYCHOTHERAPEUTIC GUIDELINES

Keep the intoxicated patient under constant supervision to prevent harm to self or others. Reorient the patient as often as necessary. Try to obtain from the patient or collateral informants an accurate history of the quantity and the type of drug ingested. When the patient is no longer intoxicated, reinterview to evaluate for additional psychopathology and suicidality. Reassure and support the patient.

EVALUATION AND MANAGEMENT

1. Evaluate the patient for medical complications, such as pneumonia, cardiac arrhythmias, heart failure, and respiratory depression.
2. Mild intoxication can generally be treated supportively and usually leads to sleep. Evaluate the patient for possible intoxication with multiple drugs. The patient may become progressively more intoxicated if multiple or long-acting drugs were taken. Keep the patient from engaging in any acts that are potentially dangerous, such as driving.
3. Barbiturate overdose is a medical emergency requiring immediate attention. Identify the type and the amount of drug taken; always suspect polyoverdose. Obtain a urine toxicology screen as part of a full battery of laboratory tests. Try to keep the patient awake. Use gastric lavage and charcoal. If the patient shows signs of coma, admit the patient to a medical intensive care unit (ICU), and be prepared to intubate. Intravenous (IV) fluids, cardiac monitoring, and other supportive treatments are indicated. Obtain the patient's blood concentration of barbiturate. In any overdose case, always evaluate the patient for suicidality.

4. If taken alone (without alcohol or other CNS depressants), benzodiazepines in overdose are much safer than are barbiturates. The lethal dose of benzodiazepines in a nondependent patient may be more than 200 times the effective dose, but the therapeutic index is less if the patient is dependent. Overdose attempts with benzodiazepines usually produce a prolonged sleep. However, benzodiazepines are often taken in combination with alcohol or other CNS depressants, and the combination may be fatal, especially in patients who are medically compromised. Blood concentrations of benzodiazepines may help determine the level of risk. Patients who have taken an overdose of benzodiazepines should be observed at least one day in an ICU, since polyoverdose is always a possibility.

DRUG TREATMENT

No medication is indicated.

Barbiturate And Similarly Acting Sedative, Hypnotic, or Anxiolytic Withdrawal

Sedative, hypnotic, or anxiolytic withdrawal is a substance-specific syndrome that follows the reduction or the termination of a regularly used psychoactive agent. Withdrawal from barbiturates, benzodiazepines, and other sedative-hypnotics is, like alcohol withdrawal, a potentially life-threatening emergency. Fortunately, withdrawal is easily treated with a slow taper of the drug on which the patient is dependent.

CLINICAL FEATURES AND DIAGNOSIS

Withdrawal is a state of CNS hyperactivity characterized by the following signs and symptoms: anxiety, insomnia, sensitivity to sound and light, tachycardia, mild hypertension, tremor, headache, sweating, abdominal distress, nausea, vomiting, hallucinations, and craving for the drug (Table 8.11-2). Untreated, the syndrome may progress to seizures, delirium, coma, and death.

TABLE 8.11–2
Diagnostic Criteria for Sedative, Hypnotic, or Anxiolytic Withdrawal

A. Cessation of (or reduction in) sedative, hypnotic, or anxiolytic use that has been heavy and prolonged.
B. Two (or more) of the following, developing within several hours to a few days after criterion A:
 (1) autonomic hyperactivity (e.g., sweating or pulse rate greater than 100)
 (2) increased hand tremor
 (3) insomnia
 (4) nausea or vomiting
 (5) transient visual, tactile, or auditory hallucinations or illusions
 (6) psychomotor agitation
 (7) anxiety
 (8) grand mal seizures
C. The symptoms in criterion B cause clinically significant distress or impairment in social, occupational, or other important areas of functioning.
D. The symptoms are not due to a general medical condition and are not better accounted for by another mental disorder.
Specify if:
 With perceptual disturbances

Table from DSM-IV, *Diagnostic and Statistical Manual of Mental Disorders*, ed 4. Copyright American Psychiatric Association, Washington, 1994. Used with permission.

The degree of withdrawal depends on the dose, the duration of use, and the drug's pharmacokinetics. Drugs with long elimination half-lives tend to produce less severe withdrawal syndromes than do drugs with short elimination half-lives. The half-life also determines whether the onset of withdrawal occurs hours to days after sedative-hypnotic consumption has ceased. Since all sedative-hypnotics have cross-tolerance, a medically supervised detoxification can be performed with any drug of that type.

INTERVIEWING AND PSYCHOTHERAPEUTIC GUIDELINES

Withdrawal patients are likely to be agitated and uncomfortable. Empathize with their discomfort, and explain that cooperating with the interview is the quickest way for them to receive relief. Emphasize that accurate information regarding the type of drug used, the frequency of use, the quantity of use, and the time of the last ingestion is crucial in determining a safe, appropriate detoxification regimen. Remind the patient that underestimation of the dose can lead to inadequate detoxification doses; overestimation can lead to an overdose during detoxification. Show the patient that the primary concern is to provide effective treatment.

EVALUATION AND MANAGEMENT

1. Monitor the patient's vital signs frequently, even while the patient is asleep.
2. Determine the patient's level of dependence with a pentobarbital challenge test (Table 8.11-3). If the patient is dependent on multiple sedative-hypnotics or alcohol, the method outlined here will treat withdrawal from all the drugs, since they show cross-tolerance.
3. After obtaining the patient's history and the results of a urine toxicology screen, identify the possible abuse of other drugs, including opioids, cocaine, and other stimulants.
4. After gradually detoxifying the patient from sedative-hypnotics and after evaluating the patient for any comorbid psychiatric disorders, refer the patient for outpatient drug dependence treatment and rehabilitation.

DRUG TREATMENT

No drugs are indicated, other than barbiturates at gradually reduced dosages as part of the protocol determined by the pentobarbital challenge test.

TABLE 8.11–3.
PENTOBARBITAL CHALLENGE TEST

1. Give pentobarbital 200 mg orally.
2. Observe for intoxication after one hour, e.g., sleepiness, slurred speech, or nystagmus.
3. If the patient is not intoxicated, give another 100 mg of pentobarbital every two hours (maximum 500 mg over six hours).
4. Total dose given to produce mild intoxication is equivalent to daily abuse level of barbiturates.
5. Substitute phenobarbital 30 mg (longer half-life) for each 100 mg of pentobarbital.
6. Decrease by about 10 percent a day.
7. Adjust rate if signs of intoxication or withdrawal are present.

For a more detailed discussion of this topic, see D A Ciraulo, D J Greenblatt: Sedative-, Hypnotic-, or Anxiolytic-Related Disorders, Sec 13.11, p 872; T W Uhde, M E Tancer: Barbiturates, Sec 32.6, p 1926, in CTP/VI.

8.12. Bromide Intoxication

Bromide intoxication is a syndrome that follows the ingestion of bromides. Bromides are drugs with a long onset of action that were once used as anticonvulsants but are now largely obsolete. They are found in some over-the-counter preparations, such as Bromo-Seltzer. Their elimination half-life is more than one week, allowing the drugs to accumulate in the body. Bromide intoxication is thought to be uncommon. However, since most clinicians do not routinely consider the disorder in the differential diagnosis, it is likely to be missed. The patient's history is always one of long-term abuse of the drugs; bromides accumulate slowly and cannot be taken in large doses because of gastric irritation.

CLINICAL FEATURES AND DIAGNOSIS

The patient's symptoms may be similar to those of a wide range of functional and organic disorders, including schizophrenia, mania, delirium, and depression. Bromide intoxication can present with almost any clinical picture and was once called the great masquerader. The differential diagnosis should include syphilis, alcoholism, encephalitis, multiple sclerosis, uremia, brain tumor, schizophrenia, mania, and depression. The symptoms may include labile affect, cognitive deficits, irritability, confusion, delusions, and hallucinations. The abuse of other sedative-hypnotics, such as benzodiazepines and barbiturates, may further complicate the evaluation. The symptoms may persist for two to three weeks, since the half-life of bromide is about 12 days.

Associated symptoms include an acneform rash, primarily on the face and the scalp, nodular lesions on the legs, incoordination, tremor, ataxia, hyperreflexia, weakness, Babinski's sign, loss of gag and corneal reflexes (also present in barbiturate intoxication), absence of nystagmus (also present in barbiturate intoxication), and presence of delirium during intoxication (also occurs during withdrawal from barbiturates). Additional signs include slurred speech, halitosis, cyanosis, papilledema, mydriasis, and furred tongue.

INTERVIEWING AND PSYCHOTHERAPEUTIC GUIDELINES

Reassure the patient that the condition is reversible and that the symptoms can be controlled.

EVALUATION AND MANAGEMENT

1. Obtain the history of the long-term abuse of over-the-counter sedatives, and, if possible, obtain a sample of the drug.

2. Obtain the history of the abuse of other drugs, especially sedative-hypnotics. Determine whether withdrawal from sedative-hypnotics is likely.
3. If the serum bromide concentration is <50 mg/dL, the patient is bromide-intoxicated; however, the clinical symptoms are not directly related to blood concentrations.
4. Correct the patient's nutritional deficiencies.

DRUG TREATMENT

Stop all bromide-containing medications, and give large doses of saline (6 to 12 g a day) either orally or intravenously (IV). Hemodialysis may be needed in severe cases.

Avoid tranquilizers if possible, although concomitant sedative-hypnotic withdrawal may require treatment. Severe agitation may be treated with a high-potency antipsychotic—for example, thiothixene (Navane), trifluoperazine (Stelazine), fluphenazine (Prolixin), or haloperidol (Haldol)—all given at 2 to 5 mg orally or intramuscularly (IM).

For a more detailed discussion of this topic, see E D Caine, H Grossman, J M Lyness: Delirium, Dementia, and Amnestic and Other Cognitive Disorders and Mental Disorders Due to a General Medical Condition, Chap 12, p 705; T C Manschreck: Delusional Disorder and Shared Psychotic Disorder, Sec 15.2, p 1031, in CTP/VI.

8.13. Caffeine Intoxication

Caffeine is an alkaloid that acts as a psychomotor stimulant. It is present in many foods, beverages, and both over-the-counter drugs and prescribed drugs. *Caffeine intoxication* (also known as caffeinism) results from the excessive ingestion of caffeine.

CLINICAL FEATURES AND DIAGNOSIS

Caffeine is the most commonly used psychoactive drug. An estimated 20 to 30 percent of all adult Americans consume more than 500 mg of caffeine a day. Tolerance and dependence occur. The most common sources of caffeine are coffee, tea, and soft drinks (Table 8.13-1).

The daily consumption of at least 250 mg of caffeine is needed to produce intoxication. Caffeine intoxication can exacerbate or cause the symptoms of a variety of psychiatric disorders, including anxiety disorders (especially panic disorder), depression, mania, and schizophrenia. The symptoms of caffeine intoxication include restlessness, nervousness, excitement, insomnia, flushed facies, diuresis, gastrointestinal disturbances, muscle twitching, rambling thoughts and speech, tachycardia or cardiac arrhythmia, periods of inexhaustibility, and psychomotor agitation (Table 8.13-2). The effects of caffeine intoxication last only several hours and can usually be managed supportively. Assess caffeine intake in patients with anxiety or insomnia.

TABLE 8.13-1
Common Sources of Caffeine and Representative Decaffeinated Products

Source	Caffeine per Unit
Beverages and foods (5–6 oz)	
Fresh drip coffee, brewed coffee	90–140 mg
Instant coffee	66–100 mg
Tea (leaf or bagged)	30–100 mg
Cocoa	5–50 mg
Decaffeinated coffee	2–4 mg
Chocolate bar or ounce of baking chocolate	25–35 mg
Soft drinks (8–12 oz)	
Pepsi, Coke, Tab, Royal Crown, Dr. Pepper, Mountain Dew	25–50 mg
Canada Dry Ginger Ale, Caffeine Free Coke, Caffeine Free Pepsi, 7-Up, Sprite, Squirt, Caffeine Free Tab	0 mg
Prescription medications (1 tablet or capsule)	
Cafergot, Migralam	100 mg
Anoquan, Aspir-code, BAC, Darvon, Florinal	32–50 mg
Over-the-counter analgesics and cold preparations (1 tablet or capsule)	
Excedrin	60 mg
Aspirin compound, Anacin, B-C powder, Capron, Cope, Dolor, Midol, Nilain, Norgesic, PAC, Trigesic, Vanquish	~30 mg
Advil, aspirin, Empirin, Midol 200, Nuprin, Pamprin	0 mg
Over-the-counter stimulants and appetite suppressants (1 tablet or capsule)	
Caffin-TD, Caffedrine	250 mg
Vivarin, Ver	200 mg
Quick-Pep	140–150 mg
Amostat, Anorexin, Appedrine, Nodoz, Wakoz	100 mg

Table adapted from table by Jerome H Jeffe, MD.

TABLE 8.13-2.
DIAGNOSTIC CRITERIA FOR CAFFEINE INTOXICATION

A. Recent consumption of caffeine, usually in excess of 250 mg (e.g., more than 2–3 cups of brewed coffee).
B. Five (or more) of the following signs, developing during, or shortly after, caffeine use:
    (1) restlessness
    (2) nervousness
    (3) excitement
    (4) insomnia
    (5) flushed face
    (6) diuresis
    (7) gastrointestinal disturbance
    (8) muscle twitching
    (9) rambling flow of thought and speech
    (10) tachycardia or cardiac arrhythmia
    (11) periods of inexhaustibility
    (12) psychomotor agitation
C. The symptoms in criterion B cause clinically significant distress or impairment in social, occupational, or other important areas of functioning.
D. The symptoms are not due to a general medical condition and are not better accounted for by another mental disorder (e.g., an anxiety disorder).

Table from DSM-IV, *Diagnostic and Statistical Manual of Mental Disorders*, ed 4. Copyright American Psychiatric Association, Washington, 1994. Used with permission.

People show a wide range of variability in susceptibility to caffeine intoxication and dependence. Dependence is usually not a clinically important condition, but withdrawal from caffeine can be an unrecognized cause of such symptoms as headache, fatigue, decreased alertness, and social withdrawal. Headaches may persist for days.

INTERVIEWING AND PSYCHOTHERAPEUTIC GUIDELINES

Focus on the assessment of caffeine intake. Reassure and educate the patient regarding the effects of caffeine on mentation and physical signs and symptoms.

EVALUATION AND MANAGEMENT

1. Perform a complete psychiatric evaluation; focus on the amount of caffeine intake. Ask about sources other than coffee (for example, soft drinks and chocolate).
2. Rule out other psychopathology that may be exacerbated by caffeine (for example, bipolar disorder). Is the patient self-medicating with caffeine to relieve depression with energy?
3. Determine if the patient is taking medications that have significant interactions with caffeine. For example, caffeine lowers lithium (Eskalith) concentrations.
4. Assess the patient for caffeine-related medical problems. Excessive intake can cause cardiac arrhythmias, hypertension, gastrointestinal upset, and, rarely, peptic ulcers.
5. Advise the patient to restrict caffeine intake or to taper and then discontinue caffeine intake.
6. Educate the patient about the effects of caffeine and the symptoms of withdrawal.

DRUG TREATMENT

Generally, no drug treatment is indicated. Severe anxiety, can be treated with benzodiazepines such as oxazepam (Serax) 10 to 30 mg by mouth, diazepam (Valium) 5 to 10 mg by mouth, chlordiazepoxide (Librium) 10 to 25 mg by mouth, alprazolam (Xanax) 0.5 to 1 mg by mouth, or lorazepam (Ativan) 1 to 2 mg by mouth. In cases of severe withdrawal, low-dose benzodiazepines can be given for several days.

For a more detailed discussion of this topic, see J F Greden, O F Pomerleau: Caffeine-Related Disorders and Nicotine-Related Disorders, Sec 13.4, p 799; L A Papp, J M Gorman: Generalized Anxiety Disorder, Sec 17.5, p 1236, in CTP/VI.

8.14. Cannabis (Marijuana) Intoxication

Cannabis intoxication is a substance related disorder that follows the ingestion of cannabis. Cannabis (also known as marijuana, pot, grass, weed, hemp, Mary Jane, hashish, and many other names) is the most commonly abused illicit drug in the United States. It is a drug found in the resin of the plant *Cannabis sativa* that induces psychic or somatic changes when smoked or ingested in sufficient quantity.

CLINICAL FEATURES AND DIAGNOSIS

Although cannabis use has been decreasing, almost one third of all adult Americans have tried marijuana. Cannabis intoxication is caused most commonly by smoking marijuana in cigarettes (joints). Other forms include hashish, hash oil, and Δ-9-tetrahydrocannabinol (THC) (the active ingredient). All of those forms may be smoked or ingested. The onset of action after smoking is immediate. Oral ingestion produces a gradual onset of effects that may last for many hours. Advanced growing techniques developed in the United States have produced a potent marijuana called sinsemilla (without seeds).

The symptoms of cannabis intoxication are given in Table 8.14-1. Additional symptoms include dose-dependent hypothermia and mild sedation. Urine toxicology testing results can remain positive for weeks.

Cannabis use usually occurs in the context of polysubstance abuse—most commonly with cigarettes, alcohol, and cocaine. Acute intoxication usually does not require any treatment, but a mild delusional disorder, usually persecutory, can occur with a brief acute state of panic. Less common symptoms are depersonalization and (rarely) hallucinations. Naive users are prone to cannabis-induced panic. Toxic delirium, usually self-limited, can occur after large doses are ingested or inhaled (Table 8.14-2).

Although some long-term users are psychologically dependent, the diagnosis of cannabis dependence is controversial; dosage escalation (tolerance) and a withdrawal syndrome—consisting of insomnia, irritability, nausea, vomiting, and diaphoresis—can occur. Long-term use may lead to syndromes of amotivation and depression. Flashbacks may occur for several months after the last drug use. Some religions (for example, Rastafarianism) consider smoking cannabis a religious practice.

Cannabis use can exacerbate schizophrenia in previously stable patients. Cannabis increases lithium (Eskalith) concentrations and the half-life of barbiturates. It has added physiological effects with amphetamines. Cannabis-opioid and cannabis-alcohol combinations can produce tachycardia.

TABLE 8.14–1
DIAGNOSTIC CRITERIA FOR CANNABIS INTOXICATION

A. Recent use of cannabis.
B. Clinically significant maladaptive behavioral or psychological changes (e.g., impaired motor coordination, euphoria, anxiety, sensation of slowed time, impaired judgment, social withdrawal) that developed during, or shortly after, cannabis use.
C. Two (or more) of the following signs, developing within 2 hours of cannabis use:
   (1) conjunctival injection
   (2) increased appetite
   (3) dry mouth
   (4) tachycardia
D. The symptoms are not due to a general medical condition and are not better accounted for by another mental disorder.

Specify if:
   With perceptual disturbances

TABLE 8.14–2
ADVERSE REACTIONS TO MARIJUANA

Type	Predisposing factors	Symptoms	Treatment
Acute panic	Inexperienced users, hysterial or obsessional characters, oral administration	Anxiety, depression, no psychotic symptoms	Reassurance; occasionally anxiolytics; episode usually short-lived
Toxic delirium	Large dose, oral use	Confusion, disorientation, hallucinations, depersonalization, delusions	Most remit in 12 to 48 hours; antipsychotics if necessary
Flashbacks	Days or weeks after last dose, prior history of hallucinogenic use	Like hallucinogenic experience except brief	Reassurance; anxiolytics if necessary
Chronic psychosis	Prolonged heavy use of very potent marijuana or hashish; rare in U.S.	Paranoia, delusions, hallucinations, panic, bizarre behavior, occasionally violence	Antipsychotics
Amotivational syndrome	Prolonged heavy use; existence of syndrome is controversial	Apathy, decreased attention span, poor judgment, poor interpersonal relations	No known treatment

Table from S M Mirin, R D Weiss: Drug use and abuse. In *Emergency Psychiatry*, E L Bassuk, A W Birk, editors, p 170. Plenum, New York, 1984. Used with permission.

INTERVIEWING AND PSYCHOTHERAPEUTIC GUIDELINES

Reassure the patient that the syndrome is drug-induced and will stop in several hours. Engage the patient in conversation and, if possible, have a trusted friend or a family member stay with the patient and provide reassurance. Provide a nonstimulating environment.

EVALUATION AND MANAGEMENT

1. Determine the route of administration. Oral ingestion produces effects lasting up to 12 hours or longer.
2. Evaluate the patient for the abuse of alcohol, cocaine, other stimulants, sedative-hypnotics, and other drugs.
3. Obtain a urine toxicology screen.
4. Evaluate the patient for underlying psychotic, mood, and personality disorders.
5. Refer the patient for appropriate outpatient treatment when indicated.

DRUG TREATMENT

Medications are usually not required, but severe anxiety may be relieved with a benzodiazepine—for example, lorazepam (Ativan) 1 to 2 mg by mouth, alprazolam (Xanax) 0.5 to 1 mg by mouth, clonazepam (Klonopin) 0.25 to 0.5 mg by mouth, or oxazepam (Serax) 10 to 30 mg by mouth—which often leads to sleep. If psychotic symptoms predominate, use haloperidol (Haldol) 1 to 2 mg by mouth or intramuscularly (IM). Repeat in 20 to 30 minutes as needed.

For a more detailed discussion of this topic, see G E Woody, W Macfadden: Cannabis-Related Disorders, Sec 13.5, p 810, in CTP/VI.

8.15. Clonidine Withdrawal

Clonidine (Catapres) is a centrally acting α_2-agonist that reduces peripheral adrenergic tone. It is often used to treat hypertension. Its psychiatric applications include mania, opioid withdrawal, cocaine intoxication, Tourette's disorder, post-traumatic stress disorder, and other conditions associated with autonomic arousal.

CLINICAL FEATURES AND DIAGNOSIS

Withdrawal from ongoing clonidine treatment can lead to anxiety, agitation, irritability, psychosis, violence, hypertension, and seizures.

INTERVIEWING AND PSYCHOTHERAPEUTIC GUIDELINES

Explain to the patient that withdrawal is a self-limiting process and that they will be given medication to deal with uncomfortable signs and symptoms. Determine (1) the reason the patient was prescribed clonidine, (2) who prescribed it, (3) the dose prescribed, and (4) the duration of the prescription.

EVALUATION AND MANAGEMENT

The elimination half-life of clonidine is about 13 hours, and a gradual reduction of the clonidine dosage may prevent withdrawal symptoms. Even untreated symptoms of clonidine withdrawal generally resolve after several days.

DRUG TREATMENT

Agitation and possible violence may require physical restraint or tranquilization with a benzodiazepine—for example, estazolam (ProSom) 0.5 to 1 mg by mouth, lorazepam (Ativan) 1 to 2 mg by mouth or intramuscularly (IM), or oxazepam (Serax) 10 to 30 mg by mouth. In psychotic or severely agitated patients, the short-term use of parenteral antipsychotics—for example, fluphenazine (Prolixin) 2 to 5 mg IM or haloperidol (Haldol) 2 to 5 mg IM—may be needed.

For a more detailed discussion of this topic, see T W Uhde, M E Tancer: Clonidine, Sec 32.13, p 1975, in CTP/VI.

8.16. Cocaine Intoxication and Withdrawal

Cocaine Intoxication

Cocaine intoxication is a substance use disorder that follows the ingestion of cocaine. It produces both physical and behavioral effects. Cocaine can be snorted, injected, smoked, or absorbed through the mucous membranes. The potential for dependence is related to the route of administration and is greatest when the drug is either injected or smoked in its pure (freebase) form. A purified form of freebase cocaine called crack is sold in small single doses and is smoked. The low cost of small doses of crack and its availability in ready-to-smoke form have led to the widespread use of cocaine in indigent urban areas. Increased urban crack use has clearly affected drug-related crimes and violence.

CLINICAL FEATURES AND DIAGNOSIS

The symptom onset is within minutes to one hour of administration (Table 8.16-1).Since the duration of action of cocaine is short (the elimination half-life is one hour), except for cases of severe overdose, most of the drug is usually gone from the body by the time the patient presents to the emergency room or the doctor's office. Both the physical and behavioral sequelae of intoxication can produce emergencies.

The behavioral signs include agitation, aggressiveness or fighting, paranoid delusions or hallucinations, delirium, excitement, and poor judgment. The physical signs include tachycardia, hypertension, mydriasis, perspiration and chills, tremor, nausea and vomiting, fever, arrhythmia, syncope, chest pain, and, in overdoses, convulsions, respiratory depression, coma, and death.

TABLE 8.16–1
DIAGNOSTIC CRITERIA FOR COCAINE INTOXICATION

A. Recent use of cocaine.
B. Clinically significant maladaptive behavioral or psychological changes (e.g., euphoria or affective blunting; changes in sociability; hypervigilance; interpersonal sensitivity; anxiety, tension, or anger; stereotyped behaviors; impaired judgment; or impaired social or occupational functioning) that developed during, or shortly after, use of cocaine.
C. Two (or more) of the following, developing during, or shortly after, cocaine use:
   (1) tachycardia or bradycardia
   (2) pupillary dilation
   (3) elevated or lowered blood pressure
   (4) perspiration or chills
   (5) nausea or vomiting
   (6) evidence of weight loss
   (7) psychomotor agitation or retardation
   (8) muscular weakness, respiratory depression, chest pain, or cardiac arrhythmias
   (9) confusion, seizures, dyskinesias, dystonias, or coma
D. The symptoms are not due to a general medical condition and are not better accounted for by another mental disorder.

Specify if:
   With perceptual disturbances

INTERVIEWING AND PSYCHOTHERAPEUTIC GUIDELINES

Reassure the patient that the symptoms are of limited duration. Provide a quiet environment. Assess the patient for the quantity, the frequency, and the route of cocaine use. Explain all actions and procedures carefully. Approach the paranoid patient with caution. If possible, enlist the aid of family members who can reassure the patient.

EVALUATION AND MANAGEMENT

1. Take the patient's vital signs. If fever is present, treat it aggressively. Frequently monitor the patient's blood pressure and pulse.
2. Reassure the patient that the symptoms are self-limiting and will resolve soon.
3. Determine if the patient also took other drugs, especially opiates (for example, a speedball of intravenous [IV] heroin and cocaine), sedative-hypnotics, and alcohol.
4. Seclusion and restraint are a last resort and are seldom necessary.
5. The psychotic symptoms usually resolve after the acute episode but may persist in heavy abusers (cocaine delusional disorder), especially in vulnerable persons.
6. Consider admitting the patient to the hospital for cocaine detoxification if necessary. A cocaine intoxication visit to the emergency room is probably the best time to convince the patient to attend a drug rehabilitation program.
7. Educate the patient about cocaine withdrawal.

DRUG TREATMENT

Severe agitation, dangerousness, or delusions can be treated with benzodiazepines—for example, oxazepam (Serax) 10 to 30 mg by mouth or lorazepam (Ativan) 1 to 2 mg intramuscularly (IM) and repeat in one hour if needed. Benzodiazepines are usually effective and are preferable to antipsychotics, because benzodiazepines raise the seizure threshold and reduce central nervous system (CNS) irritability.

If agitation persists after several doses of benzodiazepines or if signs of benzodiazepine toxicity (ataxia, dysarthria, nystagmus) develop, give a high-potency antipsychotic—for example, fluphenazine (Prolixin) or haloperidol (Haldol), both given at 2 to 5 mg by mouth or IM. Antipsychotics should generally be avoided if possible, because they lower the seizure threshold and because the self-limited course of cocaine intoxication does not usually warrant the risks of antipsychotic side effects.

Tachycardia and hypertension, if severe or persistent, can be treated with β-blockers such as propranolol (Inderal) or clonidine (Catapres). Hemodynamic instability, seizures, respiratory depression, and other signs of an overdose are indications for admission to an intensive care unit (ICU).

Cocaine Withdrawal

Cocaine withdrawal is characterized by a dysphoric mood persisting for more than 24 hours after a decrease in cocaine consumption and with at least one of the following: (1) fatigue, (2) insomnia or hypersomnia, and (3) psychomotor agitation. Patients may also have paranoid or suicidal ideation, irritability, and depressed mood.

CLINICAL FEATURES AND DIAGNOSIS

No well-defined physiological syndrome of cocaine withdrawal occurs after the discontinuation of heavy use, but the behavioral syndrome described above is common. Cocaine withdrawal implies cocaine dependence.

The most prominent symptom of cocaine withdrawal is a craving for cocaine. The severity of the withdrawal is related to the amount and the duration of use and to the route of administration. Snorting produces less dependence and withdrawal; intravenous abuse and smoking crack (freebase) produces more dependence and withdrawal (Table 8.16-2).

The symptoms peak in several days but may last for up to several weeks. An underlying or secondary major depression may be diagnosed if the symptoms persist for more than several weeks. In addition, underlying personality disorders, dependence on alcohol, and dependence on sedative-hypnotics may be obscured by cocaine use.

INTERVIEWING AND PSYCHOTHERAPEUTIC GUIDELINES

Patients with cocaine withdrawal are dysphoric, and major depression is included in the differential diagnosis. But, since personality disorders (especially borderline and antisocial personality disorders) are often present, cocaine withdrawal patients are often perceived as manipulative. The patient will probably medicate the withdrawal symptoms by returning to cocaine use; the relapse rates, even after inpatient detoxification, are high.

Reassure the patient that the syndrome is likely to resolve in one to two weeks. Determine the route, the frequency, and the quantity of cocaine use and the time of the last use. Screen the patient for dependence on other drugs. Setting limits can help educate the patient about what behaviors are acceptable.

TABLE 8.16–2
DIAGNOSTIC CRITERIA FOR COCAINE WITHDRAWAL

A. Cessation of (or reduction in) cocaine use that has been heavy and prolonged.
B. Dysphoric mood and two (or more) of the following physiological changes, developing within a few hours to several days after criterion A:
   (1) fatigue
   (2) vivid, unpleasant dreams
   (3) insomnia or hypersomnia
   (4) increased appetite
   (5) psychomotor retardation or agitation
C. The symptoms in criterion B cause clinically significant distress or impairment in social, occupational, or other important areas of functioning.
D. The symptoms are not due to a general medical condition and are not better accounted for by another mental disorder.

Table from DSM-IV, *Diagnostic and Statistical Manual of Mental Disorders*, ed. 4. Copyright American Psychiatric Association, Washington, 1994. Used with permission.

EVALUATION AND MANAGEMENT

1. Assess the suicide risk. Even though the syndrome will probably resolve in several days, suicidal patients may require psychiatric admission to the hospital.
2. Encourage the patient to attend a detoxification or rehabilitation program.
3. Refer the patient to a support group (for example, Narcotics Anonymous) or to family or group therapy.
4. Evaluate the patient for an underlying psychiatric disorder and the abuse of other drugs.

DRUG TREATMENT

Severe agitation and maladaptive behavior can be controlled with benzodiazepines (for example, estazolam [ProSom] 0.5 to 1 by mouth, oxazepam 10 to 30 mg by mouth, or lorazepam 1 to 2 mg by mouth or IM).

Antidepressants can be used for persistent symptoms of depression, but they are usually not started unless the patient has a full depressive syndrome two weeks after stopping the cocaine.

Cocaine dependence has been treated with desipramine (Norpramin), doxepin (Sinequan), and other antidepressants. Bromocriptine (Parlodel) has also been used. The goal of treatment of cocaine dependence is abstinence.

For a more detailed discussion of this topic, see J H Jaffe: Cocaine-Related Disorders, Sec 13.6, p 817, in CTP/VI.

8.17. L-Dopa Intoxication

L-Dopa (levodopa [Larodopa, Dopar]) can cause intoxication. It is commonly used to treat Parkinson's disease and parkinsonian syndromes after a head injury, manganese intoxication, carbon monoxide poisoning, encephalitis, and cerebrovascular diseases. L-Dopa is also used for dystonia musculorum deformans.

CLINICAL FEATURES AND DIAGNOSIS

The psychiatric manifestations of L-dopa intoxication consist of psychotic symptoms (for example, hallucinations and delusions) and alterations of mood (for example, mania and depression). Additional reactions include anxiety, dyskinesias, dementia, and delirium. A common preparation is a combination of L-dopa and carbidopa (Sinemet). The medical complications of L-dopa intoxication include nausea, vomiting, urinary retention, hypotension, bradycardia, and toxicity in the gastrointestinal tract, liver, bone marrow, and blood.

INTERVIEWING AND PSYCHOTHERAPEUTIC GUIDELINES

The conduct of the interview depends on the symptoms present. Contact the physician who prescribed the L-dopa, usually a neurologist or internist. Explain to the patient that symptoms are self-limited and will resolve.

EVALUATION AND MANAGEMENT

1. Determine the ingested amount of L-dopa or l-dopa-carbidopa.
2. Reduce the dosage of L-dopa or L-dopa-carbidopa if possible.
3. Consider alternatives to L-dopa, including anticholinergic drugs, amantadine (Symmetrel), and bromocriptine (Parlodel).
4. Depression is common in patients with Parkinson's disease and should be treated.

DRUG TREATMENT

Begin by reducing the dosage of L-dopa. Severe agitation or anxiety may be treated with short-acting benzodiazepines—for example, oxazepam (Serax) 10 to 30 mg by mouth, lorazepam (Ativan) 1 to 2 mg by mouth or intramuscularly (IM), or estazolam (ProSom) 0.5 to 1 mg by mouth. Avoid antipsychotics. Tricyclic antidepressants may improve the depressive symptoms of Parkinson's disease. Never give monoamine oxidase inhibitors (MAOIs) with L-Dopa.

For a more detailed discussion of this topic, see E D Caine, H Grossman, J M Lyness: Delirium, Dementia, and Amnestic and Other Cognitive Disorders and Mental Disorders Due to a General Medical Condition, Chap 12, p 705; T C Manschreck: Delusional Disorder and Shared Psychotic Disorder, Sec 15.2, p 1031; H I Kaplan, B J Sadock: Other Pharmacological Therapies, Sec 32.27, p 2122, in CTP/VI.

8.18. Drug Flashback

A *drug flashback* (also called posthallucinogen perception disorder) is a recurrence of a drug-induced effect that occurs some time after the drug was last taken. Flashbacks are common after hallucinogen use (up to 25 percent of lysergic acid diethylamide [LSD] users experience flashbacks) and rare after cannabis use. Patients typically come to clinical attention when a flashback is distressing or dysphoric.

CLINICAL FEATURES AND DIAGNOSIS

Flashbacks cannot be easily explained by the pharmacokinetics of the drug, and they may occur years after the drug was used. They may be precipitated by stress, fatigue, illness, or even by walking into a brightly lit area. Visual hallucinations, distortions, and illusions are typical symptoms, but somatic and psychological symptoms may also occur. If the symptoms are associated with distress, a diagnosis of posthallucinogen perception disorder may be made.

Hallucinogen-induced flashbacks usually resolve within hours but may last up to two days and occasionally longer. Flashback complications include severe anxiety, panic, depression, suicidal ideation, and persistent psychosis. Flashbacks may recur for months or years.

INTERVIEWING AND PSYCHOTHERAPEUTIC GUIDELINES

Usually, the patient is aware that the experience is a drug flashback, since the subjective experience is similar to what was experienced during active use of the drug. If the patients have had dysphoric or distressing trips before, they may be expecting distressing flashbacks. If the patients are not aware that they are experiencing flashbacks, they may believe that they are going insane. Reassuring the patient that the symptoms will pass is useful and is called "talking down" the patient.

EVALUATION AND MANAGEMENT

1. Obtain the patient's history of hallucinogen use and rule out acute hallucinogen intoxication.
2. Rule out other possible causes, including physical or mental disorders.
3. Reassure the patient that the episode is temporary and due to previous drug use. Provide the companionship of a family member or a close friend if possible; otherwise, have a staff member stay with the patient.

DRUG TREATMENT

Drug treatment is usually not needed, but, in cases of severe anxiety or agitation, start with a benzodiazepine—for example, estazolam (ProSom) 0.5 to 1 mg by mouth, oxazepam (Serax) 10 to 30 mg by mouth, alprazolam (Xanax) 0.5 to 1 mg by mouth, or lorazepam (Ativan) 1 to 2 mg by mouth or intramuscularly (IM), all given every four hours as needed. If that medication is ineffective, consider an antipsychotic. The choice of antipsychotic depends on the desired side-effect profile. High-potency antipsychotics—for example, fluphenazine (Prolixin), thiothixene (Navane), and haloperidol (Haldol), all given at 2 to 5 mg by mouth or IM every four hours as needed—are usually used but often produce extrapyramidal side effects. If sedation is desired and if anticholinergic side effects and reducing the seizure threshold are not concerns, a low-potency antipsychotic—for example, thioridazine (Mellaril) or chlorpromazine (Thorazine), both given at 10 to 25 mg by mouth every four hours as needed—may also be considered. If acute hallucinogen intoxication is a possibility, low-potency antipsychotics should be avoided, because of their possible exacerbation of anticholinergic side effects and their lowering of the seizure threshold.

For a more detailed discussion of this topic, see J Yager, M J Gitlin: Clinical Manifestations of Psychiatric Disorders, Chap 10, p 637; G E Woody, W Macfadden: Cannabis-Related Disorders, Sec 13.5, p 810; T J Crowley: Hallucinogen-Related Disorders, Sec 13.7, p 831, in CTP/VI.

8.19. Hallucinogen Hallucinosis

Hallucinogen hallucinosis (intoxication) is characterized by impaired perception and maladaptive behavior in an alert patient, with related physical signs, after the use of a hallucinogen.

CLINICAL FEATURES AND DIAGNOSIS

Usually, the history of hallucinogen use is available, and the patient associates the symptoms with the drug use (Table 8.19-1). Common hallucinogens include lysergic acid diethylamide (LSD), dimethoxymethylamphetamine (DOM, STP), a 4-bromo homologue of dimethoxymethylamphetamine (DOB), dimethyltryptamine (DMT), trimethoxyamphetamine (TMA), psilocybin, mescaline (peyote, tops, cactus), methylenedioxyamphetamine (MDA), methylenedioxymethamphetamine (MDMA, ecstasy), and phencyclidine (PCP) (Table 8.19-2). Often, contaminants— such as anticholinergic drugs, cocaine and other stimulants, and strychnine—have been added to the hallucinogen.

The symptoms usually begin one hour after ingestion and generally last 8 to 12 hours. The typical clinical presentation is a panic reaction (bad trip). After taking a hallucinogen, the patients have trouble in distinguishing drug-induced symptoms from reality and believe that they have gone mad. Associated fears are that the patients have done permanent damage to their brains or chromosomes and will never recover. Bad trips most often occur in first-time users and in those who are anxious or isolated.

Most hallucinogenic drugs have stimulant effects and produce increased activity, insomnia, and elevated vital signs. Other symptoms include suspiciousness, synesthesias (stimulation of one sensory modality is perceived in another sensory modality), intense anxiety, visual hallucinations, fear of losing control, and depression. Hepatotoxicity and death have been attributed to MDMA.

The patients can usually be stabilized in one to two days. Severe agitation, dangerousness, or persistent psychotic symptoms may warrant hospitalization.

INTERVIEWING AND PSYCHOTHERAPEUTIC GUIDELINES

Reassure the patient that the symptoms are drug-induced and will resolve with time. Encourage the patient with constant reassurance and orientation (for example, "You're OK; you're in the hospital; you're going to be all right; it's now Monday afternoon").

TABLE 8.19-1
DIAGNOSTIC CRITERIA FOR HALLUCINOGEN INTOXICATION

A. Recent use of a hallucinogen.
B. Clinically significant maladaptive behavioral or psychological changes (e.g., marked anxiety or depression, ideas of reference, fear of losing one's mind, paranoid ideation, impaired social or occupational functioning) that developed during, or shortly after, hallucinogen use.
C. Perceptual changes occurring in a state of full wakefulness and alertness (e.g., subjective intensification of perceptions, depersonalization, derealization, illusions, hallucinations, synesthesias) that developed during, or shortly after, hallucinogen use.
D. Two (or more) of the following signs, developing during, or shortly after, hallucinogen use:
    (1) pupillary dilation
    (2) tachycardia
    (3) sweating
    (4) palpitations
    (5) blurring of vision
    (6) tremors
    (7) incoordination
E. The symptoms are not due to a general medical condition and are not better accounted for by another mental disorder.

Table from DSM-IV, *Diagnostic and Statistical Manual of Mental Disorders*, ed 4. Copyright American Psychiatric Association, Washington, 1994. Used with permission.

TABLE 8.19–2
COMMONLY ABUSED HALLUCINOGENIC DRUGS

Drug	Source	Psychedelic Dose	Peak Symptoms	Duration of Action	Prominent Somatic Effects	Prominent Psychological Effects
D-Lysergic acid diethylamide (LSD)	Synthetic (from fungi)	50 μg	2 to 3 hrs	8 to 12 hrs undulating activity as effect declines	Increased sympathetic nervous system activity: dilated pupils, increased BP, pulse, deep tendon reflexes, temperature, blood sugar, tremor	Hypervigilance, illusions, emotional lability, loss of body boundaries, time slowing, increased intensity of all sensations
Psilocybin	Mushroom	10 mg	90 mins	4 to 6 hrs	Like LSD but milder	Like LSD but less intense, more visual, more euphoria; paranoia
Dimethyltryptamine (DMT)	Synthetic	50 mg	5 to 20 mins	30 to 60 mins	Like LSD but with more intense sympathomimetic symptoms	Like LSD but usually more intense, in part because of sudden onset; must be smoked or injected; cannot be taken orally
Mescaline	Peyote cactus	200 mg	2 to 3 hrs	8 to 12 hrs	Nausea, vomiting; otherwise like LSD, perhaps more intense sympathomimetic effects	Like LSD but perhaps more sensory and perceptual changes; euphoria prominent
Dimethoxymethyl-amphetamine (DOM, STP)	Synthetic	5 mg	3 to 5 hrs	6 to 8 hrs at doses below 5 mg; 16 to 24 hrs at high doses (10 to 30 mg)	Minimal effects at low dose; autonomic effects prominent at doses above 5 mg	May resemble amphetamine combined with LSD but long-lasting; high incidence of flashbacks, psychosis; chlorpromazine may aggravate symptoms

Table from S M Mirin, R D Weiss: Drug use and abuse. In *Emergency Psychiatry*, E L Bassuk, A W Birk, editors, p. 162. Plenum, New York, 1984. Used with permission.

EVALUATION AND MANAGEMENT

1. Place the patient in a nonstimulating environment.
2. Unless the patient seems violent, have a friend or a family member stay with the patient constantly.
3. Monitor the patient's vital signs, which may be elevated.
4. Urine toxicology screens and blood concentrations of the drug taken should be done if possible.
5. Consider intoxication with multiple drugs, particularly when the symptoms persist. The agents are frequently contaminated with other drugs, such as amphetamines and PCP.
6. If the patient is severely agitated and potentially dangerous, physical restraint may be needed. Avoid physical restraint, if possible, in PCP intoxication.
7. Organic delusional and mood disorders that last more than several days may develop in some patients.
8. Evaluate whether the psychotic symptoms preceded the use of the hallucinogen and whether other diagnoses should be considered (for example, schizophreniform disorder and mood disorder with psychotic features).

DRUG TREATMENT

If tranquilization is needed, benzodiazepines are preferred, since antipsychotics (especially low-potency antipsychotics) may produce anticholinergic effects, which can exacerbate the signs of hallucinogen intoxication. Start with oxazepam (Serax) 10 to 30 mg by mouth or lorazepam (Ativan) 1 to 2 mg by mouth or intravenously (IV), both given every four hours as needed. If that is ineffective after several doses or if the signs of benzodiazepine toxicity occur (ataxia, dysarthria), a high-potency antipsychotic may be added—for example, fluphenazine (Prolixin), thiothixene (Navane), or haloperidol (Haldol), all given at 2 to 5 mg by mouth or intramuscularly (IM) every four hours as needed.

For a more detailed discussion of this topic, see Hallucinogen-Related Disorders, Sec 13.7, p 831, in CTP/VI.

8.20. Impending Death Associated with Antipsychotic Medication

The introduction of antipsychotic medications has not increased the rate of sudden death in psychiatric patients. Patients with acute psychoses may die as a result of stresses related to the acute psychosis, rather than to the treatment. Nonetheless, antipsychotic medications do have potentially dangerous side effects, especially for the medically ill. Life-threatening complications are not more commonly associated with either high-potency or low-potency antipsychotics.

CLINICAL FEATURES AND DIAGNOSIS

The side effects of antipsychotics that may possibly contribute to sudden death include (1) ventricular fibrillation (antipsychotics are not arrhythmogenic); (2)

depressed gag reflex, leading to asphyxia from the aspiration of regurgitated food; (3) lowering of the seizure threshold, causing seizures; (4) dystonia of the larynx and pharynx, leading to asphyxiation; (5) orthostatic hypotension, leading to a cerebrovascular event or myocardial infarction; (6) neuroleptic malignant syndrome; (7) anticholinergic effects, reducing gastrointestinal (GI) motility and leading to shock in patients with acquired megacolon; (8) endobronchial mucous plugs in asthmatic patients; and (9) clozapine (Clozaril)-induced agranulocytosis, leading to opportunistic infection.

INTERVIEWING AND PSYCHOTHERAPEUTIC GUIDELINES

No evidence indicates that the use of antipsychotic medications increases the likelihood of sudden death. Carefully describe the potential side effects to the patients and their families. Instruct them to seek medical care rapidly if side effects occur, especially dystonia, severe rigidity, seizures, and hypotension. Inform patients that antipsychotics in rare cases cause agranulocytosis, so they should be evaluated for any sign of even a minor infection, such as a fever.

EVALUATION AND MANAGEMENT

Give the appropriate emergency medical care.

DRUG TREATMENT

Decrease the antipsychotic dosage or discontinue the antipsychotic if necessary to eliminate severe side effects. Many side effects can be reduced by switching to another antipsychotic drug. Extrapyramidal side effects are easily treated with anticholinergic drugs. Anticholinergic side effects, hypotension, and the lowering of the seizure threshold can be decreased by changing to a higher-potency antipsychotic.

For a more detailed discussion of this topic, see S C Schulz: Schizophrenia: Somatic Treatment, Sec 14.8, p 987; D P Van Kammen, S R Marder: Dopamine Receptor Antagonists, Sec 32.15, p 1987, in CTP/VI.

8.21. Intoxication

Intoxication is defined as maladaptive behavior—such as belligerence, impaired judgment, or impaired social or occupational functioning—associated with recent substance ingestion.

CLINICAL FEATURES AND DIAGNOSIS

A substance-specific syndrome may be observed in some patients that will help in making the diagnosis. See Table 8.21-1 for the diagnostic criteria for intoxication.

INTERVIEWING AND PSYCHOTHERAPEUTIC GUIDELINES

The mental status of intoxicated patients changes as the substance is cleared. But potentially dangerous patients require immediate evaluation, even though they may be completely different several hours later. Always consider the possibility that multiple substances have been taken. Assume that the patient is minimizing the amount of substance taken and the frequency and the duration of substance abuse.

Be reassuring and give the patient a sense that the environment is under control and that limits have been set, at least temporarily, on their use of alcohol or drugs.

Constantly consider possible medical complications of either acute or chronic intoxication. For example, central nervous system (CNS) or respiratory depression may occur after the use of opioids, barbiturates, or sedative-hypnotics; seizures and cardiac arrhythmias may follow the use of cocaine.

EVALUATION AND MANAGEMENT

1. Obtain the patient's vital signs.
2. Look for other obvious signs of intoxication, including ataxia, dysarthria, nystagmus, pupillary changes, CNS depression, and agitation.
3. Consider the possibility of an overdose. Assume that the amount of substance taken has been underrepresented. Also consider the possibility of polysubstance intoxication or overdose.
4. Look for withdrawal symptoms. Patients who are intoxicated on alcohol or a sedative-hypnotic may also have withdrawal symptoms if the amount taken on an ongoing basis has been recently decreased.
5. Rapidly assess the patient for dangerousness, and prevent harm to the patient and to others. Physical restraints and involuntary hospitalization are sometimes necessary. Restraints should be used with caution, particularly in phencyclidine (PCP) intoxication, in which patients are at risk for rhabdomyolysis.
6. Evaluate and treat the patient's medical problems.
7. Provide an environment appropriate to the substance ingested—for example, minimize stimulation after PCP use but provide interactive support after lysergic acid diethylamide (LSD) use.
8. Allow the substance to clear, and reevaluate when the patient is no longer intoxicated. A patient intoxicated on multiple substances with different pharma-

TABLE 8.21-1
CRITERIA FOR SUBSTANCE INTOXICATION

A. The development of a reversible substance-specific syndrome due to recent ingestion of (or exposure to) a substance. Note: Different substances may produce similar or identical syndromes.

B. Clinically significant maladaptive behavioral or psychological changes that are due to the effect of the substance on the central nervous system (e.g., belligerence, mood lability, cognitive impairment, impaired judgment, impaired social or occupational functioning) and develop during or shortly after use of the substance.

C. The symptoms are not due to a general medical condition and are not better accounted for by another mental disorder.

Table from DSM-IV, *Diagnostic and Statistical Manual of Mental Disorders,* ed 4. Copyright American Psychiatric Association, Washington, 1994. Used with permission.

cokinetic actions may be clearing one substance (such as alcohol) while the blood concentration of another substance (such as a barbiturate) is rising.

DRUG TREATMENT

Drug treatment depends on the substances taken and the patient's clinical needs. If tranquilization is needed, benzodiazepines are preferable to antipsychotics; benzodiazepines raise the seizure threshold, but antipsychotics lower the seizure threshold. In general, avoid medications of any type if possible.

For a more detailed discussion of this topic, see Substance-Related Disorders, Chap 13, pp 755–887, in CTP/VI.

8.22. Lithium Toxicity

Lithium toxicity is produced by an excess of lithium (Eskalith). The toxic state affects the central nervous system (CNS), thyroid, kidneys, gastrointestinal (GI) system, and metabolic system.

CLINICAL FEATURES AND DIAGNOSIS

Peak serum lithium concentrations are reached about two hours after ingestion (four hours after ingesting controlled-release preparations); consequently, the peak is usually over by the time the patient comes to clinical attention. The elimination half-life of lithium is about 22 hours, and excretion is almost completely renal.

Lithium concentrations are increased by dehydration, low salt intake, decreased fluid intake, thiazide diuretics, and many nonsteroidal anti-inflammatory drugs. Lithium side effects are common, but most do not lead to emergencies. The side effects include mild tremor, hypothyroidism, polyuria, polydipsia, nausea, vomiting, diarrhea, weight gain, leukocytosis, acne, psoriasis, hypercalcemia, elevated serum magnesium, and hyperparathyroidism. Long-term administration of lithium can cause impaired renal concentrating ability, diabetes insipidus, and possibly renal failure.

INTERVIEWING AND PSYCHOTHERAPEUTIC GUIDELINES

Reassure the patient that mild lithium toxicity is usually benign. Questions concerning fluid and salt intake may clarify the cause of mild toxicity. However, lithium overdose in a suicide attempt is a toxicological emergency that may require dialysis. Immediately estimate the dose of lithium taken. When the amount taken was considerably more than the patient's daily dose, get an immediate blood lithium concentration and a medical consultation if the concentration is more than 2.0 mEq/l or if the patient shows signs of deterioration in mental functioning.

EVALUATION AND MANAGEMENT

1. Obtain a serum lithium concentration, and test for electrolytes, blood urea nitrogen (BUN), creatinine, complete blood count, and thyroid functions, including thyroid-stimulating hormone (TSH). Obtain two blood lithium concentrations over several hours to assess whether the concentrations are rising or falling.
2. Perform a neurological examination. The acute toxic effects of lithium primarily affect the brain. The early signs include dysarthria, ataxia, a mild fine tremor, and neuromuscular irritability. Severe intoxication may produce a severe tremor, delirium, impaired consciousness, seizures, coma, and death.
3. For mild cases, consider decreasing the lithium dosage or changing the schedule of drug administration.
4. Check the results of thyroid function tests, including TSH, and examine the patient for goiter. Mild abnormalities in thyroid function without clinical hypothyroidism (chemical hypothyroidism) are common. Whether those abnormalities should be treated is controversial. Clinical hypothyroidism can be treated with supplemental thyroid hormone.
5. If polyuria is present (daily urine output greater than three liters), determine if lithium-induced diabetes insipidus is present. Maintain adequate fluid intake, decrease the lithium dosage, change the dosage schedule to a single bedtime dose, and consider treatment with a thiazide or potassium-sparing diuretic (which will treat the diabetes insipidus).
6. Hydration (intravenous normal saline) and diuresis with osmotic or loop diuretics (for example, furosemide [Lasix] or ethacrynic acid [Edecrin]) may be effective for mild cases of intoxication.
7. Hemodialysis is rapidly effective in reducing the serum lithium concentration but may need to be repeated, since tissue stores of lithium may cause a rebound in the serum lithium concentration. Clinical improvement may lag for days after hemodialysis.
8. Electrocardiographic (ECG) monitoring is indicated in severe cases. Lithium generally causes only mild and reversible ECG abnormalities (for example, inverted or isoelectric T waves), but arrhythmias and conduction delays have been reported.
9. Evaluate for lithium overdose secondary to a suicide attempt.

DRUG TREATMENT

Decrease the lithium dosage or discontinue lithium if side effects are a clinical problem. Generally, try to obtain the lowest possible lithium concentration that is still effective. Changing the drug schedule to a single dose at bedtime may create peak serum concentrations during sleep that make mild side effects less bothersome.

If thiazide diuretics are needed, use a low lithium dosage, and follow the lithium concentrations and electrolytes closely. Tremor can be treated with β-blockers—for example, propranolol (Inderal).

For a more detailed discussion of this topic, see B J Fauman: Other Psychiatric Emergencies, Sec 30.2, p 1752; J W Jefferson, J H Greist: Lithium, Sec 32.16, p 2022, in CTP/VI.

8.23. Mercury Poisoning

Mercury poisoning is a mental disorder produced by long-term exposure to mercury or the ingestion of a large quantity of mercury. Long-term exposure can lead to personality changes, such as irritability, quarrelsomeness, loss of temper, depression, and chronic fatigue.

CLINICAL FEATURES AND DIAGNOSIS

Mercury poisoning causes an encephalopathy with a predilection for the cerebellum. Ataxia, tremor, and involuntary movements may be prominent and are usually permanent. Peripheral neuritis may also appear. When ingested, mercury is highly corrosive and can produce severe inflammation of the mouth, pharynx, and larynx; abdominal cramps; nausea; vomiting; and a severe enteritis, with bloody diarrhea. Hepatic injury is a delayed effect. Poisoning can also occur after the inhalation of mercury vapors. Mercury is concentrated in the kidneys and causes renal failure. The ingestion of 0.1 g of mercury can cause toxic symptoms, and the ingestion of 0.5 g is usually fatal.

INTERVIEWING AND PSYCHOTHERAPEUTIC GUIDELINES

High-risk groups include thermometer workers, photoengravers, ore workers, laboratory workers, fingerprinters, chemical workers, repairers of electrical meters, and workers in the felt hat industry. The long-term use of mercury-containing vaginal douches is another source of exposure. Explain to the patient that appropriate treatment measures will be taken that are often effective.

EVALUATION AND MANAGEMENT

1. After ingestion, remove mercury by gastric lavage.
2. Blood mercury concentrations of more than 0.03 μg/mL or urine mercury concentrations of more than 25 μg/L are abnormal and suggest exposure to mercury. Blood concentrations of more than 1.0 μg/mL cause symptoms of acute poisoning in most patients.

DRUG TREATMENT

Chelating agents bind mercury, form nontoxic stable molecules, and are excreted safely through the kidneys. Rapidly treat acute mercury poisoning with British anti-Lewisite (BAL). In chronic mercury poisoning, N-acetylpenicillamine, which binds mercury selectively without depleting copper, is the drug of choice and can be administered orally.

For a more detailed discussion of this topic, see T C Manschreck: Delusional Disorder and Shared Psychotic Disorder, Sec 15.2, p 1031, in CTP/VI.

8.24. Nitrous Oxide Intoxication

Inhaling nitrous oxide produces euphoria. Nitrous oxide (laughing gas) is used by anesthesiologists, nurse anesthetists, and dentists as an anesthetic. It is also used to provide the pressure needed for whipped cream, so it can be inhaled from whipped cream cans, and it can be purchased at restaurant supply stores in the small pressurized canisters (whippets) used to make whipped cream. Nitrous oxide is not a controlled drug.

CLINICAL FEATURES AND DIAGNOSIS

The typical abuser of nitrous oxide usually falls into one of two categories: (1) an anesthesiologist, an anesthetist, a dentist, a nurse, or a paraprofessional who has access to nitrous oxide tanks used for anesthesia; and (2) an adolescent who inhales nitrous oxide from whippets or whipped cream cans. The abusers may use nitrous oxide occasionally, with only minimal or no impairment in functioning.

The abuser exhales as much air as possible, inhales as much nitrous oxide as possible in a full breath, and then holds it in as long as possible. Masks are used to breathe in nitrous oxide from tanks; whipped cream cans are held upright without shaking to allow the gas to be released; and whippets are opened in a special device that releases the gas into a balloon or a bottle, from which the gas is inhaled.

The onset of the euphoria is rapid and is associated with a tingling throughout the entire body and, eventually, numbness. The effects usually wear off within several minutes. Nitrous oxide is often abused with cannabis or alcohol. Repeated rapid inhalation can lead to the loss of consciousness, but that effect usually requires a constant supply from a tank, a mask, or someone to hold the mask in place as the abuser passes out.

INTERVIEWING AND PSYCHOTHERAPEUTIC GUIDELINES

Patients are rarely intoxicated by the time they come to clinical attention. Carefully evaluate the patient for the use of other drugs and alcohol. Evaluate the patient for possible personality disorders and other psychiatric disorders.

EVALUATION AND MANAGEMENT

1. Obtain the patient's history of the frequency and the quantity of nitrous oxide taken and the use of other drugs of abuse, such as alcohol, cannabis, cocaine, and intravenous drugs. Physicians and nurses should be asked about the use of pharmaceutical drugs (for example, prescription opioids, stimulants, barbiturates, and benzodiazepines), which may have been taken from the hospital's supplies.
2. Evaluate the patient for other psychiatric conditions.
3. The nitrous oxide intoxication resolves rapidly, and usually no further short-term treatment is necessary.

4. Detoxification and drug rehabilitation are usually not needed unless other drugs are also being abused.

DRUG TREATMENT

No specific drug treatment is available.

For a more detailed discussion of this topic, see J H Jaffe: Introduction and Overview, Sec 13.1, p 755, in CTP/VI.

8.25. Nutmeg Intoxication

Nutmeg contains myristicin, a hallucinogen. It may be taken by adolescents seeking intoxication. Occasionally, *nutmeg intoxication* occurs accidentally when excessive amounts of nutmeg are used in baking a pie.

CLINICAL FEATURES AND DIAGNOSIS

Nutmeg intoxication is characterized by agitation, severe headaches, hallucinations, flushing, palpitations, and numbness in the extremities that occur after the ingestion of a large amount of nutmeg.

INTERVIEWING AND PSYCHOTHERAPEUTIC GUIDELINES

Reassure the patient that the symptoms of intoxication will resolve in several hours.

EVALUATION AND MANAGEMENT

1. Take the patient's vital signs. If the results are elevated, follow the patient until the signs are normal.
2. Evaluate the patient fully for signs of the abuse of other drugs, although such signs are unlikely in cases of accidental overdose.
3. The symptoms usually resolve without treatment after several hours, but observation may be needed if the patient's vital signs do not return to normal.

DRUG TREATMENT

No specific drug treatment is available. Severe anxiety or agitation may be treated with a benzodiazepine—for example, alprazolam (Xanax) 0.5 to 1 mg by mouth, lorazepam (Ativan) 1 to 2 mg by mouth or intramuscularly (IM), oxazepam (Serax) 10 to 30 mg by mouth, or estazolam (ProSom) 0.5 to 1 mg by mouth.

For a more detailed discussion of this topic, see T J Crowley: Hallucinogen-Related Disorders, Sec 13.7, p 831, in CTP/VI.

8.26. Opioid Intoxication and Withdrawal

Opioid Intoxication

Opioid intoxication follows the recent ingestion, inhalation, or injection of an opioid. It is characterized by drowsiness, euphoria, analgesia, slurred speech, impaired attention, anorexia, decreased sex drive, and hypoactivity.

CLINICAL FEATURES AND DIAGNOSIS

Opioid intoxication can lead to opioid overdose, which can be a life-threatening emergency.

The lifetime risk of opioid dependence is 0.7 percent in the United States. The opioids include opium derivatives and synthetic drugs: opium, morphine, diacetylmorphine (heroin, smack, horse, dope), methadone, codeine, oxycodone (Percodan, Percocet), hydromorphone (Dilaudid), levorphanol (Levo-Dromoran), pentazocine (Talwin), meperidine (Demerol), and propoxyphene (Darvon). Table 8.26-1 lists the duration of action of several opioids.

The route of administration depends on the drug. Opium is smoked. Heroin is typically injected (intravenously [IV] or subcutaneously) or snorted; it may be combined with stimulants (cocaine or amphetamine) for intravenous injection (speedball) to reduce sedation and increase euphoria. When injected, opioids have an onset of action in approximately five minutes and produce symptoms for up to 30 minutes. Pharmaceutical opioids are typically taken orally. Although injectable pharmaceutical opioids are available, they are less frequently abused than are street drugs because of better monitoring and control of parenteral drug supplies.

The dose of heroin (and other street opioids) is difficult to estimate accurately because the percent concentration of heroin purchased on the street varies unpredictably. Furthermore, the subjective experience of euphoria is influenced by many factors other than drug dosage. The patient may grossly overstate the dose in order to get more methadone.

Typical patients who abuse opioids fall into several categories: the heroin addict is poorly nourished and poorly groomed, antisocial, and often dependent on cocaine,

TABLE 8.26–1
DURATION OF ACTION OF OPIOIDS

Drug	Duration of Action
Heroin	3–4 hours
Meperidine	2–4 hours
Morphine, hydromorphone	4–5 hours
Methadone	12–24 hours
Propoxyphene	12 hours
Pentazocine	2–3 hours

as well as heroin; the opium addict may have been smoking opium for years; the professional patient has gone to many doctors to receive multiple prescriptions for opioids; and the health care professional has access to pharmaceutical opioids.

INTERVIEWING AND PSYCHOTHERAPEUTIC GUIDELINES

In evaluating a patient who has possibly overdosed, initiate medical treatment immediately. When interviewing the patient or family and friends later, remember that the amount (dose) of the drug taken is very unreliable. An overdose commonly occurs when the user unknowingly obtains some heroin that is markedly more potent than were previous batches. Always consider the possibility of an overdose on multiple drugs.

EVALUATION AND MANAGEMENT

1. Take the patient's vital signs.
2. Obtain a complete drug history, including the use of alcohol, prescribed drugs, over-the-counter drugs, and street drugs.
3. Check for past and present medical problems related to drug abuse: For parenteral users, check for acquired immune deficiency syndrome (AIDS), hepatitis, sepsis, cellulitis, osteomyelitis, scars from subcutaneous or IV injection, endocarditis, pulmonary edema, and thrombophlebitis; look for old and new track marks all over the body, including all extremities. For intranasal snorters, check for nasal septum deviation and perforation, nosebleeds, and rhinitis.
4. Obtain a toxicology screen to evaluate the patient for polysubstance abuse.
5. Avoid giving opioids in the physician's office or the emergency room exclusively for the treatment of opioid withdrawal unless absolutely necessary. Distributing opioids in the office or emergency room rapidly leads to a long line of malingering patients presenting with identical symptoms.
6. Look for objective signs of opioid intoxication, including central nervous system (CNS) depression, decreased gastrointestinal (GI) motility, respiratory depression, analgesia, nausea and vomiting, slurred speech, hypotension, bradycardia, pupillary constriction, and seizures (in overdose). Tolerant patients still have pupillary constriction and constipation.
7. Consider polydrug intoxication and overdose, particularly with alcohol and such sedative-hypnotics as barbiturates and benzodiazepines. In a polydrug overdose, the opioids may be reversed by opiate receptor antagonists—for example, naloxone (Narcan)—leaving just an overdose of alcohol and sedative-hypnotics to be treated. Cocaine intoxication may complicate the clinical picture, but cocaine intoxication is usually brief (several hours).
8. Assess the patient for suicidality and resulting intentional overdose.
9. Admit the patient to an intensive care unit (ICU) for overdose. Give supportive treatments (for example, give IV fluids and maintain the patient's vital signs). If suicidal, the patient may require constant observation to prevent another attempt.

DRUG TREATMENT

If CNS depression, respiratory depression, or other signs of moderate intoxication are present, consider a possible overdose. Give naloxone 0.8 mg IV (0.01 mg per kilogram for neonates), and wait 15 minutes. If the patient shows no response, give another 1.6 mg IV, and wait 15 minutes. If the patient still shows no response, give 3.2 mg IV, and suspect another diagnosis. If the opioid overdose is successfully reversed, continue the naloxone at 0.4 mg an hour IV. If the patient is opioid-addicted, keep the dosage of naloxone to a minimum once the patient is awake to avoid precipitating withdrawal (which recedes when the naloxone wears off). An intentional heroin overdose in a suicide attempt can be potentially fatal, but a more common history is one of accidental overdose, in which the abuser received a bag that was perhaps 15 percent heroin instead of the usual 5 percent. An accidental overdose may also occur in naive users and in previously abstinent experienced users who are no longer tolerant.

Opioid Withdrawal

Opioid withdrawal occurs after a cessation or decrease in the dose of opioid taken by a long-term user. Withdrawal is characterized by a craving for the drug, pupillary dilation, piloerection, sweating, fever, hypertension, insomnia, yawning, and a flulike syndrome with nausea and vomiting, muscle aches, malaise, lacrimation and rhinorrhea, and diarrhea. The presence of opioid withdrawal implies opioid dependence.

CLINICAL FEATURES AND DIAGNOSIS

Opioid withdrawal, although uncomfortable, is not dangerous in patients who are otherwise healthy, although patients in withdrawal may vehemently and dramatically demand that they be treated with opioids.

The objective signs of opioid withdrawal include piloerection, pupillary dilation, tremor, and elevated vital signs (Table 8.26-2). The flulike symptoms of with-

TABLE 8.26-2
DIAGNOSIS AND TREATMENT OF OPIOID WITHDRAWAL

Objective signs of opioid withdrawal
Pulse 10 beats/min over baseline* or > 90 in the absence of a history of tachycardia if the baseline is unknown
Systolic blood pressure > 10 mm Hg over baseline of > 160/95 in the absence of known hypertension
Dilated pupils
Sweating, gooseflesh, rhinorrhea, or lacrimation
Treatment
Administer methadone, 10 mg by mouth every four hours as needed when two of the four criteria above are met; decrease by 5 mg/day to zero

*Baseline refers to the patient's vital signs one hour after receiving 10 mg of methadone. For a patient who has received no methadone, the baseline vital signs should be estimated according to what one would expect from the patient's age, sex, and general health.
Table from R D Weiss, S M Mirin: Intoxication and withdrawal syndromes. In *Manual of Psychiatric Emergencies,* ed 2, S E Hyman, editor, p. 234. Little, Brown, Boston, 1988. Used with permission.

TABLE 8.26-3
WITHDRAWAL FROM OPIOID PREPARATIONS

	Morphine or Heroin	Meperidine	Methadone
First onset of symptoms (anxiety, drug seeking)	6–8 hours	2–4 hours	1–3 days
Peak withdrawal symptoms	2nd or 3rd day	8–12 hours	Gradual
Duration of withdrawal	7–10 days	4–5 days	10–14 days

Table from P Gillig: Drug abuse. In *Manual of Clinical Emergency Psychiatry*. J R Hillard, editor, p 221. American Psychiatric Press, Washington, 1990. Used with permission.

drawal—myalgias, arthralgias, rhinorrhea, lacrimation, weakness, nausea, and vomiting—are easily faked and are difficult to evaluate objectively. Withdrawal symptoms are more severe for short-acting opioids (for example, heroin and meperidine) than for long-acting drugs (for example, methadone). The onset of withdrawal is directly related to the duration of action of the drug abused. For example, methadone withdrawal begins one to three days after the last dose and lasts 10 to 14 days; heroin withdrawal begins in six to eight hours, peaks at two to three days, and lasts 7 to 10 days (Table 8.26-3).

INTERVIEWING AND PSYCHOTHERAPEUTIC GUIDELINES

Patients in opioid withdrawal are agitated and may be confused and demanding. Reassure the patients that their symptoms can be controlled with appropriate medications and that they will not be allowed to suffer or experience pain. Most patients respond to such reassurance. Do not admonish or blame the addicts for bringing on the symptoms by the abuse of drugs.

EVALUATION AND MANAGEMENT

1. Rely on objective findings (for example, piloerection, pupillary changes, and hypertension), when determining whether withdrawal is present.
2. The main objectives in treating opioid withdrawal are the prevention of medical complications (for example, in medically ill patients) and the reduction of withdrawal symptoms to avoid a return to continued opioid abuse.
3. Methadone maintenance is the primary long-term treatment for opioid dependence, and most patients can be maintained on less than 60 mg a day. Blood methadone concentrations are helpful in determining the appropriate dosage. Patients taking methadone may feign symptoms of depression and request amitriptyline (Elavil), which, when taken with methadone, can produce euphoria.
4. Naltrexone (ReVia), a long-acting opioid antagonist, can be taken orally for up to two months to help patients maintain their abstinence from opioids.
5. Therapeutic communities (for example, Phoenix House), drug rehabilitation programs, and group therapy are all helpful for the rehabilitation of opioid-dependent patients.

DRUG TREATMENT

Determine that the objective signs of withdrawal are present and that the benefits of reducing those signs outweigh the risks of dispensing more opioids. If so, give methadone 10 mg by mouth, and repeat every four to six hours if the signs of withdrawal are still present. The total dosage in 24 hours should equal the dosage for the next day (seldom more than 40 mg). Decrease the dosage by 5 mg daily for heroin withdrawal. Detoxification from methadone may require a slower decrease in the dosage.

Pentazocine-dependent patients should be detoxified on pentazocine because of its mixed agonist-antagonist effects on various opioid receptors.

Clonidine (Catapres) is a centrally acting α_2-agonist that is used primarily for hypertension that may help relieve the patient's nausea, vomiting, and diarrhea. Give 0.1 to 0.2 mg every three hours as needed, but do not exceed 0.8 mg a day. Titrate according to the patient's symptoms, and taper over two weeks. Do not give clonidine if the patient's blood pressure is less than 90/60. Clonidine may cause hypotension, is short-acting, and is not habit-forming.

For a more detailed discussion of this topic, see J H Jaffe: Opioid-Related Disorders, Sec 13.9, p 842, in CTP/VI.

8.27. Phencyclidine (or Phencyclidinelike) Intoxication

Phencyclidine (PCP) intoxication consists of a constellation of signs, symptoms, and maladaptive behavior after the use of PCP.

CLINICAL FEATURES AND DIAGNOSIS

PCP is a hallucinogen belonging to the class of arylcyclohexylamines that were once called dissociative anesthetics. In addition to hallucinations and delusions, PCP produces belligerence, assaultiveness, agitation, impulsiveness, unpredictability, nystagmus (vertical or horizontal), hypertension, tachycardia, numbness or diminished response to pain, ataxia, dysarthria, muscle rigidity, hyperacusis, echolalia, staring into space, anticholinergic effects, and, in large doses, hyperthermia, seizures, extrapyramidal movement disorders, myoglobinuria, renal failure, delirium, and death. The degree of intoxication is dose-dependent.

PCP commonly causes paranoid ideation and unpredictable violence that brings the abuser to medical attention. PCP-induced psychotic states may be long-lasting in vulnerable persons. A delusional state may emerge one week after an overdose. The patient often has amnesia for the acute psychotic episode, which may be followed by an episode of depression. The psychosis can be persistent. Tolerance and a withdrawal syndrome consisting of lethargy, drug craving, and depression have been reported. Delirium can emerge up to a week after PCP is discontinued, possibly because of PCP's release from fat stores.

PCP is used as a veterinary anesthetic, and it also produces anesthesia in humans. Since PCP-intoxicated patients feel no pain, they are prone to injure themselves and those nearby. Abuse is widely prevalent because PCP is easily synthesized in illegal laboratories.

PCP may be administered orally, by sniffing, or intravenously (IV), although usually it is smoked in a tobacco or cannabis cigarette (a laced joint). Sometimes patients take PCP inadvertently by drinking PCP-containing punch at a party or by unknowingly smoking a laced joint, which can cause sudden, unpredicted behavior. Street names include PCP, peace pill, angel dust, crystal, peace, peace weed, supergrass, and superweed. A dose of PCP is impossible to assess accurately, and the dose in one cigarette may range from 1 to 250 mg. PCP is sometimes marketed as lysergic acid diethylamide (LSD), mescaline, or cannabis.

Intoxication symptoms can begin within five minutes of smoking or injecting and one hour after oral intake. Intoxication usually lasts three to six hours, although a full recovery may require one or two days. PCP is detectable in the patient's urine for more than a week after its use.

INTERVIEWING AND PSYCHOTHERAPEUTIC GUIDELINES

Do not try to talk down or reassure a PCP-intoxicated patient, who may be completely out of touch with the environment. Reduce the stimulation of the patient to a minimum. Provide psychiatric and medical treatment for potential behavioral and physiological complications.

EVALUATION AND MANAGEMENT

1. Take the patient's vital signs.
2. Assess whether PCP has been taken, using whatever history is available.
3. Determine if the patient appears to be psychotic, agitated, or out of contact with the environment.
4. Conduct a physical examination and a medical evaluation for such complications as hypertension, seizures, and vomiting.
5. Isolate the patient in a dark, quiet area—alone, if possible. Limit the number of staff members in the room unless the patient is potentially dangerous and requires physical intervention. Do not overstimulate the patient.
6. Avoid restraints if at all possible, since patients may injure themselves or others during the process of putting on the restraints and may also injure themselves in attempting to fight against limb restraints. Anesthetized PCP-intoxicated patients can break their own limbs trying to fight against limb restraints. They are also at risk for rhabdomyolysis.
7. If PCP was recently taken orally, gastric lavage may be of use in a patient who is relatively cooperative, although the risk of vomiting and aspiration should be considered.
8. Hospitalization may be needed for the medical, behavioral, or psychological sequelae of PCP intoxication.

DRUG TREATMENT

Acidification of the urine, which increases the renal excretion of PCP, is usually done with large doses (1 to 2 g) of ascorbic acid (vitamin C) or cranberry juice. However, PCP is stored in fatty tissues (including the brain), where it has usually been deposited by the time the patient comes for treatment, so increasing renal clearance may not bring about clinical improvement; nonetheless, it is common clinical practice, since it is relatively devoid of complications.

Benzodiazepines—for example, lorazepam (Ativan) 1 to 2 mg given intramuscularly (IM), diazepam (Valium) 5 to 10 mg by mouth or IV, oxazepam (Serax) 10 to 30 mg by mouth, and estazolam (ProSom) 0.5 to 1 mg by mouth—are the drugs of choice for agitation, since they raise the seizure threshold and do not cause anticholinergic effects. The dose may be repeated as necessary unless signs of benzodiazepine toxicity are present (for example, worsened dysarthria or ataxia).

Antipsychotics are also a possibility, especially after several doses of benzodiazepines have been ineffective. High-potency antipsychotics—for example, fluphenazine (Prolixin), thiothixene (Navane), and haloperidol (Haldol), all given at 2 to 5 mg IM—are preferable because they cause fewer anticholinergic effects than do low-potency antipsychotics. Since PCP itself can cause anticholinergic effects or seizures, low-potency antipsychotics should be avoided.

A combination of a benzodiazepine and an antipsychotic (for example, lorazepam 2 mg and haloperidol 5 mg) has also been used with some success. Some clinicians believe that the combination is more effective than either drug alone.

For a more detailed discussion of this topic, see T J Crowley: Phencyclidine (or Phencyclidinelike)-Related Disorders, Sec 13.10, p 864, in CTP/VI.

8.28. Phenylpropanolamine (Diet Pill) Toxicity

Agitation, paranoia, psychosis, anxiety, headache, dizziness, insomnia, restlessness, tachycardia, and hypertension may be induced by an excessive dose of phenylpropanolamine.

CLINICAL FEATURES AND DIAGNOSIS

Phenylpropanolamine is found in over-the-counter cold medications and appetite suppressants. It is most commonly used as a decongestant. Phenylpropanolamine is a sympathomimetic amine with properties similar to those of ephedrine. A moderate dose does not usually cause signs of intoxication.

INTERVIEWING AND PSYCHOTHERAPEUTIC GUIDELINES

Reassure the patient that the symptoms are induced by the drug and will resolve as the drug is cleared, usually in four to six hours. Educate the patient about the importance of avoiding an excessive dose. With patients taking phenylpropanolamine for appetite suppression, evaluate the patient for a possible eating disorder.

EVALUATION AND MANAGEMENT

1. Discontinue the medication containing the phenylpropanolamine.
2. Evaluate the patient for possible toxic drug interactions with monoamine oxidase inhibitors (MAOIs), anticholinergics, and caffeine.

DRUG TREATMENT

Benzodiazepines—for example, lorazepam (Ativan) 0.5 to 1 mg by mouth, diazepam (Valium) 5 to 10 mg by mouth, oxazepam (Serax) 10 to 30 mg by mouth, chlordiazepoxide (Librium) 10 to 25 mg by mouth, and alprazolam (Xanax) 0.5 to 1 mg by mouth, all given every three to four hours as needed—may be used for severe restlessness, anxiety, or insomnia.

For a more detailed discussion of this topic, see T C Manschreck: Delusional Disorder and Shared Psychotic Disorder, Sec 15.2, p 1031, in CTP/VI.

8.29. Psychotropic Drug Withdrawal

The symptoms of *psychotropic drug withdrawal* are associated with the abrupt discontinuation or the rapid decrease in the dosage of a psychotropic medication that has been taken steadily for weeks or longer.

CLINICAL FEATURES AND DIAGNOSIS

The common symptoms include insomnia, anxiety, agitation, weakness, chills, and pain. Withdrawal from psychotropic drugs capable of producing tolerance and dependence (for example, benzodiazepines and other sedative-hypnotics) can produce delirium and seizures. Withdrawal from antipsychotics can cause withdrawal dyskinesias and may unmask or worsen tardive dyskinesia. Withdrawal from antipsychotics or antidepressants with prominent anticholinergic effects (or from anticholinergic drugs themselves) can cause sinus tachycardia, ventricular arrhythmias, and cholinergic rebound, causing flulike symptoms.

Psychotropic drug withdrawal does not refer only to true withdrawal syndromes, like those encountered with substances that cause pharmacological dependence. Rather, the term is used to describe any syndrome that can develop when a drug is decreased or discontinued.

Discontinuation of the drug may be necessary because of side effects, allergic reactions, or other toxic effects. Although most psychotropic drugs do not cause pharmacological dependence and withdrawal, symptoms of rebound often occur. Since most psychotropic drugs are central nervous system (CNS) depressants, the most common symptoms of psychotropic drug withdrawal are insomnia and anxiety.

TABLE 8.29-1
COMMONLY OBSERVED WITHDRAWAL SYMPTOMS (BENZODIAZEPINE WITHDRAWAL SYNDROME)

Anxiety
Irritability
Insomnia
Fatigue
Headache
Muscle twitching or aching
Tremor, shakiness
Sweating
Dizziness
Concentration difficulties

*Nausea, loss of appetite
*Observable depression
*Depersonalization, derealization
*Increased sensory perception (smell, sight, taste, touch)
*Abnormal perception or sensation of movement

*Symptoms likely to represent true withdrawal, rather than an exacerbation or the return of the original anxiety.
Table from P P Roy-Byrne, D Hommer: Benzodiazepine withdrawal: Overview and implications for the treatment of anxiety. Am J Med *84:* 1041, 1988. Used with permission.

INTERVIEWING AND PSYCHOTHERAPEUTIC GUIDELINES

Reassure the patient that the symptoms of psychotropic drug withdrawal are neither proof that the drug is absolutely necessary nor proof that drug dependence has become a problem. Inform the patient that the symptoms are usually self-limited, will end in a few days, and can be reduced by a slower lowering of the drug dosage.

EVALUATION AND MANAGEMENT

1. Determine what drugs the patient is taking, including prescribed drugs, over-the-counter drugs, alcohol, and drugs of abuse.
2. Consider whether the patient is pharmacologically dependent on alcohol, benzodiazepines, barbiturates, or other sedative-hypnotics. Withdrawal from those substances is potentially dangerous and requires active intervention. The severity of the withdrawal from benzodiazepines is related to the drug's pharmacokinetics (Table 8.29-1). Dependence on benzodiazepines with short elimination half-lives can lead to abrupt and severe withdrawal symptoms.
3. Determine whether the psychotropic drug must be discontinued immediately or whether a slow taper over a period of weeks is possible. If a slow taper of the drug is possible, the withdrawal symptoms may disappear altogether.
4. If necessary, treat the withdrawal symptoms with other medications, as described below.

DRUG TREATMENT

Withdrawal from alcohol, benzodiazepines, barbiturates, and other sedative-hypnotics is usually treated with long-acting benzodiazepines, although some psychiatrists prefer to detoxify benzodiazepine-dependent patients by using the drug on which they are dependent.

Sinus tachycardia and ventricular arrhythmias after the abrupt discontinuation of antidepressants or highly anticholinergic antipsychotics can be treated with anticholinergic drugs, including atropine and oral anticholinergics—for example, benztropine (Cogentin) 1 to 2 mg by mouth twice a day.

Withdrawal syndromes that develop when antipsychotics or antidepressants are suddenly discontinued can be minimized if the drug is gradually tapered over several weeks.

For a more detailed discussion of this topic, see Biological Therapies, Chap 32, pp 1895–2150, in CTP/VI.

8.30. Inhalant Intoxication and Withdrawal

Hydrocarbon solvents occur in many products in varying combinations and concentrations (Table 8.30-1). Toluene or methylbenzene is a volatile solvent readily available in glue, paint, and shoe polish. Another commonly available and highly toxic inhalant is trichloroethane, an ingredient of liquid paper correction fluid. Persons abusing these substances will place some in a bag and inhale the fumes. The practice is known as sniffing, bagging, and huffing. The inhaled substances are rapidly absorbed, and the effects are virtually immediate. A drunken presentation is most common.

CLINICAL FEATURES AND DIAGNOSIS

Inhalant intoxication is diagnosed according to the criteria in Table 8.30-2. The symptoms begin within five minutes of intake and resolve in one to two hours.

TABLE 8.30-1
COMPOSITION OF ABUSED HYDROCARBON SOLVENTS

Inhalant	Chemical Constituents
Acrylic paint	Toluene
Aerosols	Fluorocarbons, nitrous oxide
Dyes	Acetone, methylene chloride
Gasoline	Hydrocarbons, tetraethyl lead
Glues and adhesives	Toluene, benzene, xylene, acetone, naphtha, n-hexane, trichloroethylene, tetrachloroethylene, trichloroethane, carbon tetrachloride
Lighter fuel	Butane
Nail polish remover	Acetone, amyl acetate
Paints, varnishes, and lacquers	Trichloroethylene, methylene chloride, toluene
Polystyrene cements	Acetone, toluene, trichloroethylene, hexane
Rubber cement	Benzene, hexane, trichloroethylene
Shoe polish	Chlorinated hydrocarbons, toluene
Spot remover	Trichloroethane, trichloroethylene, carbon tetrachloride
Typewriter correction fluid	Trichloroethane, trichloroethylene, perchloroethylene

Table from L R Goldfrank, A G Kulberg, EA Bresnitz: Occupational and environmental toxins. In *Goldrank's Toxicologic Emergencies*, L Goldfrank, N E Flomenbaum, N A Lewin, R S Weisman, M A Howland, editors, p 764. Appleton Lange, Norwalk, Conn, 1990.
Adapted from J A Vale, T J Meredith: Solvent abuse. In *Clinical Management of Poisoning and Overdose*, L Haddad, J Winchester, editors, p 801. Saunders, Philadelphia, 1982, and D G Wyse: Deliberate inhalation of volatile hydrocarbons: A review. *Can Med Assoc J 108:* 71, 1973. Used with permission.

Inhalants are generally not drugs of choice but are used by young persons when other drugs are not readily available or affordable. Inhalant abuse is usually a group social activity. The relatively few solitary sniffers are often heavy users who are psychologically disturbed. Schizoid features are common in those users. Some tolerance and dependence may develop with chronic use.

The physical signs include swollen, red eyes; blurred vision; tremor; ataxia; hyporeflexia; diplopia; residue on the face, the hands, and the clothes; irritation of the nose, the lungs, and the throat; a rash around the nose and the mouth; and breath odors.

The sequelae are serious and involve multiple systems. Inhalant abuse is associated with hepatic, pulmonary, muscular, cardiac, immunological, renal, and neurological damage. Static encephalopathy results from both the hydrocarbons and the lead present in some paints. The cerebellum can be damaged from long-term use. Occasional deaths by asphyxiation have occurred when the user became confused and failed to uncover the nose and the mouth.

Because of the serious acute and chronic effects of hydrocarbon inhalants, they are considered separately from the volatile nitrates (discussed in section 8.31), which follow the same route of administration but are different in their effects and treatment.

Withdrawal after long-term heavy use may produce such symptoms as delusions, agitation, disorientation, tachycardia, tremulousness, seizures, and hallucinations. Symptoms of withdrawal begin within hours to days after the discontinuation of toluene use.

INTERVIEWING AND PSYCHOTHERAPEUTIC GUIDELINES

Subtle cognitive deficits may be present in substance abusers who are not currently intoxicated. Preexisting organic conditions are common in patients who are

---

TABLE 8.30–2
DIAGNOSTIC CRITERIA FOR INHALANT INTOXICATION

A. Recent intentional use or short-term, high-dose exposure to volatile inhalants (excluding anesthetic gases and short-acting vasodilators).
B. Clinically significant maladaptive behavioral or psychological changes (e.g., belligerence, assaultiveness, apathy, impaired judgment, impaired social or occupational functioning) that developed during, or shortly after, use of or exposure to volatile inhalants.
C. Two (or more) of the following signs, developing during, or shortly after, inhalant use or exposure:
   (1) dizziness
   (2) nystagmus
   (3) incoordination
   (4) slurred speech
   (5) unsteady gait
   (6) lethargy
   (7) depressed reflexes
   (8) psychomotor retardation
   (9) tremor
   (10) generalized muscle weakness
   (11) blurred vision or diplopia
   (12) stupor or coma
   (13) euphoria
D. The symptoms are not due to a general medical condition and are not better accounted for by another mental disorder.

heavy users, and the relative contributions of the premorbid condition and heavy use may be difficult to establish without detailed testing.

If organicity is present, the physician should speak in simple terms, using repetition as needed. Simple explanations of the procedures provide support and reassurance.

EVALUATION AND MANAGEMENT

1. As with other intoxications, restraints may be necessary to prevent injury to the patient or others. Neurological sequelae are not progressive once the offending agent is removed.
2. A thorough medical evaluation—including a complete blood count, blood urea nitrogen, liver function tests, creatinine and toxicology screen—should be performed because of possible organ system damage and multiple substance abuse.
3. Abstinence is the only treatment. No services are specifically devoted to those who abuse inhalants. Inhalant abusers most often use multiple substances and qualify for placement according to the drug abused.

DRUG TREATMENT

As with other forms of intoxication, antipsychotics have no advantage and may aggravate organic presentations of inhalant abuse. Agitation may be safely managed with lorazepam (Ativan) 1 to 2 mg parenterally, repeated as necessary at 30-minute intervals until the patient is calm. Withdrawal can also be treated with lorazepam 1 to 2 mg by mouth, intramuscularly (IM), or intravenously (IV) repeated every 30 minutes as needed until the patient is calm.

For a more detailed discussion of this topic, see T J Crowley: Inhalant-Related Disorders, Sec 13.8, p 838, in CTP/VI.

8.31. Volatile Nitrates

The *volatile nitrates,* principally amyl nitrite and isobutyl nitrite (both also known as poppers), are liquid inhalants that are used as aphrodisiacs and stimulants. The desired effects are a relaxed anal sphincter, delayed ejaculation, and euphoria. Approximately half of all volatile nitrate abusers find the experience unpleasant because of the resulting throbbing headache, nausea, and lightheadedness or syncope. The effect is brief, so patients do not present with acute nitrate intoxication. However, nitrates are often used with other substances and in the setting of other high-risk behaviors. Methemoglobinemia may occur in vulnerable persons. There is no associated abstinence syndrome.

Although the route of administration is similar to that of hydrocarbon inhalants, the toxicity of hydrocarbon inhalants is much greater than that of volatile nitrates.

CLINICAL FEATURES AND DIAGNOSIS

The signs and symptoms of nitrate abuse are related to smooth muscle relaxation and include intense peripheral vasodilation, flushing, hypotension, and reflex tachycardia. Subjectively, the effect is experienced as warmth, a rapid pulse, throbbing headache, and dizziness. Cerebral vasodilation results in a pulsatile headache. Nitrates are also irritants and may cause tracheobronchitis. Crusty skin lesions may be noted around the nose and the lips. Long-term users have a yellowish facial tint. Nitrates are flammable liquids, and burns may result. Foreign bodies may be lodged in the rectum resulting from sexual activity associated with nitrate use.

In patients with defective heme-reducing systems, methemoglobinemia is a potentially fatal consequence of exposure to nitrates. Patients with methemoglobinemia present with cyanosis and respiratory distress that is unresponsive to oxygen therapy. The arterial blood appears to be chocolate brown, although the partial pressure of oxygen (pO_2) remains normal. Transient ST segment and T wave changes may be present on the electrocardiogram (ECG).

INTERVIEWING AND PSYCHOTHERAPEUTIC GUIDELINES

Nitrate abuse has declined as a result of (1) its association with unsafe-sex practices that may spread the human immunodeficiency virus (HIV) and (2) its criminalization in some jurisdictions. Nitrate abusers are at risk for other substance abuse; the patient's drug of choice may be marijuana, alcohol, stimulants, or (least likely) hallucinogens. Obtain a thorough substance-abuse history from the patient. Sexual activity involving nitrate abuse should prompt a thorough sexual history.

EVALUATION AND MANAGEMENT

1. In most patients, the symptoms pass quickly after cessation of nitrate use, and no specific treatment is indicated.
2. Drug counseling should be emphasized, taking advantage of any current adverse consequences to promote efforts to enroll the patient in rehabilitation.
3. Human immunodeficiency virus (HIV) testing and AIDS education may be indicated.

DRUG TREATMENT

Mild methemoglobinemia resolves within 24 to 72 hours with conservative management. If angina or an altered mental state occurs or if methemoglobinemia exceeds 30 percent, methylene blue 1 to 2 mg per kilogram of body weight as a 1 percent solution may be administered intravenously (IV) over five minutes.

For a more detailed discussion of this topic, see J H Jaffe: Introduction and Overview, Sec 13.1, p 755, in CTP/VI.

9

Schizophrenia and Other Psychotic Disorders

9.1 Brief Psychotic Disorder

Brief psychotic disorder is a diagnosis for patients who experience psychotic symptoms lasting for less than one month in response to some identifiable stressor.

CLINICAL FEATURES AND DIAGNOSIS

The psychotic symptoms may include disorganization, incoherence, loosening of associations, hallucinations, delusions, and catatonic behavior. Affective symptoms may be more common than the classic schizophrenic symptoms. While the patient's mental status may be indistinguishable from that of a patient with schizophrenia or a psychotic mood disorder, the diagnosis hinges on the history of brief duration and an identifiable stressor (Table 9.1-1).

Features suggesting a good prognosis are similar to those for schizophrenia a severe stressor, sudden onset, prominent mood symptoms, good premorbid functioning, the absence of schizoid traits, the absence of a family history of schizophrenia, symptoms that cause subjective distress, and little blunting of affect.

TABLE 9.1-1
DIAGNOSTIC CRITERIA FOR BRIEF PSYCHOTIC DISORDER

A. Presence of one (or more) of the following symptoms:
   (1) delusions
   (2) hallucinations
   (3) disorganized speech (e.g., frequent derailment or incoherence)
   (4) grossly disorganized or catatonic behavior
   Note: Do not include a symptom if it is a culturally sanctioned response pattern.
B. Duration of an episode of the disturbance is at least 1 day but less than 1 month, with eventual full return to premorbid level of functioning.
C. The disturbance is not better accounted for by a mood disorder with psychotic features, schizoaffective disorder, or schizophrenia and is not due to the direct physiological effects of a substance (e.g., a drug of abuse, a medication) or a general medical condition.

Specify if:
   With marked stressor(s) (brief reactive psychosis): if symptoms occur shortly after and apparently in response to events that, singly or together, would be markedly stressful to almost anyone in similar circumstances in the person's culture
   Without marked stressor(s): if psychotic symptoms do *not* occur shortly after, or are not apparently in response to events that, singly or together, would be markedly stressful to almost anyone in similar circumstances in the person's culture
   With postpartum onset: if onset within 4 weeks postpartum

Table from DSM-IV, *Diagnostic and Statistical Manual of Mental Disorders*, ed 4. Copyright American Psychiatric Association, Washington, 1994. Used with permission.

INTERVIEWING AND PSYCHOTHERAPEUTIC GUIDELINES

Take a structured empathic approach. Keep the questions simple but, initially, open-ended. Thought-disordered patients may need gentle redirection and structuring. Explore the patient's experience of the psychotic symptoms without confronting the unreality of the symptoms. Use a flexible approach to obtain essential information without adhering to a rigid interview structure; usually the psychotic patient cannot accommodate such an interview. When offering medication to patients with limited insight, indicate that the medication can help them feel calm and think clearly.

EVALUATION AND MANAGEMENT

1. Rule out any possible organic causes. A rapid change in the patient's mental status suggests organicity. Obtain the patient's vital signs, a detailed history of alcohol and drug abuse, and a history of prescribed and over-the-counter drugs. Many drugs can also cause psychosis, including hallucinogenic drugs, (especially phencyclidine [PCP] and lysergic acid diethylamide [LSD]), steroids, antidepressants, and many prescribed medications, including most psychotropic drugs. The patient's thyroid function should be evaluated: both hyperthyroidism and hypothyroidism can cause psychosis. A complete workup for delirium or dementia may also be necessary.
2. Hospitalization is usually indicated. Even if the symptoms can be controlled with medication in the physician's office, a thorough evaluation can seldom be completed without hospitalization.
3. A determination of the patient's premorbid personality traits may be helpful. Brief psychotic disorder often occurs in patients with borderline, schizotypal, narcissistic, histrionic, and paranoid personality disorders. Borderline, narcissistic, or histrionic personality disorder traits indicate that depression should be considered.
4. The patient should be referred for psychotherapy. The approach depends on the needs of the patient and often focuses on recovery in the postpsychotic period. Patients who are very upset by the psychotic episode and have lost self-confidence may benefit from supportive, cognitive, family, or group therapy.

DRUG TREATMENT

The two classes of drugs to be considered are the dopamine receptor antagonist antipsychotic drugs and the benzodiazepines. When an antipsychotic is chosen, a high-potency antipsychotic—for example, 2 to 5 mg of haloperidol (Haldol) as needed—is usually used. Especially in patients who are at high risk for the development of medication-induced movement disorders, the coadministration of an anticholinergic drug should be considered. Alternatively, benzodiazepines (for example, as-needed doses of 10 to 30 mg of oxazepam [Serax], 0.5 to 1 mg of estazolam [ProSom] or alprazolam [Xanax], or 1 to 2 mg of lorazepam [Ativan]) can be used in the short-term treatment of psychosis. Although these drugs have limited usefulness in the long-term treatment of psychotic disorders, they can be effective for a short time and are associated with fewer side effects than are the antipsychotics.

Avoid the long-term use of any medication to treat brief psychotic disorder. If maintenance medication is necessary, the clinician may have to reconsider the diagnosis.

For a more detailed discussion of this topic, see S G Siris, M R Lavin: Schizoaffective Disorder, Schizophreniform Disorder, and Brief Psychotic Disorder, Sec 15.1, p 1019, in CTP/VI.

9.2 Catatonic Schizophrenia

Catatonic schizophrenia is a type of schizophrenia characterized by muscular rigidity (catatonia), negativism, and stupor or excitement.

CLINICAL FEATURES AND DIAGNOSIS

The signs and the symptoms of catatonic schizophrenia include mutism, excitement, waxy flexibility, stupor, stupor alternating with excitement, negativism, mannerisms, and stereotypies (Table 9.2-1). Mood disorders can present as catatonia. The differential diagnosis also includes organically caused coma, toxic psychosis, antipsychotic-induced rigidity and akinesia, conversion disorder, dissociative states, malingering, and factitious disorders.

INTERVIEWING AND PSYCHOTHERAPEUTIC GUIDELINES

Remember that unresponsive catatonic patients are awake and aware. Explain all actions and procedures to them. The patients often fully remember what happened and what was said during their stupor.

EVALUATION AND MANAGEMENT

1. Rule out any medical illness presenting as catatonic decompensation (for example, neuroleptic malignant syndrome).

TABLE 9.2–1
DIAGNOSTIC CRITERIA FOR CATATONIC TYPE

A type of schizophrenia in which the clinical picture is dominated by at least two of the following:
  (1) motoric immobility as evidenced by catalepsy (including waxy flexibility) or stupor
  (2) excessive motor activity (that is apparently purposeless and not influenced by external stimuli)
  (3) extreme negativism (an apparently motiveless resistance to all instructions or maintenance of a rigid posture against attempts to be moved) or mutism
  (4) peculiarities of voluntary movement as evidenced by posturing (voluntary assumption of inappropriate or bizarre postures), stereotyped movements, prominent mannerisms, or prominent grimacing
  (5) echolalia or echopraxia

Table from DSM-IV, *Diagnostic and Statistical Manual of Mental Disorders*, ed 4. Copyright American Psychiatric Association, Washington, 1994. Used with permission.

2. Assess the patient for the side effects of medications, with particular attention to antipsychotic-induced akinesia, which can resemble catatonia. Rule out comorbid substance abuse.
3. Conduct a psychiatric evaluation to confirm the diagnosis. The patient's history obtained from collateral informants is particularly important.
4. Catatonic patients may need treatment for self-inflicted injuries, malnutrition, dehydration, exhaustion, or hyperpyrexia.
5. Provide a safe environment for the patient and for staff members because catatonic patients can unpredictably erupt into an excited, violent state. Restraint and sedation may be needed.
6. Evaluate the patient for psychosocial stressors that may have led to an exacerbation. Has the patient's living situation changed? Was the patient traumatized?
7. Evaluate the patient for depression, which may be contributing to the catatonic decompensation.
8. Hospitalization may be needed. Catatonic patients are at serious risk for impulsive violence and are often unable to meet their own basic needs.

DRUG TREATMENT

Emergency treatment consists of an antipsychotic, such as fluphenazine (Prolixin) 2 to 5 mg intramuscularly (IM), haloperidol (Haldol) 2 to 5 mg IM, thiothixene (Navane) 5 mg IM, or trifluoperazine (Stelazine) 5 mg IM, all given every 30 minutes as needed. Lorazepam (Ativan) 1 to 2 mg IM every four to six hours may also be useful for treating the patient's catatonia.

For a more detailed discussion of this topic, see A A Lipton, R Cancro: Schizophrenia: Clinical Features, Sec 14.7, p 968, in CTP/VI.

9.3 Delusional Disorder

Delusional disorder is characterized by false fixed beliefs not subject to reality testing. *Paranoia* is characterized by delusions or suspiciousness of grandeur, control, or persecution.

CLINICAL FEATURES AND DIAGNOSIS

In delusional disorder, delusions are of at least one month's duration and are well systematized as opposed to bizarre or fragmented. The patient's emotional response to the delusional system is congruent with and appropriate to the content of the delusion. The personality remains intact or deteriorates minimally. Patients often are hypersensitive and hypervigilant, which may lead, despite their high-functioning capacities, to a relatively socially isolated existence.

TABLE 9.3-1
DIAGNOSTIC CRITERIA FOR DELUSIONAL DISORDER

A. Nonbizarre delusions (i.e., involving situations that occur in real life, such as being followed, poisoned, infected, loved at a distance, or deceived by spouse or lover, or having a disease) of at least 1 month's duration.
B. Criterion A for schizophrenia has never been met. **Note:** Tactile and olfactory hallucinations may be present in delusional disorder if they are related to the delusional theme.
C. Apart from the impact of the delusion(s) or its ramifications, functioning is not markedly impaired and behavior is not obviously odd or bizarre.
D. If mood episodes have occurred concurrently with delusions, their total duration has been brief relative to the duration of the delusional periods.
E. The disturbance is not due to the direct physiological effects of a substance (e.g., a drug of abuse, a medication) or a general medical condition.

Specify type (the following types are assigned based on the predominant delusional theme):
  Erotomanic type: delusions that another person, usually of higher status, is in love with the individual
  Grandiose type: delusions of inflated worth, power, knowledge, identity, or special relationship to a deity or famous person
  Jealous type: delusions that the individual's sexual partner is unfaithful
  Persecutory type: delusions that the person (or someone to whom the person is close) is being malevolently treated in some way
  Somatic type: delusions that the person has some physical defect or general medical condition
  Mixed type: delusions characteristic of more than one of the above types but no one theme predominates
  Unspecified type

Table from DSM-IV, *Diagnostic and Statistical Manual of Mental Disorders*, ed 4. Copyright American Psychiatric Association, Washington, 1994. Used with permission.

The patients are comparatively free of psychopathology in areas other than the delusional system (Table 9.3-1). The onset is often in middle or late adult life.

INTERVIEWING AND PSYCHOTHERAPEUTIC GUIDELINES

Do not argue with or challenge the patient's delusions. A delusion may become even more entrenched if the patient feels that its defense is necessary. Examine life stresses that precipitated the patient's treatment. If treatment is indicated, explain the rationale to the patient.

The main objectives in the initial interview are to gain the patient's trust, determine the patient's level of impairment, and consider other diagnoses, such as depression, mania, schizophrenia, substance abuse (for example, cocaine), and medical conditions.

EVALUATION AND MANAGEMENT

1. The patient's drug history and a physical and neurological examination can help identify possible organic causes.
2. Patients with suicidal or homicidal ideation may require hospitalization.
3. Outpatient treatment is difficult because of poor patient cooperation, but individual psychotherapy may be helpful. An early goal is to enlist the patient's trust and then to focus on the impairments caused by the delusional system. Work toward eliminating the delusions.

DRUG TREATMENT

Treat acute agitation with benzodiazepines, such as lorazepam (Ativan) 1 to 2 mg by mouth or intramuscularly (IM), or antipsychotics, such as haloperidol (Haldol) 2 to 5 mg by mouth or IM.

Although antipsychotics are currently considered the drugs of choice for maintenance therapy, adequate proof of their efficacy is lacking. If a coexisting mood disorder exists, antidepressants, lithium (Eskalith), or carbamazepine (Tegretol) may be used. Pimozide (Orap) may also be of use.

For a more detailed discussion of this topic, see T C Manschreck: Delusional Disorder and Shared Psychotic Disorder, Sec 15.2, p 1031, in CTP/VI.

9.4 Grandiosity

Grandiosity is an exaggerated feeling of importance, power, knowledge, or identity. It can range from a mild exaggeration of a true characteristic to psychotic delusions of grandeur. The content of the delusion may be that the patient has made some important discovery or possesses some unrecognized talent or great wealth. Sometimes grandiose delusions are religious and involve beliefs that the patient has a special relationship with God or is on an important religious mission.

CLINICAL FEATURES AND DIAGNOSIS

Grandiose delusions occur in mania, schizophrenia, or delusional disorder resulting from intoxication with cocaine, amphetamine, or hallucinogens. The most important goals of evaluating grandiosity are determining the severity, the duration, and the cause.

INTERVIEWING AND PSYCHOTHERAPEUTIC GUIDELINES

Grandiose patients are often easily engaged in an interview if allowed to discuss the content of their grandiose beliefs, although some manic patients may be irritable and uncooperative. Do not challenge the patient's beliefs, even if they are obviously false. However, do not agree that they are true. If the patient asks directly "Don't you believe I can fly?", the best response that primary care physicians can make is that they do not know, that they understand the patient believes it, and that the belief will be investigated further.

The interview is an important time to try to determine the severity and the duration of the grandiose ideas. Is the patient grandiose about other areas? Explore for paranoid thoughts. Some paranoid ideas have a grandiose core—that is, paranoid patients believe that they are important enough for others to be against them. Try to assess the impairment caused by the grandiose ideas.

EVALUATION AND MANAGEMENT

1. Evaluate the degree of impairment. Delusional patients may have such impaired judgment that they are dangerous to self or others and require hospitalization, involuntarily if necessary. Does the patient plan to act on the grandiose beliefs? Has the patient fought with people who challenge the grandiose convictions? Are there homicidal plans? Is the patient at risk of self-harm because of the nature of the grandiose delusions?
2. Rule out medical causes, especially if the patient is psychotic or if the symptoms are new in a patient without a history of similar episodes. The patient's drug history, a urine drug screening, and a complete list of the medications taken are mandatory. Prescribed drugs (for example, steroids, tricyclic antidepressants, monoamine oxidase inhibitors [MAOIs], L-dopa, and phenylephrine) can cause grandiose delusions. Metabolic and endocrine disorders, withdrawal from alcohol or sedative-hypnotics, and other drug-related conditions should be considered. Are the patient's vital signs normal?
3. Make a definitive diagnosis. Focus on the severity, the duration, and the related symptoms. Mildly grandiose patients who have been that way for many years may fulfill the diagnostic criteria for narcissistic, borderline, histrionic, or paranoid personality disorder. Determine whether other long-standing maladaptive patterns are present. Patients who have a persistent and well-circumscribed grandiose delusional system, who are not depressed or manic, and who do not have either prominent hallucinations or bizarre delusions may receive a diagnosis of delusional disorder, grandiose type.
4. Disposition depends on the diagnosis, the severity of the symptoms, and the availability of treatment options. If the patient has a possible medical disorder, he or she may need hospitalization for a complete workup. A psychiatric consultation should be obtained. If the patient is psychotic, determine the likelihood that the patient will go to the psychiatrist and cooperate in evaluation and treatment. Find out if family members can supervise the patient and bring the patient to outpatient appointments.

DRUG TREATMENT

Drug treatment depends on a definitive diagnosis. Acute agitation may require tranquilization with a benzodiazepine (for example, oxazepam [Serax] 10 to 30 mg by mouth, estazolam [ProSom] 0.5 to 1 mg by mouth, lorazepam [Ativan] 1 to 2 mg by mouth or intramuscularly [IM]) or, if the patient is psychotic, an antipsychotic—for example, 2 to 5 mg by mouth or IM doses of trifluoperazine (Stelazine), thiothixene (Navane), fluphenazine (Prolixin), or haloperidol (Haldol). Focus the drug treatment of patients with personality disorders on specific symptoms. Delusional disorders are generally treated with antipsychotics. Mania and schizophrenia also require a psychopharmacological treatment plan.

For a more detailed discussion of this topic, see H S Akiskal: Mood Disorders: Clinical Features, Sec 16.6, p 1123; J G Gunderson, K A Phillips: Personality Disorders, Chap 25, p 1425, in CTP/VI.

9.5 Hallucinations

Hallucinations are false sensory perceptions occurring in the absence of any external stimulus. They are distinguished from distortions and illusions, which involve misperceptions of real stimuli. The patient perceives the hallucination, at least temporarily, as real.

CLINICAL FEATURES AND DIAGNOSIS

Clearly identify the specific sensory modalities (for example, auditory, visual, tactile, olfactory, and gustatory) in which the hallucinations occur. The duration, the circumstances, and the interpretation of the significance of the hallucinations are important. Identify the patient's past hallucinatory experiences and delusional interpretations (fixed false beliefs). Hallucinations often occur in multiple sensory modalities and are usually associated with delusions.

Hallucinations are psychotic symptoms; their presence requires a diagnosis before treatment is initiated. Visual, olfactory, and gustatory hallucinations are most common in organic disorders (for example, temporal lobe epilepsy). Tactile hallucinations of bugs crawling on or under the skin (formications) are common in cocaine intoxication and in withdrawal from alcohol and sedative-hypnotics. Hallucinations that occur only when the patient is falling asleep (hypnagogic) or waking up (hypnopompic) are generally considered nonpathological.

Intoxication with hallucinogens, cocaine, amphetamines, or other stimulants can cause hallucinations, as can withdrawal from alcohol and sedative-hypnotics. Many medications can cause hallucinations as a side effect. Organic conditions such as epilepsy are commonly associated with hallucinations. Delirium may have hallucinations as a feature. Drugs used to treat Parkinson's disease (for example, levodopa [Larodopa]) can cause hallucinations.

Hallucinations are also symptoms of several psychiatric disorders, such as schizophrenia, schizophreniform disorder, schizoaffective disorder, mania, depression with psychotic features, borderline personality disorder, brief reactive psychosis, and induced psychotic disorder. In unusual circumstances and in some cultures, certain hallucinations are normal—for example, hearing the voice or seeing an image of a deceased loved one during grief and bereavement. Typically, though, the patient recognizes that those hallucinations are not real. Patients may pretend to have hallucinations in certain situations (for example, to escape prosecution).

INTERVIEWING AND PSYCHOTHERAPEUTIC GUIDELINES

As with any psychotic patient, do not directly challenge the symptom, even if the patient seems uncertain about whether it is real. Do not say, for example, "You know those voices aren't real, don't you?" Observe whether the hallucination distresses the patient. Is it an extremely foreign experience, or is it something that the patient seems familiar with? If the patient seems to be responding to internal stimuli during the interview, ask what the patient is seeing or hearing. Is the content of the hallucination congruent with the patient's mood? Focus on obtaining a history that provides most of the information necessary for a diagnosis. Ask about command hallucinations—whether auditory hallucinations come from inside or outside the patient's head—since true auditory hallucinations are usually perceived as coming from outside one's head. Ask how the patient copes with the hallucinations.

EVALUATION AND MANAGEMENT

1. Evaluate the patient for possible medical and neurological conditions: for example, delirium, hyperthyroidism or hypothyroidism, epilepsy, or a central nervous system (CNS) infection. Identified medical conditions should be reversed or treated accordingly.
2. A drug history (including prescribed, over-the-counter, and drugs of abuse) and a urine drug test will help in determining whether drug intoxication or withdrawal is the cause or whether the hallucination is a drug side effect.
3. Does the patient have a history of a primary psychiatric condition of which the hallucinations are a symptom? If so, what has been the course of the disorder? Have previous episodes been characterized by similar hallucinations? Is the patient coming to treatment attention because the hallucinations have increased in frequency or intensity?
4. Dangerous psychiatric patients require hospitalization, even involuntary commitment. A patient might contemplate a dangerous act in response to the hallucinations (for example, committing suicide to obey the voices).
5. Severely psychotic patients and those who are unable to care for themselves may also require hospitalization. Consider whether the patient is participating in and compliant with outpatient treatment, whether such resources as family, friends, and shelter are available, and whether other aspects of the case (for example, withdrawal from alcohol or drugs, medical complications, and neurological conditions) warrant hospital admission.
6. Refer patients who are not dangerous or severely disorganized to outpatient psychiatric treatment.

DRUG TREATMENT

Hallucinations expected to resolve rapidly (for example, hallucinogen intoxication and hallucinations during grief and bereavement) may be treated with benzodiazepines. The tranquilization of agitated patients can be achieved with benzodiazepines or antipsychotics, both of which produce rapid behavioral control.

Antipsychotics, lithium (Eskalith), and anticonvulsants are usually not initiated in the primary care setting and should, instead, be started when the patient is in ongoing psychiatric treatment, since the effective use of those drugs requires time and compliance.

For a more detailed discussion of this topic, see E D Caine, H Grossman, J M Lyness: Delirium, Dementia, and Amnestic and Other Cognitive Disorders and Mental Disorders Due to a General Medical Condition, Chap 12, p 705; Substance-Related Disorders, Chap 13, pp 755–1018; A A Lipton, R Cancro: Schizophrenia: Clinical Features, Sec 14.7, p 968, in CTP/VI.

9.6 Ideas of Reference

Ideas of reference occur when patients misinterpret external events, as directly related to themselves.

CLINICAL FEATURES AND DIAGNOSIS

Although ideas of reference may occur occasionally in anyone, they are common in paranoid patients and may be the initial nidus for a paranoid delusional system. If the ideas of reference are severe or persistent or become organized into a well-formed system, they become delusions of reference. Typical ideas of reference include "People are talking about me" and "The news on television is about me."

Ideas of reference often occur in schizophrenia; delusional disorder; and schizoid, borderline, and paranoid personality disorders. They may also occur in other conditions, including mania, psychotic depression, substance-related disorders, and body dysmorphic disorder.

INTERVIEWING AND PSYCHOTHERAPEUTIC GUIDELINES

Do not challenge ideas of reference directly. The clinician should explore the degree to which the referential thinking is fixed: Does the patient firmly believe something that is not possible? Evaluate the patient for delusions, particularly paranoid thoughts, thought control, thought insertion, thought broadcasting, and mind reading. How do people around the patient react to the referential ideas? Does the patient avoid talking about those ideas with others? Does the patient plan to take action against the objects of the referential thinking?

Reassure the patient that the material can be discussed in confidence. Primary care physicians must not do not do anything that may make the patient more suspicious, lest they become incorporated into a paranoid delusional system.

EVALUATION AND MANAGEMENT

1. A definitive diagnosis is crucial. All the disorders discussed earlier should be considered in the differential diagnosis.
2. Drugs, especially such hallucinogens as lysergic acid diethylamide (LSD) and phencyclidine (PCP) and such psychostimulants as cocaine and amphetamine,

can cause psychotic symptoms, including ideas of reference. The patient's vital signs and the results of a urine toxicology screen may help rule out substance-induced ideas of reference.

3. Assess the degree to which the patient responds to referential thinking. Dangerous patients should be hospitalized.

DRUG TREATMENT

Drug treatment depends on the diagnosis and the severity of the impairment. Depression, schizophrenia, and mania—all require different approaches to drug treatment, so the proper diagnosis is critical.

If well-formed, systematized referential delusions are present in the context of a delusional disorder, antipsychotic medications may be only minimally helpful. Patients with delusional disorder often refuse treatment, and their delusions are often refractory to antipsychotic medications.

For a more detailed discussion of this topic, see J Yager, M J Gitlin: Clinical Manifestations of Psychiatric Disorders, Chap 10, p 637; A A Lipton, R Cancro: Schizophrenia: Clinical Features, Sec 14.7, p 968; T C Manschreck: Delusional Disorder and Shared Psychotic Disorder, Sec 15.2, p 1031, in CTP/VI.

9.7 Illusions

Illusions are perceptual misinterpretations of real external stimuli. For example, a person might mistake a door closing as a gun shot. Hallucinations, by contrast, have their origin in internal stimuli.

CLINICAL FEATURES AND DIAGNOSIS

Illusions are much less significant symptoms than are hallucinations. Illusions often occur in normal people, especially when they are falling asleep, tired, or overstimulated. The important clinical task is to determine when illusions are symptoms of psychotic disorders, such as schizophrenia. In psychotic patients, distinguishing illusions from hallucinations may be difficult. The clinician must also determine whether the illusions are secondary to delirium, intoxication, or withdrawal.

In normal people, sensory deprivation can produce illusions, particularly in the elderly who have decreased sensory acuity. Physical and psychological stress can also precipitate illusions.

INTERVIEWING AND PSYCHOTHERAPEUTIC GUIDELINES

If hallucinations are also present, the interview should include a full evaluation for psychotic disorders. If the illusions are mild, reassure the patient that illusions are often normal and do not necessarily indicate a major psychiatric problem, especially when the illusions occur only after sensory deprivation or when the patient is under stress.

EVALUATION AND MANAGEMENT

1. Focus initially on whether such frank psychotic symptoms as hallucinations and delusions are present.
2. Perform a complete mental status examination and obtain the patient's history. The cognitive examination should evaluate the patient for such disorders as schizophrenia, depression, mania, anxiety disorders, psychoactive substance abuse, and organic mental disorders. Assess the patient medically, since illusions may be related to underlying medical illnesses.
3. Identify the course of the illusions and what impairment, if any, is present. Illusions are usually transitory. The presence of persistent illusions and of any impairment caused by the illusions suggests serious psychopathology.
4. In the elderly who experience illusions after sensory deprivation, the restoration of an appropriately stimulating environment usually resolves the symptoms.

DRUG TREATMENT

No specific drug treatment is indicated. If the symptom has extremely upset the patient benzodiazepines—such as diazepam (Valium) 5 to 10 mg by mouth one or two times a day, clonazepam (Klonopin) 0.25 to 0.5 mg by mouth one or two times a day, or lorazepam (Ativan) 1 to 2 mg by mouth one to three times a day—may be helpful for short-term use. If the illusion is a symptom of another disorder, such as psychosis, antipsychotics may be indicated.

For a more detailed discussion of this topic, see H I Kaplan, B J Sadock: Typical Signs and Symptoms of Psychiatric Illness, Sec 9.3, p 535; J Yager, M J Gitlin: Clinical Manifestations of Psychiatric Disorders, Chap 10, p 637, in CTP/VI.

9.8 Neologisms (New Words)

A *neologism* is a new word created by the patient. Neologisms are often condensations of two or more other words.

CLINICAL FEATURES AND DIAGNOSIS

Neologisms occur in patients with schizophrenia and other psychotic disorders and in patients with aphasia. Neologisms sometimes also sometimes occur in patients with mental retardation, with communication or learning disorders, and with pervasive developmental disorders.

Neologisms are a single symptom and must be placed in the context of a complete mental status examination. Usually, neologisms are not a specific complaint of the patient but instead are noticed by others. Schizophrenic patients often have fixed and consistent neologisms. The error in language may reflect a fixed delusional system and may not be associated with other language abnormalities. In contrast, a patient with Wernicke's aphasia frequently develops new neologisms and has other language comprehension impairments.

INTERVIEWING AND PSYCHOTHERAPEUTIC GUIDELINES

The patient's overall language functioning should be evaluated. The clinician should perform a mental status examination and assess the patient for psychotic symptoms, such as hallucinations and delusions, which may help confirm a diagnosis of a psychotic disorder.

EVALUATION AND MANAGEMENT

1. Are the neologisms and any associated psychotic symptoms new or old?
2. If the symptoms are new, is there an identifiable stressor or precipitant?
3. Is there reason to suspect a medical cause? Drug intoxication, head trauma, central nervous system lesion, or epilepsy are possible etiologies.
4. Are there other signs of a psychotic disorder?

DRUG TREATMENT

Pharmacotherapy treatment depends on the definitive diagnosis.

For a more detailed discussion of this topic, see H I Kaplan, B J Sadock: Typical Signs and Symptoms of Psychiatric Illness, Sec 9.3, p 535, in CTP/VI.

9.9 Paranoia

Paranoia is a general term used to describe a range of thinking and behavior, from normal suspiciousness to systematized persecutory delusions.

CLINICAL FEATURES AND DIAGNOSIS

Paranoia is a nonspecific symptom that can be present in personality disorders, delusional disorder, schizophrenia, mania or depression with psychotic features, brief psychotic disorder, and substance-related disorders. Paranoid patients are potentially dangerous, since they may act out violently against someone they perceive to be a threat.

The primary care physician should determine the course and the severity of the paranoid ideation. Paranoid personality disorder and delusional disorder of the persecutory type typically have paranoid ideation that has been relatively constant over long periods. The absence of delusions in paranoid personality disorder and the prominent delusions that are the major defining clinical feature in delusional disorder differentiate those two diagnoses. Paranoia in mania or depression is present only during acute episodes. Schizophrenia is usually identified by the presence of other symptoms, such as hallucinations and thought disorders.

The objectives in treating the paranoid patient are to evaluate immediately the patient's potential dangerousness, to make a definitive psychiatric diagnosis, and to initiate an appropriate treatment plan based on the diagnosis.

INTERVIEWING AND PSYCHOTHERAPEUTIC GUIDELINES

The primary care physician should not directly challenge the paranoid patient's beliefs, no matter how implausible they seem. When testing the extent of the patient's paranoid ideation, the clinician must be cautious and avoid alienating the patient. For example, the physician may ask, "What do other people say when you tell them that the FBI is against you?" and "How do you respond to that?" Paranoid patients may have already encountered surprise or disbelief from others, so that line of questioning may be less threatening than directly challenging their beliefs.

The patient may be paranoid about the interviewing physician. Therefore, the physician should maintain a formal stance, as paranoid patients view overfamiliarity with suspicion. Do not interview the patient in a potentially dangerous situation, such as alone in an office with the door closed; security should be readily available if the patient becomes violent.

EVALUATION AND MANAGEMENT

1. The patient's vital signs and laboratory tests may provide clues to a possible organic (that is, medical or substance-related) disorder. Laboratory screening tests should include a complete blood count (CBC); a complete chemistry profile, including electrolytes, liver function tests, renal function tests, and tests for calcium and magnesium; a urine drug test; thyroid function tests; and blood concentrations of any medications being taken.
2. If substance-related disorders and general medical conditions are ruled out, then a complete psychiatric evaluation should lead to a diagnosis. Neuropsychological testing, electroencephalography (EEG), and structural brain imaging by a computed tomography (CT) scan or magnetic resonance imaging (MRI) may help identify any underlying organic conditions.
3. The dangerous patient may need hospitalization, even involuntary commitment. Question the patient in detail about any plans for suicide or homicide. Directly ask what the patient may do to those perceived to be against him or her. Ask about previous acts of violence, including suicide attempts.

DRUG TREATMENT

In the emergency room or office, anxiety or agitation in paranoid patients is treated according to the diagnosis. If the patient is already taking an antipsychotic medication, give another dose of that drug. In general, psychotic paranoid patients can be given haloperidol (Haldol), thiothixene (Navane), fluphenazine (Prolixin), or trifluoperazine (Stelazine), all at a dose of 2 to 5 mg by mouth or intramuscularly (IM) as needed. Paranoid conditions caused by intoxication or withdrawal from drugs can be managed with lorazepam (Ativan) 1 to 2 mg by mouth or IM. Severely anxious paranoid patients can also be treated with lorazepam. Paranoia with agitation caused by delirium or dementia can be managed with haloperidol 1 to 5 mg by mouth or IM.

For a more detailed discussion of this topic, see E D Caine, H Grossman, J M Lyness: Delirium, Dementia, and Amnestic and Other Cognitive Disorders and Mental Disorders Due to a General Medical Condition, Chap 12, p 705; A A Lipton, R Cancro: Schizophrenia: Clinical Features, Sec 14.7, p 968; T C Manschreck: Delusional Disorder and Shared Psychotic Disorder, Sec 15.2, p 1031; in CTP/VI.

9.10 Postpartum or Puerperal Psychosis

Postpartum or *puerperal psychosis* is an acute psychotic episode in a woman that appears shortly after she has given birth.

CLINICAL FEATURES AND DIAGNOSIS

Postpartum psychosis can occur within one year after giving birth, but most often it begins within the first week of childbirth. While many of those affected have no previous psychiatric problems, the incidence is greatest in patients with a history of bipolar disorder, previous postpartum psychiatric disorders (psychotic and depressive disorders), and a family history of postpartum psychiatric disorders. The disorder occurs after 0.1 to 0.2 percent of all pregnancies.

Manic symptoms are the most common; depression with psychotic features is also common. Typical symptoms include agitation, restlessness, and a labile mood, including elation, insomnia, crying spells, confusion, and eventually the development of a full-blown psychotic episode with features of mania and delirium. Suicide or infanticide occurs in up to 10 percent of untreated cases. Obsessions are common and often focus on an impulse to hurt or kill the infant.

Postpartum psychosis should not be confused with the so-called postpartum blues, a normal condition that occurs in up to 50 percent of women after childbirth. Postpartum blues is self-limited, lasts only a few days, and is characterized by tearfulness, fatigue, anxiety, and irritability that begin shortly after childbirth and lessen in severity over the course of a week.

INTERVIEWING AND PSYCHOTHERAPEUTIC GUIDELINES

Postpartum psychotic patients may wish to harm their infant, so arrange to prevent their flight or any sudden violence. Often, new mothers are discharged from the postpartum obstetric ward a day or two after giving birth, and they experience the onset of postpartum psychosis days or weeks after the hospital stay ends. Be alert for the condition, and use the family to provide the patient's history.

If hospitalization is indicated, reassure the patient and her family that most often the condition is brief and that she can expect recovery. Involve the family in the evaluation and treatment, exploring the effects that the episode is having, especially on the father, siblings, and grandparents.

EVALUATION AND MANAGEMENT

1. Consider the high risk for infanticide or suicide, and be prepared to hospitalize the patient.
2. Conduct a full medical workup for possible organic causes.
3. Follow-up counseling is important and should include help with child rearing and observing the patient for subsequent mania, depression, or other psychiatric syndromes.
4. Family therapy can help explore and process the effects that the episode had on the family and can help the family cope with possible subsequent episodes. The patient may need the family to provide child care.
5. Antipsychotics, alone or in combination with electroconvulsive therapy (ECT), are often needed. Brief psychotic disorder, manic episode, and mixed episode— all can occur with postpartum onset and should be considered in the differential diagnosis.

DRUG TREATMENT

The patient may require a brief course of antipsychotic medication, such as haloperidol (Haldol) or fluphenazine (Prolixin), both given at 2 to 5 mg by mouth three times a day. For agitation, the patient may require 2 to 5 mg intramuscularly (IM) of a high-potency antipsychotic. Breast-feeding should be prohibited during drug treatment. Because of the high incidence of postpartum psychosis in women with bipolar disorder, lithium (Eskalith) prophylaxis during the third trimester or shortly after giving birth should be considered. Antidepressants should be used in patients with suicidal depression.

For a more detailed discussion of this topic, see B J Parry: Postpartum Psychiatric Syndromes, Sec 15.4, p 1059, in CTP/VI.

9.11 Schizoaffective Disorder

Schizoaffective disorder has been understood in various ways. (1) It may be a type of either schizophrenia or a mood disorder. (2) It may be a combination of both schizophrenia and a mood disorder. (3) It may be completely distinct from

TABLE 9.11-1
DIAGNOSTIC CRITERIA FOR SCHIZOAFFECTIVE DISORDER

A. An uninterrupted period of illness during which, at some time, there is either a major depressive episode, a manic episode, or a mixed episode concurrent with symptoms that meet criterion A for schizophrenia.

    Note: The major depressive episode must include criterion A1 (see Table 10.2-1): depressed mood.

B. During the same period of illness, there have been delusions or hallucinations for at least 2 weeks in the absence of prominent mood symptoms.

C. Symptoms that meet criteria for a mood episode are present for a substantial portion of the total duration of the active and residual periods of the illness.

D. The disturbance is not due to the direct physiological effects of a substance (e.g., a drug of abuse, a medication) or a general medical condition.

Specify type:

    Bipolar type: if the disturbance includes a manic or a mixed episode (or a manic or a mixed episode and major depressive episodes)

    Depressive type: if the disturbance only includes major depressive episodes

Table from DSM-IV, *Diagnostic and Statistical Manual of Mental Disorders*, ed 4. Copyright American Psychiatric Association, Washington, 1994. Used with permission.

either of those disorders. (4) Perhaps most likely, it may comprise a heterogeneous group of disorders that include all three possibilities.

Schizoaffective disorder is less common than either schizophrenia or mood disorders. Manic energy, irritability, and a reduced need for sleep may coexist with bizarre ideation or behavior and constricted or inappropriate affects.

CLINICAL FEATURES AND DIAGNOSIS

The clinical signs and symptoms of schizoaffective disorder include all the signs and symptoms of schizophrenia, mania, and depression. Patients with schizoaffective disorder have psychotic symptoms consistent with an acute episode of schizophrenia, and those symptoms are frequently (although not always) accompanied by prominent mood symptoms. The diagnosis may be appropriate when psychotic symptoms have persisted without prominent mood symptoms for at least two weeks but the duration of all symptoms is less than that required for the diagnosis of schizophrenia. The diagnostic criteria for schizoaffective disorder are listed in Table 9.11-1.

The course can vary from one of exacerbations and remissions to a steadily deteriorating course. Patients with schizoaffective disorder, bipolar type, have a prognosis similar to those with bipolar disorder; those with schizoaffective disorder, depressive type, are prognostically similar to schizophrenia patients. Regardless of type, the same factors that suggest a poor prognosis in schizophrenia are also ominous in schizoaffective disorder: poor premorbid functioning; an insidious onset; the lack of a precipitant; the predominance of psychotic symptoms, particularly negative and deficit symptoms; an early onset; an unremitting course; and a family history of schizophrenia indicate a poor outcome.

INTERVIEWING AND PSYCHOTHERAPEUTIC GUIDELINES

In interviewing all patients with a history of psychotic symptoms, elicit a history of affective symptoms as well, as they have important treatment implications.

However, flight of ideas, distractibility, impulsivity, and intrusiveness can compromise the examination. The schizoaffective disorder patient may be more bizarre or paranoid than the typical mood disorder patient and, consequently, more difficult to interview.

The best approach is a firm, insistent style. Outline explicitly for the patient the structure of the setting and be prepared to periodically remind the patient of that structure.

Reduce stimulation as much as possible. Manic patients are sociable and may respond well to the structure provided by the staff and the psychiatrist, but may do much less well in less structured situations.

Patients are likely to be unrealistic about their abilities and prospects, minimizing the consequences of inappropriate behavior and exaggerating their chances of success. Consult the patient's family; they probably know best what the patient can tolerate outside the hospital.

Schizoaffective disorder patients are often suicidal, and suicidal ideas may be present even when the patient's mood appears to be elated. Furthermore, the patient's mood is often unstable, and a depressive affect may quickly descend on the patient, carrying with it pessimistic or nihilistic thoughts and attendant suicidal ideation. The patient's acting on suicidal thoughts in a vulnerable moment if the means are available is a significant risk and must be explored.

EVALUATION AND MANAGEMENT

The major treatment modalities for schizoaffective disorder are hospitalization, medication, and psychosocial interventions.

DRUG TREATMENT

The basic principles underlying pharmacotherapy for schizoaffective disorder are that antidepressant and antimanic protocols be followed if at all indicated and that antipsychotics be used only as needed for short-term control. If the protocols are not effective in the ongoing control of those symptoms, antipsychotic medication may be indicated. Patients with schizoaffective disorder, bipolar type, should receive trials of lithium (Eskalith), carbamazepine (Tegretol), valproate (Depakene), or some combination of those drugs if one drug alone is not effective. Patients with schizoaffective disorder, depressive type, should be given trials of antidepressants and electroconvulsive therapy (ECT) before they are determined to be unresponsive to antidepressant treatment.

For a more detailed discussion of this topic, see S G Siris, M R Lavin: Schizoaffective Disorder, Schizophreniform Disorder and Brief Psychotic Disorder, Sec 15.1, p 1019, in CTP/VI.

9.12 Schizophrenia

Schizophrenia is a chronic, relapsing, remitting psychotic disorder with protean manifestations. The premorbid adjustment, the symptoms, and the course are all variable; in fact, schizophrenia is probably a heterogeneous group of disorders. Common office presentations include distressing hallucinations (which may be loud and distracting, derogatory, or threatening), bizarre behavior, incoherence, agitation, and neglect.

Although the prevalence is only 1 per 1,000 persons in the United States, schizophrenia is overrepresented in the emergency room because of the severity of its symptoms, the inability of patients to care for themselves, their lack of insight, and their gradual social deterioration and disaffiliation.

CLINICAL FEATURES AND DIAGNOSIS

No symptom found in schizophrenia is pathognomonic for the disorder. What distinguishes schizophrenia is the course: at least six months of continuous signs of the disturbance, failure to return to the previous level of functioning, and continuing vulnerability to stress. Table 9.12-1 lists the diagnostic criteria for schizophrenia.

Patients with schizophrenia are driven to seek help for various reasons at different points during the illness. Initially, in cases with a sudden onset, patients are frightened by the confusion of their thought processes; their bizarre, alien thoughts; novel perceptual disturbances; and either a welter of emotions or a deadening of emotional responses. Patients may explicitly wonder if they are losing their minds. Cases with a gradual or insidious onset may present because of school failure, social withdrawal, or bizarre behavior.

As the illness progresses and the psychosocial consequences mount, secondary depression may result in suicidal ideation. Such patients are at high risk not because of the psychosis but from their understandable demoralization.

Most patients reach a plateau, become knowledgeable about their illness, and do not require hospitalization for exacerbations if good outpatient care is available. However, a disruption in their support system, such as the departure of their therapist or the death of a parent, may result in severe relapses.

Some patients, despite the best of care, follow a downhill course, become totally and permanently disabled, and require custodial care to maintain the basic nutrition and hygiene. A minority lose insight into the fact of their illness or the psychological nature of their illness and may wander from doctor to doctor or from hospital to hospital, seeking treatment for bizarre somatic complaints. A few patients shun all human contact, are lost to their families, and eke out an existence by eating refuse as they gradually deteriorate physically. The authorities may ultimately bring them to the emergency room because of the threat of exposure in winter or obvious medical illness, such as cellulitis of the extremities.

Substance abuse affects as many as half of schizophrenic patients and accelerates their deterioration in both direct and indirect ways.

INTERVIEWING AND PSYCHOTHERAPEUTIC GUIDELINES

Begin by talking with patients about their premorbid conditions, rather than their florid symptoms, to put the patients at ease and to establish a benchmark by which current functioning is measured.

TABLE 9.12–1
DIAGNOSTIC CRITERIA FOR SCHIZOPHRENIA

A. *Characteristic symptoms:* Two (or more) of the following, each present for a significant portion of time during a 1-month period (or less if successfully treated):

    (1) delusions
    (2) hallucinations
    (3) disorganized speech (e.g., frequent derailment or incoherence)
    (4) grossly disorganized or catatonic behavior
    (5) negative symptoms, i.e., affective flattening, alogia, or avolition

    Note: Only one criterion A symptom is required if delusions are bizarre or hallucinations consist of a voice keeping up a running commentary on the person's behavior or thoughts, or two or more voices conversing with each other.

B. *Social/occupational dysfunction:* For a significant portion of the time since the onset of the disturbance, one or more major areas of functioning such as work, interpersonal relations, or self-care are markedly below the level achieved prior to the onset (or when the onset is in childhood or adolescence, failure to achieve expected level of interpersonal, academic, or occupational achievement).

C. *Duration:* Continuous signs of the disturbance persist for at least 6 months. This 6-month period must include at least 1 month of symptoms (or less if successfully treated) that meet criterion A (i.e., active-phase symptoms) and may include periods of prodromal or residual symptoms. During these prodromal or residual periods, the signs of the disturbance may be manifested by only negative symptoms or two or more symptoms listed in criterion A present in an attenuated form (e.g., odd beliefs, unusual perceptual experiences).

D. *Schizoaffective and mood disorder exclusion:* Schizoaffective disorder and mood disorder with psychotic features have been ruled out because either (1) no major depressive, manic, or mixed episodes have occurred concurrently with the active-phase symptoms, or (2) if mood episodes have occurred during active-phase symptoms, their total duration has been brief relative to the duration of the active and residual periods.

E. *Substance/general medical condition exclusion:* The disturbance is not due to the direct physiological effects of a substance (e.g., a drug of abuse, a medication) or a general medical condition.

F. *Relationship to a pervasive developmental disorder.* If there is a history of autistic disorder or another pervasive developmental disorder, the additional diagnosis of schizophrenia is made only if prominent delusions or hallucinations are also present for at least a month (or less if successfully treated).

Classification of longitudinal course (can be applied only after at least 1 year has elapsed since the initial onset of active-phase symptoms):

    Episodic with interepisode residual symptoms (episodes are defined by the reemergence of prominent psychotic symptoms); *also specify if:* **with prominent negative symptoms**
    Episodic with no interepisode residual symptoms
    Continuous (prominent psychotic symptoms are present throughout the period of observation); *also specify if:* **with prominent negative symptoms**
    Single episode in partial remission; *also specify if:* **with prominent negative symptoms**
    Single episode in full remission
    Other or unspecified pattern

Table from DSM-IV, *Diagnostic and Statistical Manual of Mental Disorders,* ed 4. Copyright American Psychiatric Association, Washington, 1994. Used with permission.

Next, approach the patient's history chronologically to establish the earliest manifestation that suggested a prodrome, followed by the active-phase symptoms. Thought disorders, lack of motivation, paranoid thinking, and poor insight may all contribute to a difficulty eliciting an adequate history. Collateral contacts may be more revealing than the patient.

Ask in detail about unusual experiences of any kind. If the patient cannot describe any, ask about specific experiences, beginning with such prepsychotic experiences as déjà vu, numbness, derealization, and depersonalization—matters that are not immediately identified with being psychotic. Florid hallucination may then be the logical next symptom to investigate. If the patient protests the line of questioning, defuse the issue by stating that these are routine medical questions. If necessary, abandon the history of the patient's psychotic symptoms and shift to questions of mood and cognition, which may be less threatening.

Ask about suicidal ideation; 10 percent of schizophrenic patients die by suicide, usually early in the disorder.

Cognitive examination is also important, as many medical conditions may present with signs of schizophrenia, at least early in their course, but do not usually involve cognitive impairment.

EVALUATION AND MANAGEMENT

1. Because of the need for a thorough medical evaluation and the demonstrated efficacy of the psychoeducational aspects of hospitalization, all schizophrenic patients should probably be admitted to the hospital if possible during their first presentation. The hospital can be a supportive environment that provides exposure to others with similar conditions receiving similar treatment. Peers and staff members can answer many questions quickly.
2. However, if the patient is strongly opposed to hospitalization, weigh the adverse effects of forcible treatment on any future relationship against the risks of outpatient treatment or no treatment. Supervision by the patient's family may make outpatient treatment viable, but it also complicates treatment and may increase the stresses on the patient. No family should be relied on for constant observation. Conditions warranting that degree of concern require hospitalization.
3. Hospital admission late in the illness may be prompted by severe distress related to loud, continuous, derogatory, or threatening voices. Simple, repetitive commands are not typical and probably indicate malingering. In such cases, find out from others the variables not related to illness that are motivating the patient.
4. Paranoia may keep the patient from sleeping and may result in dangerous defensive behavior. Patients sometimes say that they would rather kill themselves than be captured by others. Activity at both extremes, severe apathy and agitation, may require hospital admission.
5. Threatening patients are often chronically ill, do not benefit from treatment, and can be released only if they are not a danger to themselves or others. Somatic delusions may result in self-mutilation, autoamputation, or enucleation. However, suicidal ideation in schizophrenic patients is usually a result of depression, rather than psychosis, and in most respects is similar to the suicidal ideation of other people with real losses, failures, and hopelessness about the future.
6. Unpredictability is the rule, and a high level of vigilance is indicated. In the hospital, contracts, periodic checks, and constant observation are used.

DRUG TREATMENT

Antipsychotic drugs ameliorate and reduce the signs and symptoms of schizophrenia. Consider low potency antipsychotic drugs, such as chlorpromazine (Thorazine), if the patient is hyperactive or agitated. Consider high potency antipsychotic drugs, such as trifluoperazine (Stelazine) if the patient is withdrawn or lethargic.

Start with 25 mg by mouth or intramuscularly (IM) of chlorpromazine and raise the dosage to 300 to 1,800 mg daily for acute attacks. Titrate the dosage upward until the therapeutic effect is achieved. Haloperidol (Haldol) may be used for rapid tranquilization (1 to 10 mg by mouth or IM over 30 to 60 minutes); its daily dosage may go as high as 100 mg. Long-acting depot fluphenazine (Prolixin) concentrate/decanoate (25 mg IM) can be effective for 14 to 21 days and is helpful in increasing compliance.

Risperidone (Risperdal), a drug with significant antagonist activity at the serotonin (5-hydroxytryptamine) type 2 (5-HT$_2$) receptor and at the dopamine type 2 (D$_2$) receptor, may be more effective than other available dopamine receptor antagonists at treating both the positive and the negative symptoms of schizophrenia. It may also be associated with significantly less severe neurological adverse effects than are the typical dopaminergic antagonist drugs.

Clozapine (Clozaril) is an effective antipsychotic drug and a clear second-line drug for patients who either do not respond to other available drugs or have severe tardive dyskinesia. Unfortunately, clozapine is associated with a 1 to 2 percent incidence of agranulocytosis, an adverse effect that necessitates the weekly monitoring of the blood indexes.

For a more detailed discussion of this topic, see Schizophrenia, Chap 14, pp 889–1018, in CTP/VI.

10
Mood Disorders

10.1 Agitation

Agitation is a state of increased mental excitement and motor activity that may occur in a wide range of conditions (Table 10.1-1): delirium or dementia, medical disorders, such as hypoxia, hyperthyroidism, and acidosis; drug or alcohol intoxication or withdrawal (especially adverse effects of sympathomimetics, anticholinergics, or digitalis); and many other disorders.

CLINICAL FEATURES AND DIAGNOSIS

Make a definitive diagnosis so that a treatment plan can be developed. Distinguishing between an organic and a psychological cause has implications for the subsequent treatment and course of action. Conduct a full medical examination; abnormal vital signs in an agitated patient may be the first clues of an organic medical disorder.

Keep these questions in mind during the evaluation: Is the patient paranoid and psychotic, with impaired reality testing? If the patient is psychotic and agitated, medication may be indicated immediately. Has there been recent violence? Is the patient impulsive, with poor judgment? If so, and if agitation persists, more violence may occur. Is there a treatable medical cause? Does the patient suffer from a personality disorder that may induce impulsivity or from excessive anxiety in response to stress?

INTERVIEWING AND PSYCHOTHERAPEUTIC GUIDELINES

If conversation is possible, try to quiet the patient. It is important to remain nonconfrontational, without expressing overt anger or hostility. Do not be punitive. Let the patient know that angry complaints and concerns will be listened to empathically. Limits and treatment should be honestly and clearly defined. Reassure patients that the interview is confidential, that they are in a safe place, and that everyone there is trying to help. Stay as calm and straightforward as possible. If talking is not effective, isolate the patient, and prevent excessive stimulation by staff members and other patients. If the patient appears to be at risk of losing control, let the patient know that the staff will maintain control decisively and emphatically. Even if a patient requires medication for sedation, try to determine the psychological issues involved in the agitation. If possible, correct the distortions and diminish the irrational fears to decrease panic, anxiety, and agitation. Patients using phencyclidine (PCP) cannot be quieted or reassured and should be isolated immediately.

TABLE 10.1–1
SUBSTANCE INTOXICATION VERSUS OTHER MENTAL DISORDERS IN AGITATED PATIENTS

	Physical Examination	Probable Cause	Treatment
Agitation with blank stare[1], anxiety, stupor, aggression, panic, bizarre behavior	Elevated blood pressure and heart rate, vertical and horizontal nystagmus, analgesia to pinprick, muscular rigidity, salivation, vomiting	Phencyclidine (PCP)	Minimal intervention (no talking down) Sensory deprivation with observation at a distance Diazepam for intoxication Haloperidol for psychosis No phenothiazines Diazepam for seizures α-Blockers or diazoxide for severe hypertension
Agitation with persecutory delusions or euphoria with irritability	Sympathetic signs; blood pressure elevation, tachycardia, tachypnea, mydriasis, diaphoresis, motor restlessness, tremor	Amphetamine, cocaine, or other sympathomimetics	Controlled environment Acidify urine Control hyperpyrexia, seizures (diazepam), behavior (haloperidol) No sedatives
	No sympathetic signs	Consider schizophrenia, schizophreniform disorder, delusional disorder, bipolar disorder, brief psychotic disorder, atypical psychosis	
Sensory distortion, hypersensitivity of all senses, euphoria, hallucinations, pseudohallucinations	Sympathetic excess	Epinephrine-type hallucinogens; STP, mescaline, nutmeg	Controlled environment, support and reassurance (talking down); haloperidol for behavior control
	Minimal changes	Indole-type hallucinogens; LSD, psilocytin	
Undistinguishable acute delirium	Muscarinic blockade: dilated and sluggishly reactive pupils, blurred vision, flushed face, paralytic ileus, constipation, urinary retention, fever, and hyperreflexia	Pilocarpine or methacholine	Physostigmine
	Muscarinic blockade not present	Reclassify patient by physical examination; If the findings are not clear, consider mixed or unusual presentation; consider polydrug ingestion when psychological and physical presentations are contradictory or confusing	Conservative, with observation and protection as needed

Table adapted from A DiSclafani, R C Hall, E R Gardner: Drug-induced psychosis: Emergency diagnosis and management. Psychosomatics 22: Oct, 1981.
[1]The patient with moderate-dose or high-dose PCP ingestion may present with stupor or coma and later exhibit low-dose signs and symptoms.

EVALUATION AND MANAGEMENT

1. Avoid situations in which assault of health care personnel is possible (for example, in a small office with the door closed). Have sufficient staff members present to restrain the patient if necessary.
2. Physical restraint should be used if medications are ineffective and if violence or flight is impending. Be sure to have sufficient staff members who are trained in physical restraint. Be careful to avoid restraints if PCP intoxication is suspected; instead, isolate the patient in a nonstimulating environment. If restraints are absolutely necessary, do not use limb restraints, since PCP has anesthetic effects, and the patients may injure themselves by fighting against the restraints without feeling any pain (Table 10.1-2).
3. Pay attention to any clues of impending violence. In particular, maintain vigilance for any changes in behavior, mood, speech, or affect—any of which may signal an imminent loss of control.
4. Maintain consistency among the staff members regarding the treatment plan. Give the patient a clear and unconflicted message about what behavior can and cannot be tolerated in the physician's office; however, the staff members first must agree among themselves.
5. If the patient is threatening to sign out of the hospital against medical advice, the clinician must decide if the patient can make that decision and whether leaving the hospital would pose a life-threatening danger to the patient. The patient's capacity depends on whether a psychotic, dementing, or delirious process is occurring. If the patient's capacity is deemed to be significantly impaired and if there is increased risk, the patient must be prevented from leaving. Full documentation is warranted. Consultation with hospital counsel may be helpful in borderline cases. When the patient's capacity is not impaired, but a serious medical risk is evident, the clinician must make every effort to convince the patient to remain in the hospital. Generally, the most effective approach is a nonconfrontational sympathetic stance that involves helping the patient feel in control.

TABLE 10.1–2
EMERGENCY PHYSICAL MANAGEMENT

---

1. Develop specific protocols, describing methods of restraint.
2. Determine the composition of the team (optimally, six persons, although five is safe).
    a. One person directs the restraint procedure and controls the patient's head.
    b. One person restrains a limb (four persons in all).
    c. One person administers the medication.
3. Review the specific plan for restraint, including the assignment of roles.
4. Have the necessary equipment and medication available.
5. Inform the patient about the treatment options.
6. Ask the patient to lie down so that you can apply the restraints.
7. Apply the restraints and, perhaps, medicate the patient.
8. Continue to talk with the patient about feelings and procedural issues.
9. Never leave the patient alone.
10. Convene a meeting of caretakers to discuss continuing patient observation and subsequent plans, including removal of the restraints, medication, and disposition.
11. Remove the restraints, one limb at a time.

Table from E L Bassuk: Management of the acutely ill psychiatric patient. In *Textbook of General Medicine and Primary Care*, J Noble, editor, p 27. Little, Brown, Boston, 1984. Used with permission.

DRUG TREATMENT

For escalating or severe agitation, tranquilization may be necessary. Usually, either sedative-hypnotics (for example, benzodiazepines) or antipsychotics are used.

First, check the patient's vital signs if possible. Low-potency antipsychotics, such as chlorpromazine (Thorazine), should be avoided if the patient is hypotensive. If fever is present, avoid antipsychotics, since they cause poikilothermia and can interfere with a fever workup.

If intoxication or withdrawal from alcohol or sedative-hypnotics is suspected, benzodiazepines are the drugs of choice, since antipsychotics may precipitate withdrawal seizures.

If stimulant intoxication is suspected, benzodiazepines are indicated.

If the patient is not psychotic, benzodiazepines are indicated to avoid the risk of antipsychotic side effects.

If the patient is psychotic, consider antipsychotics. Although psychotic patients can be tranquilized with benzodiazepines, that is not considered a definitive treatment for psychosis. However, using benzodiazepines to tranquilize a psychotic patient in the physician's office or the emergency room has the advantage of allowing the physician to evaluate the patient free of antipsychotics the next day.

Drug Choice

If the patient is taking a specific drug or has a history of responding to a specific drug, use that drug again. If there is no available history of drug response, any benzodiazepine is as effective as any other, and the same is true for the antipsychotics.

Benzodiazepines The drug choice is based on the available routes of administration (for example, intramuscularly [IM]), the metabolic pathway, the rate of onset of the effects, and the elimination half-life. Lorazepam (Ativan), 1 to 2 mg orally or IM, is the usual choice because it has an intermediate elimination half-life, is available in a parenteral form with rapid delivery to the central nervous system (CNS), and is metabolized by hepatic conjugation that is not delayed by liver disease. Repeat the dose hourly as needed unless signs of toxicity (for example, ataxia, dysarthria, cerebellar signs, nystagmus) are present. Benzodiazepines can reportedly cause disinhibition, which may be difficult to differentiate from worsening agitation. If disinhibition or benzodiazepine side effects are present, the benzodiazepine must be stopped and an antipsychotic started.

Antipsychotics The drug choice is based on the available routes of administration, potency, and the side-effect profile. High-potency antipsychotics are the usual drugs of choice, although they often cause extrapyramidal side effects; those effects are easily treated with anticholinergic drugs (for example, benztropine [Cogentin] 2 mg IM). Low-potency antipsychotics, although more sedating, can cause anticholinergic side effects and hypotension. The usual choice is haloperidol (Haldol),

5 mg orally or IM, which may be repeated if necessary in one hour. Akathisia (restlessness) is a common side effect of high-potency antipsychotics and may be indistinguishable from worsening agitation.

Combined Benzodiazepine-Antipsychotic   A combination of the two drugs is safe and is often used. Typically, the combination is lorazepam 2 mg and haloperidol 5 mg given together intramuscularly, although thiothixene (Navane) 5 mg may be used instead of haloperidol. Those combinations are safe and may be more effective than either drug alone, although that has not been conclusively proved. Furthermore, antipsychotics may reduce the risk of benzodiazepine disinhibition, and benzodiazepines may reduce the risk of akathisia. The disadvantage of such a combination is that, if the patient responds, it is impossible to tell which drug was effective or whether only the combination was effective.

For a more detailed discussion of this topic, see H I Kaplan, B J Sadock: Typical Signs and Symptoms of Psychiatric Illness, Sec 9.3, p 535; E D Caine, H Grossman, J M Lyness: Delirium, Dementia, and Amnestic and Other Cognitive Disorders and Mental Disorders Due to a General Medical Condition, Chap 12, p 705, in CTP/VI.

10.2 Depression

Depression is a period of impaired functioning associated with sad or irritable mood and related symptoms, including sleep and appetite changes, anhedonia (loss of interest from regular and pleasurable activities), psychomotor changes, impaired concentration, fatigue, feelings of hopelessness and helplessness, and thoughts of suicide. Most depressed persons never seek professional treatment.

CLINICAL FEATURES AND DIAGNOSIS

A depressive episode may be isolated or may occur in the course of either major depressive disorder (Table 10.2-1) or a bipolar disorder. Other diagnoses to consider are mood disorder due to a general medical condition, substance-related disorders (including intoxication, dependence, and withdrawal), dysthymic disorder, cyclothymic disorder, personality disorders, bereavement (grief), and adjustment disorders. *Bereavement* is a normal, although painful, response to a major loss; it is responsive to support and empathy and improves over time. If a bereaved patient's symptoms do not resolve, it is important to look for major depression.

Depressed patients do not always complain of sadness. They may be irritable or somatically preoccupied. Evaluate the patient for all associated signs and symptoms of depression, even in the absence of overt sadness. Any patient complaining of memory loss and depression must be evaluated for pseudodementia, a condition

TABLE 10.2-1
CRITERIA FOR MAJOR DEPRESSIVE EPISODE

A. Five (or more) of the following symptoms have been present during the same 2-week period and represent a change from previous functioning; at least one of the symptoms is either (1) depressed mood or (2) loss of interest or pleasure.

   Note: Do not include symptoms that are clearly due to a general medical condition, or mood-incongruent delusions or hallucinations.

   (1) depressed mood most of the day, nearly every day, as indicated by either subjective report (e.g., feels sad or empty) or observation made by others (e.g., appears tearful).
      Note: In children and adolescents, can be irritable mood.
   (2) markedly diminished interest or pleasure in all, or almost all, activities most of the day, nearly every day (as indicated by either subjective account or observation made by others)
   (3) significant weight loss when not dieting or weight gain (e.g., a change of more than 5% of body weight in a month), or decrease or increase in appetite nearly every day.
      Note: In children, consider failure to make expected weight gains.
   (4) insomnia or hypersomnia nearly every day
   (5) psychomotor agitation or retardation nearly every day (observable by others, not merely subjective feelings of restlessness or being slowed down)
   (6) fatigue or loss of energy nearly every day
   (7) feelings of worthlessness or excessive or inappropriate guilt (which may be delusional) nearly every day (not merely self-reproach or guilt about being sick)
   (8) diminished ability to think or concentrate, or indecisiveness, nearly every day (either by subjective account or as observed by others)
   (9) recurrent thoughts of death (not just fear of dying), recurrent suicidal ideation without a specific plan, or a suicide attempt or a specific plan for committing suicide
B. The symptoms do not meet criteria for a mixed episode.
C. The symptoms cause clinically significant distress or impairment in social, occupational, or other important areas of functioning.
D. The symptoms are not due to the direct physiological effects of a substance (e.g., a drug of abuse, a medication) or a general medical condition (e.g., hypothyroidism).
E. The symptoms are not better accounted for by bereavement, i.e., after the loss of a loved one, the symptoms persist for longer than 2 months or are characterized by marked functional impairment, morbid preoccupation with worthlessness, suicidal ideation, psychotic symptoms, or psychomotor retardation.

Table from DSM-IV, *Diagnostic, and Statistical Manual of Mental Disorders,* ed 4. Copyright American Psychiatric Association, Washington, 1994. Used with permission.

that resembles dementia but usually results from depression rather than a brain dysfunction.

INTERVIEWING AND PSYCHOTHERAPEUTIC GUIDELINES

Engage the patients by being empathic and supportive. Many depressed patients feel isolated and hopeless. Be reassuring and inform them that they will be helped and that depression is readily treatable. Avoid glib, empty optimism ("Cheer up" or "It's not so bad"), which patients perceive as a lack of empathy. Address any ambivalence that the patients have about seeking treatment. Inform them that depression is common. Help identify specific stressors to make the patients feel less guilty and self-deprecating. Help reduce guilt by using a medical model, emphasizing that depression is an illness, like hypertension, that requires medical treatment. A collateral history from family members or friends is valuable in the assessment of depressed patients.

EVALUATION AND MANAGEMENT

The evaluation and treatment of patients with mood disorders must be directed toward three goals:

1. A guarantee of patient safety involves evaluating and treating possible suicidal ideation. Any acute medical problems that have resulted from suicide attempts or gestures should also be treated. If the patient has taken a drug overdose, emergency medical and toxicological evaluations must be obtained immediately.
2. A complete diagnostic evaluation will rule out medical, neurological, and pharmacological causes of depressive symptoms (Table 10.2-2).
3. A treatment plan should address not only the immediate symptoms but also the patient's prospective well-being. Although the current emphasis is on pharmacotherapy and psychotherapy addressed to the individual patient, stressful life events are also associated with increases in relapse rates among patients with mood disorders. Thus, treatment must reduce the number and the severity of the stressors in patients' lives. A history of manic or hypomanic episodes suggests a bipolar disorder. The diagnosis of bipolar disorder has implications for treatment and prognosis that are different from the implications for depression without mania.

Overall, the treatment of mood disorders is rewarding for physicians. Specific treatments are now available for depressive episodes, and the data suggest that prophylactic treatment is also effective. The physician should engage the patient in the treatment process, and provide reassurance that the episode is treatable and will eventually be over. Because the prognosis for each episode is good, optimism is always warranted and welcomed by both the patient and the patient's family, even if initial treatment results are not promising. However, mood disorders are chronic, and the patient and the family must be advised about future treatment strategies.

Hospitalization

The first and most critical decision the physician must make is whether to attempt inpatient or outpatient treatment. Clear indications for hospitalization are the need for diagnostic procedures, the risk of suicide or homicide, and the patient's grossly reduced ability to get food and shelter. Any adverse changes in the patient's symptoms or behavior or the attitude of the patient's support system may be sufficient to warrant hospitalization.

Patients with mood disorders are often unwilling to enter a hospital voluntarily, necessitating involuntary commitment. Patients with major depressive disorder are often incapable of making decisions because of their slowed thinking, negative *Weltanschauung* (world view), and hopelessness.

Psychosocial Therapies

Although most studies indicate—and most clinicians and researchers believe— that combined psychotherapy and pharmacotherapy is the most effective treatment

TABLE 10.2-2
NEUROLOGICAL, MEDICAL, AND PHARMACOLOGICAL CAUSES OF DEPRESSIVE SYMPTOMS

Neurological
Cerebrovascular diseases
Dementias (including dementia of the
 Alzheimer's type)
Epilepsy*
Fahr's disease*
Huntington's disease*
Hydrocephalus
Infections (including HIV and neurosyphilis)*
Migraines*
Multiple sclerosis*
Narcolepsy
Neoplasms*
Parkinson's disease
Progressive supranuclear palsy
Sleep apnea
Trauma*
Wilson's disease*
Endocrine
Adrenal (Cushing's*, Addison's diseases)
Hyperaldosteronism
Menses-related*
Parathyroid disorders (hyper- and hypo-)
Postpartum*
Thyroid disorders (hypothyroidism and apathetic
 hyperthyroidism)*
Infectious and Inflammatory
Acquired immune deficiency syndrome (AIDS)*
Chronic fatigue syndrome
Mononucleosis
Pneumonia—viral and bacterial
Rheumatoid arthritis
Sjögren's arteritis
Systemic lupus erythematosus*
Temporal arteritis
Tuberculosis
Miscellaneous Medical
Cancer (especially pancreatic and other GI)
Cardiopulmonary disease
Porphyria
Uremia (and other renal diseases)*
Vitamin deficiencies (B$_{12}$, C, folate, niacin,
 thiamine)*
Pharmacological (representative drugs)
Analgesics and anti-inflammatory
 Ibuprofen
 Indomethacin
 Opioids
 Phenacetin
Antibacterials and antifungals
 Ampicillin
 Cycloserine
 Ethionamide
 Griseofulvin
 Metronidazole
 Nalidixic acid

Pharmacological (continued)
 Nitrofurantoin
 Streptomycin
 Sulfamethoxazole
 Sulfonamides
 Tetracycline
Antihypertensives and cardiac drugs
 β-Adrenergic receptor antagonists
  (propranolol)
 Alphamethyldopa
 Bethtanidine
 Clonidine
 Digitalis
 Guanethidine
 Hydralazine
 Lidocaine
 Prazosin
 Procainamide
 Quanabenzacetate
 Rescinnamine
 Reserpine
 Veratrum
Antineoplastics
 C-Asparaginase
 6-Azauridine
 Bleomycin
 Trimethoprim
 Vincristine
 Zidovudine
Neurological and psychiatric
 Amantadine
 Antipsychotics (butyrophenones,
  phenothiazines, oxyindoles)
 Baclofen
 Bromocriptine
 Carbamazepine
 Levodopa
 Phenytoin
 Sedatives and hypnotics (barbiturates,
  benzodiazepines, chloral hydrate)
 Tetrabenazine
Steroids and hormones
 Corticosteroids (including ACTH)
 Danazol
 Oral contraceptives
 Prednisone
 Triamcinolone
Miscellaneous
 Acetazolamide
 Choline
 Cimetidine
 Cyproheptadine
 Diphenoxylate
 Disulfiram
 Methysergide
 Stimulants (amphetamines, fenfluramine)

*These conditions are associated with manic symptoms.

for major depressive disorder, some data suggest that either pharmacotherapy or psychotherapy alone is effective, at least in patients with mild major depressive episodes. The regular use of combined therapy adds to the cost of treatment and exposes patients to unnecessary side effects.

Three types of short-term psychotherapies—cognitive therapy, interpersonal therapy, and behavior therapy—have been studied regarding their efficacy in the treatment of major depressive disorder. Psychoanalytically oriented psychotherapy, although its efficacy has not been as well researched, has long been used for depressive disorders; many clinicians use the technique as their primary method. What differentiates the three short-term psychotherapy modalities from the psychoanalytically oriented approach are the active and directive roles of the therapist, the directly recognizable goals, and the endpoints for short-term therapy.

DRUG TREATMENT

Although the specific, short-term psychotherapies have influenced the treatment of major depressive disorder, the pharmacotherapeutic approach to mood disorders has revolutionized their treatment and has dramatically affected their course and reduced their inherent costs to society.

The physician must integrate pharmacotherapy with psychotherapeutic interventions. If physicians view mood disorders as fundamentally evolving from psychodynamic issues, their ambivalence about the use of drugs may result in a poor response, noncompliance, and probably inadequate dosages for too short a treatment period. Alternatively, if physicians ignore the psychosocial needs of the patient, the outcome of pharmacotherapy may be compromised.

Effective and specific treatments (for example, tricyclic drugs) have been available for the treatment of major depressive disorder for 40 years. The use of specific pharmacotherapy approximately doubles the chance that a depressed patient will recover in one month. Several problems remain in the treatment of major depressive disorder: some patients do not respond to the first treatment; all currently available antidepressants take three to four weeks to exert significant therapeutic effects, although they may begin to show their effects earlier; and, until relatively recently, all available antidepressants have been toxic in overdoses and have had adverse effects. However, the introduction of bupropion (Wellbutrin), venlafaxine (Effexor), and the serotonin-specific reuptake inhibitors (SSRIs)—for example, fluoxetine (Prozac), paroxetine (Paxil), sertraline (Zoloft), and fluvoxamine (Luvox)—gives primary care physicians drugs that are much safer and much better tolerated than previous drugs but that are equally effective. Recent indications (for example, eating disorders and anxiety disorders) for antidepressant medications make the grouping of those drugs under the single label of antidepressants somewhat confusing.

The principal indication for antidepressants is a major depressive episode. The first symptoms to improve are often poor sleep and appetite patterns, although that may be less true when SSRIs are used than when tricyclic drugs are used. Agitation, anxiety, depressive episodes, and hopelessness are the next symptoms to improve. Other target symptoms include low energy, poor concentration, helplessness, and decreased libido.

TABLE 10.2-3
CURRENTLY USED ANTIDEPRESSANT DRUGS

Drug/Class	Trade Name	Typical Therapeutic Dosage (mg/day)
Tricyclics		
Tertiary amines		
Amitriptyline	(Elavil)	150–300
Doxepin	(Sinequan)	150–300
Clomipramine*	(Anafranil)	25–250
Imipramine	(Tofranil)	150–300
Trimipramine	(Surmontil)	150–300
Secondary amines		
Desipramine	(Norpramin)	150–300
Nortriptyline	(Pamelor)	75–150
Protriptyline	(Vivactil)	15–30
Tetracyclics		
Secondary amines		
Amoxapine	(Asendin)	200–300
Maprotiline	(Ludiomil)	100–225
Monocyclic		
Buproplon	(Wellbutrin)	300–450
Serotonin-specific reuptake inhibitors		
Fluoxetine	(Prozac)	20–60
Sertraline	(Zoloft)	50–200
Paroxetine	(Paxil)	20–50
Fluvoxamine*	(Luvox)	50–300
Serotonin-norepinephrine reuptake inhibitor		
Venlafaxine	(Effexor)	75–300
Phenylpiperazines		
Trazodone	(Desyrel)	300–600
Nefazodone	(Serzone)	300–500
Monamine oxidase inhibitors		
Tranylcypromine	(Parnate)	20–60
Phenelzine	(Norall)	30–90

*Approved for the treatment of obsessive-compulsive disorder.

Available Drugs

Table 10.2-3 lists drugs available for antidepressant therapy. The tricyclic drugs, the tetracyclic drugs, and the monoamine oxidase inhibitors (MAOIs) are the classic antidepressants. Although those drugs are usually used, the antidepressant armamentarium has been significantly augmented by the addition of the SSRIs and bupropion. Those drugs (especially the SSRIs) are generally much safer than either tricyclic drugs or MAOIs, and they have been shown to be equally effective in studies of depressed outpatients. Other atypical antidepressants include venlafaxine, trazodone (Desyrel), nefazodone (Serzone), and alprazolam (Xanax). The sympathomimetics (for example, amphetamines) are also indicated for the treatment of depressive disorders in special therapeutic situations (for example, depression due to human immunodeficiency virus [HIV] disease).

General Clinical Guidelines

The most common clinical mistake leading to an unsuccessful trial of an antidepressant drug is the use of too low a dosage for too short a time. Unless adverse events prevent it, the dosage of an antidepressant should be raised to the maximum recommended level and maintained at that level for at least four weeks before a drug trial can be considered unsuccessful. Alternatively, if a patient is improving clinically on a low dosage of the drug, that dosage should not be raised unless clinical improvement stops before the maximal benefit is obtained. If a patient does not begin to respond to appropriate dosages of a drug after two or three weeks, the clinician may decide to obtain a plasma concentration of the drug if the test for that particular drug is available. The test may show either noncompliance or particularly unusual pharmacokinetic disposition of the drug, thereby suggesting an alternative dosage.

Duration and Prophylaxis

Antidepressant treatment should be maintained for at least six months or the length of the previous episode, whichever is greater. Several studies show that prophylactic treatment with antidepressants is effective in reducing the number and the severity of recurrences. One study concluded that, if episodes are less than $2^1/_2$ years apart, prophylactic treatment for five years is probably indicated. Another factor suggesting prophylactic treatment is the seriousness of previous depressive episodes. Episodes that have involved significant suicidal ideation or impairment of psychosocial functioning may indicate prophylactic treatment. When antidepressants are stopped, they should be tapered gradually over one to two weeks, depending on the half-life of the particular compound.

Failure of Drug Trial

If the first antidepressant drug has received an adequate trial and, if appropriate, the clinician is confident of the plasma concentrations obtained, the two available options are (1) augmenting the drug with lithium, liothyronine (sometimes called or L-triiodothyronine) (Cytomel), or L-tryptophan or (2) switching to an alternative primary agent. When switching agents, the clinician should switch a patient who has been taking a tricyclic or tetracyclic drug to an SSRI (or possibly an MAOI) and should switch a patient who has been taking an SSRI to a tricyclic or tetracyclic drug (or possibly an MAOI). At least two weeks should elapse between the use of an SSRI and the use of an MAOI, and the two drugs should never be used concurrently.

Venlafaxine is an effective antidepressant drug that may have unique efficacy properties, including a faster than usual onset of action and demonstrated efficacy in seriously depressed patients (for example, patients with melancholic features). The clinician can also consider switching a first-line drug nonresponder to trazodone, nefazodone, or bupropion.

For a more detailed discussion of this topic, see Mood Disorders, Chap 16, pp 1067–1190; A Roy: Suicide, Sec 30.1, p 1739; Psychotherapies, Chap 31, pp 1767–1894; T W Uhde, M E Tancer: Benzodiazepine Receptor Agonists and Antagonists, Sec 32.7, p 1933; N Sussman: Bupropion, Sec 32.8, p 1951; J M Himmelhoch: Monoamine Oxidase Inhibitors, Sec 32.18, p 2038; Serotonin-Specific Reuptake Inhibitors, Sec 32.19, pp 2054–2072; J C Nelson: Sympathomimetics, Sec 32.20, p 2073; A J Prange Jr, R A Stern: Thyroid Hormones, Sec 32.22, p 2083; J J Barry, A F Schatzberg: Trazodone and Nefazodone, Sec 32.23, p 2089; J B Kessel, G M Simpson: Tricyclic and Tetracyclic Drugs, Sec 32.24, p 2096; J A Grebb: Venlafaxine, Sec 32.26, p 2120; S L Dubovsky: Electroconvulsive Therapy, Sec 32.28, p 2129; B J Sadock, H I Kaplan: Other Biological Therapies, Sec 32.30, p 2144; G A Carlson, S F Abbott: Mood Disorders and Suicide, Chap 44, p 2367; G S Alexopoulos: Mood Disorders, Sec 49.6b, p 2566 in CTP/VI.

10.3 Grief and Bereavement

Grief is the characteristic feeling precipitated by the death of a loved one or by some other significant loss. *Bereavement* is the state of being deprived of a loved one by death and implies a state of mourning through which grief may be relieved.

CLINICAL FEATURES AND DIAGNOSIS

Grief is frequently seen in doctor's offices and may be present in either identified patients or their family members or friends. Usually, grief is a normal, self-limiting process that can be managed with supportive, common-sense measures. The course of grief is affected by the patient's preparation for the loss, the abruptness of the loss, and its significance to the patient.

The clinician must look for signs of complications, including major depression, psychotic features, agitation, suicidality, alcohol abuse, and drug abuse. Persistent visual hallucinations or dreams that beckon the patient to reunite with the deceased are particularly ominous.

Although symptoms of grief and depression overlap, the symptoms of the grieving patient are generally considered appropriate for the circumstances. The depressed patient has inappropriate symptoms, such as prolonged functional impairment, morbid preoccupation with feeling worthless, and marked psychomotor retardation (Table 10.3-1).

Although grief is generally described as occurring after the death of a loved one, other major losses can also precipitate grief—divorce, the death of a pet, the loss of a job, the loss of a body part, and the loss of status. The clinical presentation of grief varies with cultural background. The clinician must determine what is considered an appropriate response in the patient's culture.

The clinical symptoms of normal grief include depressed mood, insomnia, anxiety, poor appetite, loss of interest, guilt feelings about what could have been done

TABLE 10.3–1
GRIEF VERSUS DEPRESSION

Grief	Depression
Normal identification with deceased. Little ambivalence toward deceased	Abnormal overidentification with deceased
	Increased ambivalence and unconscious anger toward deceased
Crying, weight loss, decreased libido, withdrawal, insomnia, irritability, decreased concentration and attention	Similar to grief
Suicidal ideas rare	Suicidal ideas common
Self-blame relates to how deceased was treated	Self-blame is global
No global feelings of worthlessness	Person thinks he or she is generally bad or worthless
Evokes empathy and sympathy	Usually evokes interpersonal annoyance or irritation
With time, symptoms abate; self-limited; usually clears within 6 months	Symptoms do not abate and may worsen; may still be present after years
Vulnerable to physical illness	Vulnerable to physical illness
Responds to reassurance, social contacts	Does not respond to reassurance, pushes away social contacts
Not helped by antidepressant medication	Helped by antidepressant medication

TABLE 10.3–2
STAGES OF GRIEF AND BEREAVEMENT

Stage	John Bowlby	Stage	C. M. Parkes
1	**Numbness or protest.** Characterized by distress, fear, and anger. Shock may last moments, days, weeks, or months	1	**Alarm.** A stressful state characterized by physiological changes, e.g., rise in blood pressure and heart rate; similar to Bowlby's first stage
2	**Yearning and searching for the lost figure.** World seems empty and meaningless, but self-esteem remains intact. Characterized by preoccupation with lost person, physical restlessness, weeping, and anger. May last several months or even years	2	**Numbness.** Person appears superficially affected by loss but is actually protecting himself or herself from acute distress
3	**Disorganization and despair.** Restlessness and aimlessness. Increase in somatic preoccupation, withdrawal, introversion, and irritability. Repeated reliving of memories	3	**Pining (searching).** Person looks for or is reminded of the lost person. Similar to Bowlby's second stage
		4	**Depression.** Person feels hopeless about future, cannot go on living, and withdraws from family and friends
4	**Reorganization.** With establishment of new patterns, objects, and goals, grief recedes and is replaced by cherished memories. Healthy identification with deceased occurs	5	**Recovery and reorganization.** Person realizes that his or her life will continue with new adjustment and different goals

to prevent the loss (survivor guilt), dreams about the deceased, irritability, anger at medical professionals who were treating the deceased, poor concentration, focus on objects or activities that are reminiscent of the deceased (linkage objects), sensations that the deceased is still present (identification phenomena), shortness of breath, difficulty in talking, and other somatic symptoms. Psychological states encountered in grieving patients include shock, denial, yearning and searching for the deceased, depression, and reorganization. The active symptoms generally last from three to six months, followed by several months in which normal functioning and behavior are restored.

Table 10.3-2 lists the stages of grief and bereavement.

INTERVIEWING AND PSYCHOTHERAPEUTIC GUIDELINES

No less effort should be expended in managing grieving patients because grief is considered a normal reaction. Clinicians can help patients through the painful process. Treating a patient with an acute grief reaction may prevent the development of major depression.

Encourage grieving patients to express their feelings about the deceased and to review the relationship, describing its positive and negative aspects. Many patients are angry at the deceased for dying and should be encouraged to express that anger, although they feel guilty about it.

Reassure patients that the symptoms are normal and will pass and that they are not psychiatrically ill. However, avoid simplistic reassurances that suppress patients' abilities to express their feelings, such as, "It's destiny." Some patients with unresolved grief present with repeated somatic complaints and should be encouraged to talk about their losses. Providing a quiet place may make grieving patients comfortable.

EVALUATION AND MANAGEMENT

1. The goals of treatment are to facilitate a normal grieving process and to identify and treat any pathological process.
2. Determine the details of the loss. What was the importance of the relationship? How sudden or unpredicted was the loss? What is the significance of the loss to the patient? Does the patient feel responsible for causing the death?
3. Does the patient have a history of major depression? If so, the risk of depression as a complication of grief is increased. How has the patient dealt with losses in the past?
4. Evaluate the patient for psychotic symptoms, agitation, increased activity, alcohol abuse, drug abuse, and suicidality. Look for severe depression, insomnia, appetite changes, and somatic symptoms. Has the patient done anything destructive or shown uncharacteristic poor judgment? Does the patient have the same symptoms of the deceased's illness? The presence of such symptoms indicates complicated or unresolved grief and requires appropriate intervention.
5. Do not overlook patients who do not express significant grief after a major loss. Those patients may have an increased risk of subsequent complicated or unresolved grief. The patients may be in shock or may have cultural or personality features that cause limited emotional expression. Encourage patients to express their emotions, and explore why it is difficult for them to do so. Delayed grief reactions may occur, typically, on the anniversary of the death.
6. Encourage patients to spend time with families and friends to help fill the space vacated by the deceased. Returning to work or school may help the patients' sense of self-esteem. Group therapy and self-help groups are also beneficial for the grieving. Give patients simple structured tasks, such as getting up and dressing before noon every day, writing down feelings for a specified period each day, and scheduling daily chores and free time.
7. Complicated grief reactions require significant interventions. Suicidal or severely depressed patients may require hospitalization. Refer patients with unresolved grief to supportive outpatient psychotherapy. Those patients may come to the emergency room or doctor's office with somatic or depressive complaints while denying the significance of their losses. Unresolved grief may result from family conflicts, ambivalent feelings toward the deceased, or traumatic loss. The presence of psychosis, severe agitation, or alcohol or substance abuse requires appropriate intervention. Allow patients to see the deceased to say goodbye.

DRUG TREATMENT

Most grieving patients should not be medicated, especially since they may later feel that medications interfered with the mourning process. Severe insomnia or anxiety may be treated with benzodiazepines. For example, estazolam (ProSom) or lorazepam (Ativan), are both given at 0.5 to 1 mg by mouth every four hours as needed for anxiety; flurazepam (Dalmane) or temazepam (Restoril) are both given at 15 to 30 mg by mouth at bedtime as needed for insomnia. Patients with major depression may require a course of antidepressants. Patients dependent on alcohol or drugs may require detoxification. Antipsychotics are not required unless the patient has an underlying psychotic disorder or the grief reaction is complicated by psychotic depression.

For a more detailed discussion of this topic, see S Zisook: Death, Dying, and Bereavement, Sec 29.6, p 1713, in CTP/VI.

10.4 Mania

Mania is a distinct episode of abnormally and persistently elevated, expansive, or irritable mood, which has led to impaired judgment and caused a marked impairment in the patient's functioning.

The most important tasks in treating a manic episode are to recognize it and to make an appropriate referral to a psychiatrist.

CLINICAL FEATURES AND DIAGNOSIS

If psychotic symptoms are present, delusions are often grandiose or paranoid and may also be mood-incongruent. The criteria for manic episode are given in Table 10.4-1.

TABLE 10.4-1
CRITERIA FOR MANIC EPISODE

A. A distinct period of abnormally and persistently elevated, expansive, or irritable mood, lasting at least 1 week (or any duration if hospitalization is necessary).
B. During the period of mood disturbance, three (or more) of the following symptoms have persisted (four if the mood is only irritable) and have been present to a significant degree:
 (1) inflated self-esteem or grandiosity
 (2) decreased need for sleep (e.g., feels rested after only 3 hours of sleep)
 (3) more talkative than usual or pressure to keep talking
 (4) flight of ideas or subjective experience that thoughts are racing
 (5) distractibility (i.e., attention too easily drawn to unimportant or irrelevant external stimuli)
 (6) increase in goal-directed activity (either socially, at work or school, or sexually) or psychomotor agitation
 (7) excessive involvement in pleasurable activities that have a high potential for painful consequences (e.g., engaging in unrestrained buying sprees, sexual indiscretions, or foolish business investments)
C. The symptoms do not meet criteria for a mixed episode.
D. The mood disturbance is sufficiently severe to cause marked impairment in occupational functioning or in usual social activities or relationships with others, or to necessitate hospitalization to prevent harm to self or others, or there are psychotic features.
E. The symptoms are not due to the direct physiological effects of a substance (e.g., a drug of abuse, a medication, or other treatment) or a general medical condition (e.g., hyperthyroidism).

Note: Maniclike episodes that are clearly caused by somatic antidepressant treatment (e.g., medication, electroconvulsive therapy, light therapy) should not count toward a diagnosis of bipolar I disorder.

Table from DSM-IV, *Diagnostic and Statistical Manual of Mental Disorders,* ed 4. Copyright American Psychiatric Association, Washington, 1994. Used with permission.

Mania usually occurs in the context of bipolar I disorder, schizoaffective disorder, mood disorder due to a general medical condition, and substance-related disorders. Patients with bipolar I disorder usually also have major depressive episodes. Electroconvulsive therapy, antidepressant medications, and other medications can precipitate mania. In a single clinical evaluation of a psychotic patient, mania may be indistinguishable from schizophrenia; the proper diagnosis must be based on the patient's history.

The lifetime prevalence of bipolar disorder is about 1 percent, divided equally between men and women. Without treatment, a manic episode usually lasts from three to six months.

INTERVIEWING AND PSYCHOTHERAPEUTIC GUIDELINES

Manic patients may be initially entertaining and charming, but they can become annoying, irritating, and inescapable. Their behavior may be unpredictable, and sometimes it may include violence. Set firm limits early with manic patients, and do not allow them to exploit or take advantage of the situation. Provide a nonstimulating environment for the interview, as manic patients are highly distractible.

EVALUATION AND MANAGEMENT

1. Maintain a secure environment that will prevent flight, and be sure that enough staff members are available if restraint is required. Manic episodes are psychiatric emergencies and usually require hospitalization.
2. Observe the patient for signs of general medical conditions, not only because the poor judgment of manic patients predisposes them to comorbidity, but also because agitation from other organic causes may be mistaken for mania.
3. Evaluate the patient for signs of drug intoxication, alcohol withdrawal, or the side effects of prescribed medications. Neuroleptic-induced akathisia may cause restlessness or agitation.
4. Order laboratory tests, including a complete blood count (CBC), thyroid function tests, a urine toxicology screen, a chemistry profile, hepatic and renal function tests (blood urea nitrogen [BUN] and creatinine), and an electrocardiogram (ECG).
5. Correct thyroid problems and other medical problems if present. Perform a complete, detailed physical examination as soon as the patient can cooperate.

DRUG TREATMENT

Lithium (Eskalith, Lithobid) is usually the treatment first used for manic episodes. However, lithium requires 7 to 10 days before it is effective. Carbamazepine (Tegretol) and divalproex (Depakote) are also effective. Antipsychotics are rapidly effective and commonly used, but their use should be discouraged because of side effects, such as tardive dyskinesia. Carbamazepine has an onset of action comparable to that of the antipsychotics. Benzodiazepines—for example, lorazepam (Ativan) and clonazepam (Klonopin)—are also effective and may be used for acute agitation or to augment the antipsychotics.

If agitation or hyperactivity requires tranquilization, avoid antipsychotics. Start with a benzodiazepine—for example, lorazepam 1 to 2 mg by mouth or intramuscularly (IM) as needed or clonazepam 1 to 2 mg by mouth as needed. Repeat the benzodiazepine as needed until the patient's agitation is reduced or until the signs of benzodiazepine intoxication occur (ataxia, slurred speech, nystagmus). Disinhibition caused by benzodiazepines may be indistinguishable from worsening mania. If the patient becomes increasingly agitated, discontinue the benzodiazepine immediately. Manic patients who are also substance abusers may be particularly unresponsive to benzodiazepines or may require very high doses.

If the patient is benzodiazepine-intoxicated and still agitated or otherwise appears to be unresponsive to the benzodiazepine, discontinue that drug and give an antipsychotic. All the antipsychotics are equal in their eventual antimanic efficacy. Many psychiatrists prefer to use high-potency antipsychotics because those drugs cause few anticholinergic and hypotensive side effects; typical regimens are fluphenazine (Prolixin) or haloperidol (Haldol), both given at 5 mg by mouth three times a day or 5 mg IM every four hours as needed. Titrate the dosage according to the patient's response. Antipsychotics, other than clozapine (Clozaril), may be augmented with benzodiazepines for acute agitation to avoid exposure to high dosages of antipsychotics. If the patient is already taking lithium and is in outpatient treatment, check with the outpatient physician. If a current or recent lithium level is below the therapeutic level, consider discharging the patient back to outpatient care after raising the lithium dosage and giving the patient adjunctive medication—for example, lorazepam 1 to 2 mg by mouth every four to six hours. Use that treatment only in patients who are firmly engaged in outpatient follow-up and who have adequate support systems.

For a more detailed discussion of this topic, see Mood Disorders, Chap 16, pp 1067–1189, in CTP/VI.

10.5 Self-Mutilation

Self-mutilation is an action that can be used to manipulate others but may genuinely reflect an intent to do self-harm. Self-mutilation is most commonly accomplished with a sharp object, such as a knife. In severe cases, patients cut-off their own ears, genitals, or other body parts. Burning oneself with cigarettes and inserting objects under the skin are other methods. Head banging, nail biting, and hair pulling are variants sometimes seen in children.

CLINICAL FEATURES AND DIAGNOSIS

Usually, the problem is long-term, but it can occur impulsively in psychotic patients. The intent is typically not suicide, although self-injurious patients are also prone to suicide attempts, and self-mutilation may precede a suicide attempt. Self-mutilation is more common in females than in males and is more common in patients in their 20s than in older patients.

The common sites of self-injury include the wrists, the arms, and the thighs. The breasts, the face, and the abdomen are less typical sites.

The reasons for self-cutting include anger at self or others, tension, a wish to die, and the need to feel pain to feel alive. Many patients who cut themselves claim that the experience is painless. Self-mutilating behavior is also effective in gaining attention. The behavior may be used to manipulate and elicit specific responses. Patients who are malingering may injure themselves to obtain either psychiatric or medical-surgical treatment. Patients with factitious disorders may injure themselves to create evidence supporting their need to maintain the sick role.

The most common diagnosis among self-mutilating patients is severe personality disorder, often borderline or antisocial personality disorder. Substance abuse and dependence are commonly associated features.

Self-mutilation in a child who is a victim of child abuse may be an act of aggression intended for the abuser directed instead toward the self.

Psychotic patients may injure themselves. The self-mutilating behavior in psychotic patients is sometimes bizarre and may be based on a somatic delusion (for example, that a part of the body is contaminated). In psychotic patients, the self-mutilating act may be unpredictable and impulsive. Patients who are psychotic because of phencyclidine (PCP) intoxication may injure themselves with total disregard for the pain, since the drug causes not only psychosis but also analgesia.

Other types of self-mutilating behavior with typical onset during childhood include head banging and nail biting. Scratching and hair pulling are less common. All may occur as circumscribed stereotypy and habit disorders or in the course of pervasive disorders, such as schizophrenia, mental retardation, autistic disorder, other pervasive developmental disorders, and organic disorders. Lesch-Nyhan syndrome is an X-linked recessive developmental disorder associated with metabolic derangements that can lead to persistent self-mutilating behavior. Ongoing physical restraint may be required.

INTERVIEWING AND PSYCHOTHERAPEUTIC GUIDELINES

Suspect self-mutilation if other explanations do not easily account for the patient's injuries. Try to determine early in the evaluation whether the patient is psychotic. Explore the possible secondary gain that the self-mutilation provides the patient. If the patient is a child, look for a possible history of child abuse.

Distinguish patients who admit to self-mutilating behavior from patients who are mutilating themselves but deny it. Although the distinction does not always lead to specific interventions, the admitted self-mutilator can be addressed directly, but the denying self-mutilator may be unpredictable and should be treated cautiously.

Consider self-mutilating patients highly dangerous. Maintain clear and firm control of the situation, and clearly inform the patient that continued self-injurious behavior will not be tolerated.

Try to determine whether the self-mutilating behavior is under voluntary control and thus likely to respond to a nonsomatic intervention. Self-mutilating behavior in patients with psychotic disorders, organic disorders, autistic disorder, and other pervasive developmental disorders is less under voluntary control than is self-mutilating behavior in patients with personality disorders.

EVALUATION AND MANAGEMENT

1. Perform a complete evaluation, including a medical and psychiatric history, a complete mental status examination, a history of drug and alcohol use, and a physical examination. Examine the patient's body for scars from previous self-mutilating acts.
2. If the patient is a child, look carefully for evidence of possible child abuse.
3. Try to assess the purpose of the self-mutilating behavior: Was it a suicide attempt or is it due to psychosis? Does it reflect aggression toward another, or is it being used to manipulate the environment and elicit a response from others?
4. Make a definitive psychiatric diagnosis. Self-destructive behavior is a sign of many different diagnoses.
5. If the patient is clearly not psychotic and if the behavior is intended to elicit some specific response from others, use crisis-intervention techniques to reduce the patient's motivation to manipulate others.
6. If the self-mutilation is a suicide gesture, be conservative, and respond to all acts of self-injury as potentially life-threatening. Any other response may deliver a message that the patient must escalate the dangerousness of the self-destructive acts to elicit a definitive intervention.
7. If the patient is psychotic, hospitalization is necessary.
8. Hospitalize nonpsychotic patients if the self-mutilating behavior is likely to continue.
9. During psychiatric hospitalization, maintain one-to-one constant observation to prevent further self-mutilating behavior.
10. To prevent continued self-mutilation, use drug treatment and physical restraints only as interventions of last resort.

DRUG TREATMENT

The drug treatment plan should focus on long-term management, since self-mutilating behaviors are usually chronic. Drug choice should be based on a definitive diagnosis and a specific treatment of that disorder.

A sufficient dose of an antipsychotic will eliminate all purposeful behavior, including self-mutilation. However, if the only target symptom is the self-mutilating behavior, tranquilization with antipsychotics, benzodiazepines, or barbiturates is not appropriate for purposes other than providing immediate behavioral control.

Antipsychotics are indicated if the patient is chronically psychotic. Anticonvulsants such as carbamazepine (Tegretol) may be useful in some organic conditions and in impulse-control disorders. β-Blockers, such as propranolol (Inderal)—are also helpful in reducing violence.

For a more detailed discussion of this topic, see J Yager, M J Gitlin: Clinical Manifestations of Psychiatric Disorders, Chap 10, p 637; E D Caine, H Grossman, J M Lyness: Delirium, Dementia, and Amnestic and Other Cognitive Disorders and Mental Disorders Due to a General Medical Condition, Chap 12, p 705; A A Lipton, R Cancro: Schizophrenia: Clinical Features, Sec 14.7, p 968, in CTP/VI.

10.6 Suicide

Suicide is intentional, self-inflicted death. Suicidal ideation and attempted suicide are among the most common emergency presentations. Common themes in suicide include a crisis that causes intense suffering and feelings of hopelessness and helplessness, conflicts between survival and unbearable stress, a narrowing of the patient's perceived options, and the wish to escape. Suicidal ideation occurs in vulnerable persons in response to many kinds of stressors at any age and may be present for long periods without resulting in an attempt.

CLINICAL FEATURES AND DIAGNOSIS

Identifying suicidal patients is crucial but difficult. Studies reveal that male sex, white race, advancing age, and social isolation increase the risk of completed suicide. Patients with family histories of suicide attempts or completions are at increased risk, as are patients with histories of chronic pain, recent surgery, or chronic physical illness. Also at increased risk are patients who are unemployed, live alone, or have an anniversary of a loss. High risk factors for suicide are listed in Table 10.6-1.

Eighty percent of patients who commit suicide have a mood disorder and 25 percent are alcohol dependent. Suicide is the cause of death for 15 percent of people in those two groups. The risk for alcoholic persons is particularly high in the six months after a major loss. Schizophrenia is a less common disorder and, therefore, accounts for a lower number of suicides, but 10 percent of persons with schizophrenia die by suicide.

The best hope for suicide prevention lies in the early detection and treatment of those contributory psychiatric disorders.

The role of prior suicide attempts in suicide risk assessment is complex. The majority of completed suicide victims have made no prior attempts; they are success-

TABLE 10.6-1
HIGH-RISK FACTORS FOR SUICIDE

Personal and Social Factors	Clinical Features and Symptoms
Male sex	Depressive illness, especially at onset or toward end of illness
Age > 55 yr	
Recent separation, divorce, or widowhood	Marked motor agitation, restlessness, and anxiety
Social isolation with real or imagined unsympathetic attitude of relatives or friends	Marked feelings of guilt, inadequacy, and hopelessness, self-denigration or nihilistic delusion
Impulsive, hostile personality	Severe hypochondriacal preoccupations: delusion or near-delusional conviction of physical disease, e.g., cancer, heart disease, or sexually transmitted disease
Personally significant anniversaries	
History of suicide in family, or of affective disorder	
Unemployment or financial difficulties, particularly if causing a drastic fall in economic status	Command hallucinations
	Alcohol or drug abuse
Previous suicide attempt	Physical illness that is chronic, painful, or disabling, especially in patients who have previously enjoyed good health
Detailed planning and taking precautions against being discovered	Use of drugs (e.g., reserpine) that can cause severe depression

Table from *Merck Manual*, ed 16, p 1626. Merck Sharp & Dohme Research Laboratories, Rahway, NJ 1992. Used with permission.

ful the first time. Although anyone who has made a prior suicide attempt has a demonstrated capacity for self-destructive behavior, only 10 percent of persons who attempt suicide are successful within 10 years.

A substantial number of deliberately self-aggressive persons cut or burn themselves in a clearly nonlethal manner with no intention of killing themselves. A variety of motives may be present, including deliberate manipulation and unconscious rage at significant others. Diagnostically, the patients may meet the criteria for antisocial or borderline personality disorder, or the behavior may coexist with other bizarre ideation and behavior in schizophrenia.

Especially disturbing and medicolegally challenging are parasuicides, who repeatedly and, to some extent, predictably engage in near-lethal behavior while denying suicidal ideation. The most common variant is the patient who takes repetitive, unintentional drug overdoses. Such patients appear to have personality disturbances without major psychiatric symptoms. They often demand their release from the hospital as soon as they recover from the acute intoxication, sometimes sooner, and it is difficult to justify treating them coercively. However, detaining such persons involuntarily is wise if the frequency of their parasuicidal behavior escalates.

INTERVIEWING AND PSYCHOTHERAPEUTIC GUIDELINES

There is no truth to the myth that talking about suicide in a clinical setting induces it. Patients may spontaneously describe suicidal ideation. If they do not, question them directly.

Start by asking if the patients have ever felt like giving up or have felt that they would be better off dead. That approach carries little stigma and can be accepted by most people. Then talk about exactly what thoughts the patients have had and document the thoughts. Once the subject has been broached, use words like "killing" and "dying," rather than "hurting" since some patients are confused about the point of the question: most do not want to hurt themselves, even if they do want to kill themselves.

Ask the following questions: How frequent are your suicidal thoughts? Has your preoccupation with suicidal ideas increased? Have you simply had morbid thoughts, or have you thought about exactly how you might kill yourself? Have you thought casually or seriously about killing yourself? Have you considered any particular method?

Compare the patient's age and sophistication with how well the stated intentions match the methods. A woman of normal intelligence who insists that she wants to die and would take six to eight aspirin tablets to do so provokes less concern than does a child who makes the same statement.

Are the chosen means of committing suicide available to the patients? Have they taken any active steps, such as accumulating pills and settling their affairs? How pessimistic are they? Can they imagine any way in which things might improve?

That last question assists with both assessment and treatment, as patients may suggest some avenues of escape from their dilemma. If they do not, are they hopeless about the future? If so, are their fears realistic or delusional? A young man who is hopeless because his wife has left him is at less risk than a man who is convinced without foundation that he is dying of cancer and that everyone is withholding the truth.

Obtain a history from significant others if the patient is uncooperative.

EVALUATION AND MANAGEMENT

1. When evaluating suicidal patients, do not leave them alone; remove any potentially dangerous objects from the room.
2. When evaluating a patient who has just made a suicide attempt, assess whether the attempt was planned or impulsive. Determine the lethality, the patient's chance of discovery (for example, was the patient alone, and did the patient notify anyone?), the patient's reactions to being saved (is the patient disappointed or relieved?), and whether the factors that led to the attempt have changed.
3. Management depends largely on the diagnosis. Patients with severe depression may be treated as outpatients if their families can supervise them closely and if treatment can be initiated rapidly. Otherwise, hospitalization may be necessary.
4. The suicidal ideation of alcoholic patients generally remits with abstinence in a few days. No specific treatment is required in most cases. Depression that persists after the physiological signs of alcohol withdrawal have resolved warrants a high suspicion of major depression. All suicidal patients who are intoxicated by alcohol or drugs must be reassessed when they are sober.
5. Suicidal ideas in schizophrenic patients must be taken seriously, as they tend to use violent and sometimes bizarre methods of high lethality.
6. Patients with personality disorders benefit mostly from empathic confrontation to resolve the crisis that led to the attempted suicide. Assist them to resume a rational, responsible approach to the problem that precipitated the crisis and to which they have usually contributed. The involvement of family or friends and environmental manipulation may be helpful.
7. Long-term hospitalization is recommended for the conditions that contribute to self-mutilation, but brief hospitalization does not usually affect such habitual behavior. Parasuicides may also benefit from long-term rehabilitation, and a brief period of stabilization may be necessary from time to time, but no short-term treatment can be expected to alter their course significantly.

DRUG TREATMENT

A patient in crisis because of a death or other event with a limited course may function better after receiving mild sedation as needed, particularly if sleep has been disturbed. Benzodiazepines are the drugs of choice, and a typical regimen is lorazepam (Ativan) 1 mg one to three times a day for two weeks. The regular use of a benzodiazepine may increase the patient's irritability, and irritability is a risk factor for suicide, so benzodiazepines should be used with caution in hostile patients. Only provide small quantities of the medication, and see the patient again within days.

Antidepressants are an essential part of the treatment for patients who present with suicidal ideas. If prescribed, a definite follow-up appointment should be made, preferably on the following day.

For a more detailed discussion of this topic, see A Roy: Suicide, Sec 30.1, p 1739, in CTP/VI.

11

Anxiety and Dissociative Disorders

11.1 Anxiety

Anxiety is a feeling of dread accompanied by somatic signs indicative of a hyperactive autonomic nervous system. Anxiety is a common nonspecific symptom that is often a normal emotion. Pathological anxiety is disproportionate to any real threat and is maladaptive.

CLINICAL FEATURES AND DIAGNOSIS

Anxiety and anxiety disorders can present with any number of physical and psychological signs and symptoms, including those outlined in Table 11.1-1. Patients who present to the primary care physician's office with anxiety may have any of the medical disorders delineated in Table 11.1-2, all of which must be considered in the differential diagnosis. The anxiety disorders are specific illnesses characterized by pathological anxiety that is not secondary to an organic factor or another psychiatric diagnosis; they include panic disorder (see Section 11.3), phobias (Section 11.4), obsessive-compulsive disorder (Section 11.5), posttraumatic stress disorder (Section 11.6), and generalized anxiety disorder. Patients with generalized anxiety disorder have ongoing worry and anxiety with associated motor tension, autonomic hyperactivity, and vigilance. A significant proportion of the patients experience panic attacks and depression.

INTERVIEWING AND PSYCHOTHERAPEUTIC GUIDELINES

Anxious patients often feel helpless, frightened, and out of control. Remain calm and reassuring; encourage patients to express their ideas and concerns. Reassure

TABLE 11.1-1
SIGNS AND SYMPTOMS OF ANXIETY

Physical Signs	Psychological Symptoms
Trembling, twitching, feeling shaky	Feeling of dread
Backache, headache	Difficulty in concentrating
Muscle tension	Hypervigilance
Shortness of breath, hyperventilation	Insomnia
Fatigability	Decreased libido
Startle response	Lump in the throat
Autonomic hyperactivity	Butterflies in the stomach
Flushing and pallor	
Tachycardia, palpitations	
Sweating	
Cold hands	
Diarrhea	
Dry mouth (xerostomia)	
Urinary frequency	
Paresthesia	
Difficulty in swallowing	

239

TABLE 11.1–2
MEDICAL DISORDERS ASSOCIATED WITH ANXIETY

Gastrointestinal system	Neurological system
Colitis	Acquired immune deficiency syndrome (AIDS)
Crohn's disease	Dementia and delirium
Irritable bowel syndrome	Epilepsy
Peptic ulcer disease	Essential tremor
Cardiovascular system	Huntington's chorea
Cardiac arrhythmias	Lupus cerebritis
Cardiomyopathies	Multiple sclerosis
Congestive heart failure	Parkinson's disease
Coronary insufficiency	Vestibular dysfunction
Mitral valve prolapse	Wilson's disease
Postmyocardial infarction	Endocrine system
Respiratory system	Adrenal insufficiency
Asthma	Carcinoid syndrome
Chronic obstructive pulmonary disease	Cushing's syndrome
Hyperventilation syndrome	Hyperparathyroidism
Pneumothorax	Hyperthyroidism
Pulmonary edema	Hypoglycemia
Pulmonary embolism	Hypokalemia
	Hypothyroidism

Table from W R Dubin, K J Weiss: *Handbook of Psychiatric Emergencies,* p 157. Springhouse, Springhouse, Pa, 1991. Used with permission.

patients about the nature of their symptoms; for example, tell panic disorder patients that they are not having a heart attack or going insane.

When obtaining the patient's history, focus on precipitants, avoidance behavior, medical problems, obsessions, compulsions, and the time, course, and nature of the symptoms.

Discuss your diagnostic formulation in a clear and realistically hopeful fashion. Anxious patients may take comfort in hearing about the cause of their anxiety and the available treatment options.

EVALUATION AND MANAGEMENT

1. Rule out substance-related disorders and medical conditions before considering other diagnoses. Does the patient with classic panic attacks have a cardiac arrhythmia or hyperthyroidism? Obtain a full medical history. Is the patient taking medications that cause anxiety? Does the patient drink large quantities of caffeinated beverages? Consider a thorough neurological examination, blood and urine screening tests (including a toxicology screen), and a computed tomography (CT) scan of the head if a brain lesion is suspected.

2. Precipitating events, the severity and the duration of the anxiety, the patient's history of anxiety, such associated symptoms as insomnia and depression, and the anxiety's diurnal variation must be determined. Does the patient have an impairment caused by the anxiety?

3. Before making a definitive diagnosis, consider the following questions: Does the patient have a major depressive disorder, a psychotic disorder, or a panic disorder? Is the disorder situational anxiety? Does the patient have a substance use disorder, a personality disorder, or a medical condition? Does the patient have hyperventilation syndrome?

4. Any life stress can produce anxiety, and may result in situational disorders. Supportive and cognitive psychotherapies are helpful.
5. Anxiety is a common symptom of depression. Depression with anxiety is the appropriate diagnosis if other depressive symptoms are present: depressed mood, changes in appetite and sleep, diurnal variation, anhedonia, feelings of hopelessness and helplessness, guilt feelings, death thoughts, psychomotor agitation or retardation, and impaired concentration. Cognitive and supportive psychotherapies are useful.
6. Anxiety is a prominent symptom in panic disorder (with or without agoraphobia), agoraphobia without a history of panic disorder, specific phobia, social phobia, obsessive-compulsive disorder, posttraumatic stress disorder, and generalized anxiety disorder. The definitive treatment of those disorders includes psychotherapy, usually behavior and cognitive therapy.
7. Psychotic patients often experience anxiety in association with their psychotic symptoms. Psychotherapy is critical in helping patients to understand and to deal with their psychotic experiences. Supportive therapy, which may include advice, reassurances, education, modeling, limit setting, and reality testing, is generally the therapy of choice. Behavior therapy, group therapy, and family therapy can also be of use.

DRUG TREATMENT

Benzodiazepines are usually the anxiolytic drugs of choice; however, evaluate the anxiety and the associated symptoms thoroughly before prescribing a benzodiazepine.

For patients with generalized anxiety disorder, not only are the benzodiazepines useful in treatment, but also helpful are buspirone (BuSpar) and tricyclic antidepressants. Benzodiazepines are particularly effective for the somatic manifestations of generalized anxiety.

Since situational disorders are usually time-limited, benzodiazepines are useful for the relief of the anxiety or insomnia. For repeated anxiety in relation to specific situations (for example, stage fright), β-blockers such as propranolol (Inderal) are useful when taken before exposure to the situation and do not have the risks of sedation and dependence.

For psychotic or depressed patients, an antipsychotic or an antidepressant may be more appropriate than an anxiolytic. Benzodiazepines are useful temporarily to relieve the anxiety accompanying depression, but they are not a definitive treatment. Antidepressants are indicated in depressive disorders and can be combined with cognitive and supportive psychotherapy. If medication is needed in psychotic disorders, the question of whether the symptoms should be treated with a benzodiazepine or an antipsychotic is controversial. In general, giving an antipsychotic represents a decision to initiate an ongoing plan to continue treatment with that antipsychotic. Antipsychotics have a relatively long elimination half-life (about one day) and are typically used in the maintenance of chronically psychotic patients. If a chronically psychotic patient responds to an antipsychotic, the antipsychotic is usually continued. Akathisia may be the cause of anxiety in patients who are already taking antipsychotics.

The drug treatment of the anxiety disorders are discussed later in this chapter: panic disorder (Section 11.3), phobias (Section 11.4), obsessive-compulsive disorder (Section 11.5), and posttraumatic stress disorder (Section 11.6). Drugs used include benzodiazepines, tricyclic antidepressants, serotonin-specific reuptake inhibitors (SSRIs), monoamine oxidase inhibitors (MAOIs), β-blockers, and clonidine (Catapres). Benzodiazepines are indicated only for short-term treatment; however, treatment often continues for prolonged periods, which raises the question of drug dependence.

For a substance-abusing patient, benzodiazepines may be contraindicated. For a patient with panic disorder or posttraumatic stress disorder, consider antidepressants. Antihistamines such as diphenhydramine (Benadryl) 25 to 50 mg or hydroxyzine (Atarax, Vistaril) 25 to 50 mg are sometimes used as an alternative to benzodiazepines.

In general, benzodiazepines should be used for short-term symptom relief—that is, not more than several months. They are not usually considered a definitive treatment, although some evidence suggests that they are effective in the long-term treatment of anxiety disorders when combined with psychotherapy. Benzodiazepines are drugs with a potential for abuse. They are often taken by cocaine abusers, who use them to come down after using cocaine. In emergency room situations where the patient is not well known, benzodiazepines should not be prescribed if there is any suspicion of malingering or substance abuse. Giving benzodiazepines in that situation may reinforce drug-seeking behavior.

When prescribing benzodiazepines, give only a several days' supply to tide the patients over until they can be seen in ongoing treatment. All benzodiazepines are effective anxiolytics, and the drug choice is based on metabolic pathway (oxidation or conjugation), desired route of administration, and elimination half-life (Table 11.1-3).

Identify the diurnal pattern of the target symptoms, including both daytime and nighttime patterns. Prescribe a drug according to the desired pharmacokinetic profile. For example, a long-acting benzodiazepine best treats daytime anxiety with insomnia at night; daytime anxiety without insomnia suggests the use of a short-acting benzodiazepine.

All benzodiazepines are well absorbed after oral administration, but diazepam (Valium) and triazolam (Halcion) are absorbed especially rapidly. For intramuscular injection, lorazepam is rapidly and predictably absorbed. Benzodiazepines that are oxidized can have a prolonged elimination half-life in the elderly and in those with liver disease.

For a more detailed discussion of this topic, see Anxiety Disorders, Chap 17, pp 1191–1249, in CTP/VI.

11.2   Hyperventilation

Hyperventilation occurs when a person breathes rapidly and deeply for several minutes, producing hypocapnia and respiratory alkalosis. When the voluntary hyperventilation stops, the hypocapnia reduces the normal drive to breathe, which leads to a mild hypoxia.

TABLE 11.1–3
BENZODIAZEPINES

Drug	Approximate Dose Equivalents[1]	Dosage Forms	Benzodiazepines Rate of Absorption	Major Active Metabolites	Average Half-Life of Metabolites (hrs)	Short-Acting/ Long-Acting[3]	Usual Adult Dosage Range (mg per day)
Alprazolam (Xanax)	0.5	0.25, 0.5, 1, 2 mg tablets	Medium	α-Hydroxyalprazolam, 4-hydroxyalprazolam	12	Short	0.5–6
Chlordiazepoxide (Librium)	10	5, 10, 25 mg tablets; 5, 10, 25 mg capsules; 100 mg parenteral	Medium	Desmethylchlordiazepoxide, demoxepam	100	Long	15–100
Clonazepam (Klonopin)	0.25	0.5, 1, 2 mg tablets	Rapid	None	34	Long	0.5–10
Clorazepate (Tranxene)	7.5	3.75, 7.5, 11.25, 15, 22.5 mg tablets; 3.75, 7.5, 15 mg capsules	Rapid	Desmethyldiazepam, oxazepam	100	Long	7.5–60
Diazepam (Valium)	5	2, 5, 10 mg tablets; 15 mg capsules (extended release); 5 mg/mL parenteral	Rapid	Desmethyldiazepam, oxazepam	100	Long	2–60
Estazolam (ProSom)	0.33	1, 2 mg tablets	Rapid	4-Hydroxy estazolam, l-oxo-estazolam	17	Short	1–2
Flurazepam (Dalmane)	5	15, 30 mg tablets	Rapid	Desalkylflurazepam, N-1-hydroxyethylflurazepam	100	Long	15–30
Halazepam (Paxipam)	20	20, 40 mg tablets	Medium	Desmethyldiazepam, oxazepam	100	Long	60–160
Lorazepam (Ativan)[2]	1	0.5, 1, 2 mg tablets; 2 mg/mL, 4 mg/mL parenteral	Medium	None	15	Short	2–6
Midazolam (Versed)[2]	1.25–1.7	1 mg/mL, 5 mg/mL parenteral	N/A	1-Hydroxymethylmidazolam	2.5	Short	1–5
Oxazepam (Serax)	15	15 mg tablets; 10, 15, 30 mg capsules	Slow	None	8	Short	30–120
Prazepam (Centrax)	10	10 mg tablets; 5, 10, 20 mg capsules	Slow	Desmethyldiazepam, oxazepam	100	Long	20–60
Quazepam (Doral)	5	7.5, 15 mg tablets	Rapid	2 oxoquazepam, N-desalkyl-2-oxoquazepam, and 3-hydroxy-2-oxoquazepam glucuronide	100	Long	7.5–30
Temazepam (Restoril)	5	15, 30 mg tablets	Medium	None	11	Short	15–30
Triazolam (Halcion)	0.1–0.03	0.125, 0.25 mg tablets	Rapid	None	2	Short	0.125–0.25

[1]High-potency drugs have an approximate close equivalent of under 1.0; 1.0–10—medium potency; over 10—low potency.
[2]Used only by anesthesiologists.
[3]Short-acting benzodiazepines have a half-life of under 25 hrs.

CLINICAL FEATURES AND DIAGNOSIS

The symptoms of hyperventilation include dizziness, light-headedness, fainting, paresthesias, and carpopedal spasm. The differential diagnosis includes seizures, hysteria, hypoglycemia, vasovagal attacks, myocardial ischemia, asthma, porphyria, pheochromocytoma, and Mèniére's disease. The psychiatric conditions associated with hyperventilation include panic disorder, phobia, obsessive-compulsive disorder, histrionic and borderline personality disorders, schizophrenia, and other syndromes in which anxiety is prominent.

INTERVIEWING AND PSYCHOTHERAPEUTIC GUIDELINES

Help the patient relax. Inform the patient that the symptoms are due to hyperventilation and will pass. Show them that they can hold their breath during an attack, despite their complaints of suffocation.

EVALUATION AND MANAGEMENT

1. If the patient is still hyperventilating, have the patient blow into a paper bag and rebreathe the air from the bag to counter the hypocapnia.
2. Rule out possible medical causes.
3. Obtain a full psychiatric evaluation. If the problem is chronic, hyperventilation may be a symptom of personality or anxiety disorders.[2] Refer the patient to appropriate outpatient treatment.

DRUG TREATMENT

Drug treatment is usually not necessary, but, if the patient is severely anxious, a single dose of a benzodiazepine—for example, lorazepam (Ativan) 1 mg by mouth or intramuscularly (IM) or alprazolam (Xanax) 0.5 to 1 mg by mouth—usually relieves the symptoms.

For a more detailed discussion of this topic, see A J Fyer, S Mannuzza, J D Coplan: Panic Disorders and Agoraphobia, Sec 17.1, p 1191; L Vachon: Respiratory Disorders, Sec 26.5, p 1501, in CTP/VI.

11.3 Panic Disorder

Panic disorder is an anxiety disorder characterized by spontaneous, episodic, and intense periods of anxiety (*panic attacks*), usually lasting about 30 minutes. The panic attacks usually occur twice a week.

CLINICAL FEATURES AND DIAGNOSIS

The symptoms of panic attacks include palpitations, sweating, shaking, dizziness, shortness of breath, and fear of dying, going crazy, or losing control (Table 11.3-1).

The lifetime prevalence of panic disorder is between 1.5 and 2 percent of the population; the disorder is more common in women than in men. The onset is typically in young adulthood.

Agoraphobia, the fear of being in situations from which escape may be difficult if symptoms of anxiety develop, commonly occurs after repeated panic attacks have left the patient incapacitated or embarrassed. Agoraphobia is described in more detail in Section 11.4.

Mitral valve prolapse is an associated cardiac condition that often presents with symptoms similar to panic disorder. Physical findings in mitral valve prolapse include a midsystolic click and murmur. Mitral valve prolapse is present in up to 50 percent of panic disorder patients.

Panic disorder can be disabling. It may lead to agoraphobia so severe that the patient cannot leave the home. Repeated unsuccessful attempts to seek treatment can lead to depression and a feeling of hopelessness and can place panic disorder patients at increased risk for suicide.

Identify panic disorder as early as possible when patients present with physical symptoms. In the typical case the patient has repeatedly presented to emergency rooms or a doctor's office with physical complaints (for example, chest pain and fainting) only to be told that the findings of the medical workup were normal, no definitive diagnosis can be made, and no treatment is recommended.

Panic attacks are believed to be biological events related to excessive noradrenergic discharge from the locus ceruleus. Panic attacks can be provoked by the infusion of lactate, the inhalation of carbon dioxide (CO_2), the administration of yohimbine (Yocon), and other physiological maneuvers. Panic disorder has a genetic component, and first-degree relatives of panic disorder patients have about a 10 times greater chance of having panic disorder than do the general population.

The first few panic attacks are often spontaneous and are not related to any identified stressor, although increased stress during the period preceding the onset of symptoms can often be identified. The panic attack begins with a rapid onset of physical symptoms, leading to a crescendo of overwhelming fear and subsequent

TABLE 11.3–1
CRITERIA FOR PANIC ATTACK

Note: A panic attack is not a codable disorder. Code the specific diagnosis in which the panic attack occurs (e.g., panic disorder with agoraphobia).

A discrete period of intense fear or discomfort, in which four (or more) of the following symptoms developed abruptly and reached a peak within 10 minutes:

(1) palpitations, pounding heart, or accelerated heart rate
(2) sweating
(3) trembling or shaking
(4) sensations of shortness of breath or smothering
(5) feeling of choking
(6) chest pain or discomfort
(7) nausea or abdominal distress
(8) feeling dizzy, unsteady, lightheaded, or faint
(9) derealization (feelings of unreality) or depersonalization (being detached from oneself)
(10) fear of losing control or going crazy
(11) fear of dying
(12) paresthesias (numbness or tingling sensations)
(13) chills or hot flushes

Table from DSM-IV, *Diagnostic and Statistical Manual of Mental Disorders,* ed 4. Copyright American Psychiatric Association, Washington, 1994. Used with permission.

behavior to leave the situation and seek help. The entire attack is usually over in about 30 minutes.

After multiple attacks, the patient learns to anticipate the attacks and avoids situations that may precipitate panic (agoraphobia). The avoidance can become crippling, since many of the situations avoided are necessary for normal work and social functioning. Panic disorder patients eventually suffer from the triad of panic attacks, anticipatory anxiety (that is, worrying about having another attack), and agoraphobic avoidance. Patients end up being anxious most of the time.

INTERVIEWING AND PSYCHOTHERAPEUTIC GUIDELINES

Reassure the patient that a diagnosis and a treatment plan can be made. The patients are often demoralized from repeated unsuccessful efforts to seek help. Inform them that help is forthcoming and that the disorder is not imaginary. Emphasize the need for compliance with medication and the benefit from behavioral and other therapies. Encourage the patients to limit or decrease their avoidant behavior, which can escalate rapidly, leading to increased dysphoria.

EVALUATION AND MANAGEMENT

Figure 11.3-1 provides an overview of the treatment of panic disorder in primary care.

1. Rule out possible medical causes for panic symptoms (Table 11.3-2). Include a detailed physical examination; electrocardiogram (ECG); a complete chemistry profile, including electrolytes, calcium, and magnesium; thyroid function tests; a urine toxicology screen; a complete blood count; and liver and renal function tests. An echocardiogram may help diagnose mitral valve prolapse. Order other tests as indicated.
2. Obtain a detailed history of all the patient's medications and drugs, especially caffeine, alcohol, sedative-hypnotics, nicotine, and bronchodilators. Drugs that are central nervous system (CNS) stimulants can precipitate panic attacks, as can withdrawal from drugs that are CNS depressants. Many panic disorder patients also self-medicate with alcohol or sedative-hypnotics.
3. Obtain a full psychiatric evaluation with special attention to the symptoms of depression and for other anxiety disorders (for example, phobias, generalized anxiety disorder, obsessive-compulsive disorder, and posttraumatic stress disorder).
4. Refer the patient for appropriate treatment. If panic disorder is the definitive diagnosis, make a referral to a psychiatrist experienced in the treatment of anxiety disorders (Table 11.3-3). Many approaches are effective.

Behavior therapy is an effective treatment for panic disorder, but some patients do not choose it: the modality requires high level of commitment and induces a high degree of anxiety during the treatment. Behavior therapy involves repeatedly

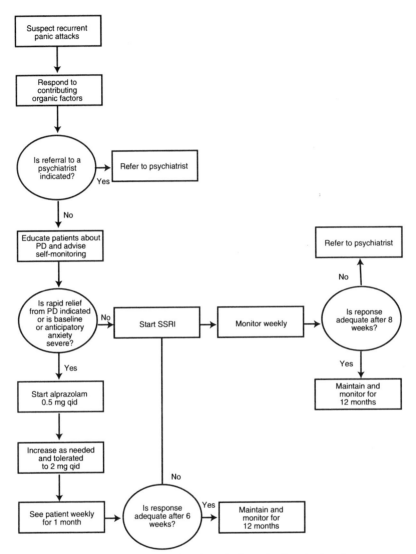

Figure 11.3-1. Algorithm for the treatment of panic disorder in primary care. (From R L Elliot: Panic Disorder in Primary Care. Prim Psychiatry 2: 58, 1995. Used with permission.)

exposing the patient to those situations that provoke the panic (in vivo exposure) and having the patient endure the symptoms to learn that panic is self-limited. The patient learns coping strategies other than fleeing the situation. Relaxation techniques may also help.

Insight-oriented psychotherapy, group therapy, and family therapy are often helpful.

TABLE 11.3–2
ORGANIC DIFFERENTIAL DIAGNOSIS FOR PANIC DISORDER

Cardiovascular diseases	Endocrine diseases (continued)
Anemia	Hypoglycemia
Angina	Hypoparathyroidism
Congestive heart failure	Menopausal disorders
Hyperactive β-adrenergic state	Pheochromocytoma
Hypertension	Premenstrual syndrome
Mitral valve prolapse	Drug intoxications
Myocardial infarction	Amphetamine
Paradoxical atrial tachycardia	Amyl nitrite
Pulmonary diseases	Anticholinergics
Asthma	Cocaine
Hyperventilation	Hallucinogens
Pulmonary embolus	Marijuana
Neurological diseases	Nicotine
Cerebrovascular disease	Theophylline
Epilepsy	Drug withdrawal
Huntington's disease	Alcohol
Infection	Antihypertensives
Ménière's disease	Opiates and opioids
Migraine	Sedative-hypnotics
Multiple sclerosis	Other conditions
Transient ischemic attack	Anaphylaxis
Tumor	B_{12} deficiency
Wilson's disease	Electrolyte disturbances
Endocrine diseases	Heavy metal poisoning
Addison's disease	Systemic infections
Carcinoid syndrome	Systemic lupus erythematosus
Cushing's syndrome	Temporal arteritis
Diabetes	Uremia
Hyperthryoidism	

TABLE 11.3–3
INDICATIONS FOR PSYCHIATRIC REFERRAL IN PANIC DISORDER

- Depression associated with suicidal thoughts or hopelessness
- Alcohol or substance abuse
- Phobic or avoidant behaviors impairing functioning
- Poor response to minor tranquilizers and SSRIs

Table from R L Elliot: Panic Disorder in Primary Care. Prim Psychiatry 2: 56, 1995. Used with permission.

DRUG TREATMENT

Benzodiazepines such as alprazolam (Xanax), clonazepam (Klonopin), and lorazepam (Ativan) are effective in stopping the panic attacks. Start with a low dosage (for example, alprazolam 0.25 to 0.5 mg or lorazepam 1 to 2 mg, both given by mouth every four hours), and increase the dosage as needed until it is clearly effective.

Show the patient early that an effective treatment is available. Many patients carry a benzodiazepine tablet with them and derive considerable relief from simply knowing that it is there, even if they never take it.

The dosage range needed for the long-term treatment of panic disorder may be relatively higher than the range needed for other conditions (for example, alprazolam 4 to 6 mg a day for panic disorder). Tricyclic antidepressants—for example, imipramine (Tofranil)—are effective, as are monoamine oxidase inhibitors (MAOIs)—for example, phenelzine (Nardil)—and serotonergic agents. Those medications are usually initiated in an ongoing outpatient treatment program, rather than in the emergency room. Buspirone (BuSpar) is not effective for panic disorder.

For a more detailed discussion of this topic, see A J Fyer, S Mannuzza, J D Coplan: Panic Disorders and Agoraphobia, Sec 17.1, p 1191, in CTP/VI.

11.4 Phobias

A *phobia* is an irrational fear of a specific object, activity, or situation that leads to avoidance. The failure to avoid the stimulus causes severe anxiety. The patient realizes that the fear is unrealistic, and the entire experience is dysphoric. Two of the more common phobias, agoraphobia and claustrophobia, are highlighted in this section.

CLINICAL FEATURES AND DIAGNOSIS

The patient experiences severe anxiety or panic related to a specific object, activity, or situation. Specific types of phobias include social phobia and agoraphobia. In social phobia the patient fears public humiliation, such as what may be encountered when speaking or performing in public, eating alone in a restaurant, or urinating in a public bathroom. In agoraphobia the patient is afraid of being in public places or situations where escape may be difficult or embarrassing or if help would not be available should an embarrassing or incapacitating symptom suddenly develop. In social phobia the focus of the fear is on public humiliation; in agoraphobia the focus of the fear is on the inability to escape.

Specific phobias are unrealistic fears of specific stimuli, such as spiders, snakes, animals, heights, storms, illness, injury, being alone, death, and contamination.

Phobic symptoms may be caused by intoxication with psychostimulants or hallucinogens and, rarely, by an organic disorder, such as a small brain tumor or a cerebrovascular disease. A physical examination and laboratory tests can usually identify those causes.

Alcohol dependence is common in phobic patients, who may medicate their anxiety with alcohol. Subsequent withdrawal from alcohol may exacerbate the anxiety.

Schizophrenic patients may have delusional fears about specific stimuli, but unlike phobic patients they do not realize that the fear is unrealistic and have other signs of schizophrenia.

Phobic disorders may be difficult to differentiate from obsessive-compulsive disorder, in which obsessive thoughts about the stimulus may lead to compulsive behavior to relieve the anxiety.

The severe anxiety that is present in patients with phobias may produce physiological symptoms, as well as psychological symptoms. Manifestations of anxiety include restlessness, diarrhea, dizziness, palpitations, hyperhidrosis, tremor, syncope, tachycardia, and urinary symptoms.

Some patients show counterphobic behavior, in which the feared stimulus is sought out intentionally and encountered repeatedly in an attempt to overcome the fear, for example, going sky diving to conquer a fear of heights.

TABLE 11.4-1
CRITERIA FOR AGORAPHOBIA

Note: Agoraphobia is not a codable disorder. Code the specific disorder in which the agoraphobia occurs (e.g., panic disorder with agoraphobia or agoraphobia without history of panic disorder).

A. Anxiety about being in places or situations from which escape might be difficult (or embarrassing) or in which help may not be available in the event of having an unexpected or situationally predisposed panic attack or panic-like symptoms. Agoraphobia fears typically involve characteristic clusters of situations that include being outside the home alone; being in a crowd or standing in a line; being on a bridge; and traveling in a bus, train, or automobile.

  Note: Consider the diagnosis of specific phobia if the avoidance is limited to one or only a few specific situations, or social phobia if the avoidance is limited to social situations.

B. The situations are avoided (e.g., travel is restricted) or else are endured with marked distress or with anxiety about having a panic attack or panic-like symptoms, or require the presence of a companion.

C. The anxiety or phobic avoidance is not better accounted for by another mental disorder, such as social phobia (e.g., avoidance limited to social situations because of fear of embarrassment), specific phobia (e.g., avoidance limited to a single situation like elevators), obsessive-compulsive disorder (e.g., avoidance of dirt in someone with an obsession about contamination), posttraumatic stress disorder (e.g., avoidance of stimuli associated with a severe stressor), or separation anxiety disorder (e.g., avoidance of leaving home or relatives).

Table from DSM-IV. *Diagnostic and Statistical Manual of Mental Disorders,* ed 4. Copyright American Psychiatric Association, Washington, 1994. Used with permission.

Agoraphobia

Agoraphobia is the fear of suffering severe anxiety in places where the possibilities for escape are perceived to be limited. Agoraphobic patients fear being in open places and leaving their homes (Table 11.4-1). Agoraphobia is associated in at least two thirds of patients with panic attacks or panic disorder. Patients often give childhood histories of shyness, separation anxiety, and school phobia and give a family history of anxiety, panic, and phobias. Most patients describe experiencing anticipatory anxiety in the face of situations deemed potentially threatening, such as thinking about or going to a restaurant or other public places. The anxiety then intensifies into a full-blown panic attack. The patient is much more likely to visit the hospital emergency room during a panic attack than with complaints of agoraphobia only; however, the patient may call the primary care physician on the telephone to report agoraphobic symptoms. Agoraphobia seldom requires hospitalization, although it can be severely incapacitating, as the patient becomes increasingly unable to function. Untreated, panic disorder with agoraphobia has a high rate of depression and places the affected person at risk for suicide. Patients may present with symptoms that can be mistaken for borderline personality disorder, such as intense anger, feelings of isolation, suicidal gestures, and manipulativeness. Borderline personality disorder can coexist with a diagnosis of agoraphobia, so it is important not to miss either diagnosis. Obtaining a psychiatric consultation for patients with agoraphobia is advisable.

Claustrophobia

Claustrophobia is a fear of enclosed places. For the claustrophobic patient, exposure to enclosed spaces provokes immediate anxiety. Although the patient recognizes that the fear is unrealistic, the fear and the avoidance interfere with functioning. The symptoms of anxiety when in enclosed spaces include panic, tachycardia, sweating, palpitations, and dyspnea.

Claustrophobia is considered a specific phobia. Its onset is usually in the patient's 30s. It may be related to panic disorder and agoraphobia but should be differentiated from posttraumatic stress disorder and obsessive-compulsive disorder. Simple phobias are common (six-month prevalence is between 5 and 12 percent) and affect women more often than men. Although claustrophobic patients may be able to successfully avoid the phobic stimulus and function well, in adulthood the phobia seldom resolves without treatment.

INTERVIEWING AND PSYCHOTHERAPEUTIC GUIDELINES

Since patients realize that the phobia is irrational, address the fear directly. Inquire about the severity of the avoidant behavior and how impaired patients' functioning has become from trying to avoid the phobic stimulus. Also ask about other anxiety symptoms—including panic, symptoms of posttraumatic stress disorder (for example, flashbacks and startle reactions), obsessions, and other associated phobias—and about depression, psychosis, and substance abuse. The patients may be embarrassed, feel foolish, or believe that they are going crazy. Take their fears seriously, and reassure them. Tell them about the availability of effective treatments.

Agoraphobia

Explore prior attempts to seek help. Agoraphobic patients may have made many unsuccessful attempts to get treatment and may become progressively frustrated and hopeless. Be calm and reassuring. Inform the patient that, although the symptoms are treatable, some time may pass before they are eliminated and that the treatment process is a gradual but effective one. If the patient comes to the physician's office with a companion, interview that person also, both individually and with the patient. Any successful treatment of an agoraphobic patient requires the close cooperation of trusted people in the patient's life. Evaluate the suicide risk and the use of alcohol or other drugs.

Claustrophobia

Claustrophobic patients are often embarrassed about their irrational fears. Reassure them, and take their fears seriously. Allow the patients to express their fears while taking a history of the specific phobia-stimulating circumstances and a history of the illness. Explain to patients that phobias are treatable.

EVALUATION AND MANAGEMENT

General Principles

1. Take the patient's vital signs.

2. Order a urine toxicology screen, a detailed physical examination, thyroid function tests, and routine laboratory screening tests.
3. Obtain a detailed history of the specific phobic stimulus, the duration and severity of the impairment, and the presence of other associated phobic stimuli. Obtain a history of any environmental changes that have made avoidance difficult or impossible.
4. Obtain a psychiatric evaluation to identify the presence of other anxiety disorders (for example, obsessive-compulsive disorder, panic disorder, generalized anxiety disorder), depression, psychotic disorders, and drug or alcohol use.
5. The primary treatment is behavior therapy (for example, systematic desensitization and imaginal or in vivo flooding), but such therapy requires considerable effort and a commitment by the patient. The patient must repeatedly encounter the phobic stimulus without the possibility of avoiding it and must learn to cope with the consequent anxiety. The treatment may begin by desensitizing the patient progressively to ever more anxiety-provoking stimuli. For example, patients who are phobic about elevators may start by imagining that they are in an elevator and slowly and repeatedly imagine that the elevator is going to higher and higher floors. The imagining is then replaced by actually getting into an elevator and then gradually going to higher and higher floors.
6. Refer the patient to supportive psychotherapy and family therapy to help both the patient and the patient's family cope with any impairments related to the phobia.
7. Refer the patient to group therapy, especially if the members of a group have a common phobia that they can help each other overcome together (for example, flying in airplanes).
8. Consider hypnosis as an adjunct to psychotherapy.

Agoraphobia

1. Determine whether panic attacks are present; if they are, determine their frequency and severity. Eliciting a history of frequent, severe, recurrent panic attacks essentially confirms the diagnosis and is critical in helping to establish the treatment.
2. Rule out substance-related disorders and medical conditions (for example, thyrotoxicosis, hypoglycemia, pheochromocytoma, temporal lobe epilepsy, stimulant intoxication, and withdrawal from alcohol or sedative-hypnotics). Obtain an electrocardiogram (ECG). Mitral valve prolapse is present in about half of all patients with panic disorder. ECGs are also helpful in reassuring patients that they are not having a heart attack during the panic attack.
3. Generally, panic attacks must be treated with medications before any psychotherapeutic techniques can be used. Once the panic attacks are controlled with medication, the most effective psychotherapeutic approach is behavior therapy (desensitization or exposure). Psychodynamic issues, although important to all patients with agoraphobia, may be of particular significance in patients who experience the agoraphobia without panic attacks. Family therapy, group therapy, and insight-oriented psychotherapy may also be helpful.

Claustrophobia

1. Obtain a complete psychiatric evaluation to rule out additional phobias and other psychiatric diagnoses that require treatment (for example, schizophrenia, personality disorders, and panic disorder).
2. Evaluate the patient for substance abuse; phobic patients may self-medicate to overcome their fears.
3. Assess the patient for any recent environmental change that no longer allows phobic avoidance (for example, the patient's workplace may have moved to a high floor in an office building that requires the use of an elevator).
4. Refer the patient for appropriate outpatient treatment, such as behavior therapy, hypnosis, relaxation techniques, and insight-oriented psychotherapy.

DRUG TREATMENT

Benzodiazepines, tricyclic antidepressants, and monoamine oxidase inhibitors (MAOIs) are all helpful for phobic patients, although most of the available research is on the treatment of social phobia. The patient can also take β-blockers—for example, propranolol (Inderal)—before encountering the phobic stimulus; β-blockers are helpful for social phobia (for example, stage fright). Extremely anxious phobic patients can be given a small supply of lorazepam (Ativan) 1 to 2 mg by mouth three times a day, oxazepam (Serax) 10 to 30 mg a day by mouth, or clonazepam (Klonopin) 0.5 to 1 mg by mouth in the morning and at bedtime—to be taken until their first outpatient appointment.

Premedication with lorazepam 1 to 2 mg by mouth, intramuscularly (IM), or intravenously (IV) or diazepam (Valium) 5 to 10 mg by mouth, IM, or IV may be needed before initiating fearful medical procedures (for example, a claustrophobic patient undergoing magnetic resonance imaging [MRI] or venipuncture in a patient with a needle phobia).

Agoraphobia

If panic disorder is present, treatment of the panic attacks with benzodiazepines (for example, alprazolam [Xanax] and clonazepam), tricyclic antidepressants (for example, imipramine [Tofranil]), monoamine oxidase inhibitors (MAOIs) (for example, phenelzine [Nardil]), and serotonin-specific reuptake inhibitors (for example, fluoxetine [Prozac]) can be considered, although those medications should be initiated only in an ongoing therapeutic relationship. An acutely anxious patient can be given lorazepam 1 to 2 mg by mouth or IM and a small supply of 1 or 2 mg tablets to be taken three times a day until the patient can be seen for follow-up. Cautiously probe for a history of substance abuse before carrying out such a treatment plan.

Claustrophobia

If the patient is acutely anxious or must undergo an anxiety-provoking medical procedure, give a short-acting benzodiazepine, such as estazolam (ProSom) 0.5 to

1 mg by mouth, lorazepam 1 to 2 mg by mouth or IM, or oxazepam 10 to 30 mg by mouth, one hour before the procedure. Benzodiazepines should be given only as a single dose or a limited several-day prescription until the patient can be seen in outpatient treatment. MAOIs and β-blockers can also be of some help.

For a more detailed discussion of this topic, see E D Caine, H Grossman, J M Lyness: Delirium, Dementia, and Amnestic and Other Cognitive Disorders and Mental Disorders Due to a General Medical Condition, Chap 12, p 705; A A Lipton, R Cancro: Schizophrenia: Clinical Features, Sec 14.7, p 968; A J Fyer, S Mannuzza, J D Coplan: Panic Disorders and Agoraphobia, Sec 17.1, p 1191; D H Barlow, M R Liebowitz: Specific Phobia and Social Phobia, Sec 17.2, p 1204, in CTP/VI.

11.5 Obsessive-Compulsive Disorder

An *obsession* is a pathological, persistent, recurrent, and irresistible idea, thought, or impulse that cannot be eliminated from consciousness by logic or reasoning. A *compulsion* is a pathological, repetitive, and unwanted need to perform an act, often in response to an obsession. The failure to perform a compulsive act leads to anxiety. The obsessive-compulsive patient will exhibit obsessions, compulsions, or both, which interfere with the patient's functioning.

CLINICAL FEATURES AND DIAGNOSIS

Common obsessions include disgust with bodily wastes and secretions, dirt, germs, contamination, or toxins; the fear that something terrible may happen; the need for symmetry, order, or exactness; excessive praying or religious thoughts; the belief in lucky and unlucky numbers; and forbidden sexual thoughts. Common compulsions include excessive hand washing, showering, bathing, toothbrushing, and grooming; repeated rituals; checking doors, locks, stove, and car brakes; cleaning to remove contaminants; touching; ordering and arranging; counting; hoarding and collecting; and measures to prevent harm to oneself or others.

Table 11.5-1 lists the diagnostic criteria for obsessive-compulsive disorder.

INTERVIEWING AND PSYCHOTHERAPEUTIC GUIDELINES

Focus on the patient's specific obsessional thoughts and compulsive behaviors. Ask about the frequency of the compulsive behavior, the time spent obsessing, and the consequent impairments. Inquire about related obsessions and compulsions that are different from the one initially identified; many patients have multiple related obsessions and compulsions. Patients recognize the irrationality of their obsessions and compulsions and see them as a source of anxiety, so address the patients directly and openly. Reassure the patients that they are not going crazy and that treatment is available.

EVALUATION AND MANAGEMENT

1. Quantify the obsessions and the compulsions in terms of their type, number, and frequency; the time spent obsessing or doing compulsive behaviors; and the impaired functioning.

TABLE 11.5–1
DIAGNOSTIC CRITERIA FOR OBSESSIVE-COMPULSIVE DISORDER

A. Either obsessions or compulsions:
   Obsessions as defined by (1), (2), (3), and (4):
   (1) recurrent and persistent thoughts, impulses, or images that are experienced, at some time during the disturbance, as intrusive and inappropriate and that cause marked anxiety or distress
   (2) the thoughts, impulses, or images are not simply excessive worries about real-life problems
   (3) the person attempts to ignore or suppress such thoughts, impulses, or images, or to neutralize them with some other thought or action
   (4) the person recognizes that the obsessional thoughts, impulses, or images are a product of his or her own mind (not imposed from without as in thought insertion)

   Compulsions as defined by (1) and (2):
   (1) repetitive behaviors (e.g., hand washing, ordering, checking) or mental acts (e.g., praying, counting, repeating words silently) that the person feels driven to perform in response to an obsession, or according to rules that must be applied rigidly
   (2) the behaviors or mental acts are aimed at preventing or reducing distress or preventing some dreaded event or situation; however, these behaviors or mental acts either are not connected in a realistic way with what they are designed to neutralize or prevent or are clearly excessive

B. At some point during the course of the disorder, the person has recognized that the obsessions or compulsions are excessive or unreasonable. **Note:** This does not apply to children.

C. The obsessions or compulsions cause marked distress, are time consuming (take more than 1 hour a day), or significantly interfere with the person's normal routine, occupational (or academic) functioning, or usual social activities or relationships.

D. If another Axis I disorder is present, the content of the obsessions or compulsions is not restricted to it (e.g., preoccupation with food in the presence of an eating disorder; hair pulling in the presence of trichotillomania; concern with appearance in the presence of body dysmorphic disorder; preoccupation with drugs in the presence of a substance use disorder; preoccupation with having a serious illness in the presence of hypochondriasis; preoccupation with sexual urges or fantasies in the presence of a paraphilia; or guilty ruminations in the presence of major depressive disorder).

E. The disturbance is not due to the direct physiological effects of a substance (e.g., a drug of abuse, a medication) or a general medical condition.

Specify if:
   With poor insight: if, for most of the time during the current episode, the person does not recognize that the obsessions and compulsions are excessive or unreasonable

Table from DSM-IV, *Diagnostic and Statistical Manual of Mental Disorders*, ed 4. Copyright American Psychiatric Association, Washington, 1994. Used with permission.

2. Complete a mental status evaluation to screen for other disorders, including depression (present in 50 percent of patients with obsessive-compulsive disorder), schizophrenia, and phobias. The differential diagnosis between phobias and obsessive-compulsive disorder is often difficult, but phobic patients are usually much more successful at avoiding the stimulus than are obsessive-compulsive patients.

3. Behavior therapy is thought to be the treatment of choice for obsessive-compulsive disorder. It is successful in 60 to 75 percent of all patients. Possible behavioral therapeutic choices include in vivo exposure (flooding), desensitization, thought stopping, implosion therapy, and aversive conditioning. Behavior therapy requires considerable commitment by the patient. Often, the patient is forcibly prevented from carrying out the compulsive act and learns that the consequent anxiety or panic will eventually lessen.

4. Some clinicians use insight-oriented psychotherapy for obsessive-compulsive disorder but usually in combination with medication.

5. Family therapy helps the patient's family cope with the patient's impaired functioning and can reduce the usual marital stress.

6. For patients who do not respond to any other treatments, psychosurgery (bilateral leukotomies that produce lesions in the thalamofrontal connections) may be effective.

DRUG TREATMENT

Clomipramine (Anafranil), fluvoxamine, (Luvox), and fluoxetine (Prozac) are potent inhibitors of serotonin reuptake and are drugs of first choice. Paroxetine (Paxil) and sertraline (Zoloft) are also effective. Those medications should be prescribed in connection with ongoing treatment. If the patient comes to the emergency room or doctor's office in an acutely anxious state, a benzodiazepine—for example, alprazolam (Xanax) 0.25 to 1 mg by mouth, clonazepam (Klonopin) 0.5 to 1 mg by mouth, or lorazepam (Ativan) 1 to 2 mg by mouth, all given every four hours as needed—may help reduce the acute anxiety.

For a more detailed discussion of this topic, see M A Jenike: Obsessive-Compulsive Disorder, Sec 17.3, p 1218; J G Gunderson, K A Phillips: Personality Disorders, Chap 25, p 1425, in CTP/VI.

11.6 Posttraumatic Stress Disorder

Posttraumatic stress disorder occurs in response to an extraordinary trauma (for example, combat or rape) (Table 11.6-1). The event is reexperienced (for example, through flashbacks); stimuli associated with the event are avoided (for example, avoiding elevators after an attack in an elevator); or the patient has a generalized numbing of responsiveness (for example, a restricted range of affect) and persistent symptoms of arousal (hypervigilance). Substance abuse can complicate the disorder.

CLINICAL FEATURES AND DIAGNOSIS

The principal clinical features of posttraumatic stress disorder are the painful reexperiencing of the event, a pattern of avoidance and emotional numbing, and fairly constant hyperarousal. The disorder may not develop until months or even years after the event. The mental status examination often reveals feelings of guilt, rejection, and humiliation. The patient may also describe dissociative states and panic attacks. Illusions and hallucinations may be present. Associated symptoms can include aggression, violence, poor impulse control, depression, and substance-related disorders.

A major consideration in the diagnosis of posttraumatic stress disorder is the possibility that the patient also incurred a head injury during the trauma. Other organic considerations that can both cause and exacerbate the symptoms are epilepsy, alcohol use disorders, and other substance-related disorders. Acute intoxication or withdrawal from some substances may also present a clinical picture that is difficult to distinguish from posttraumatic stress disorder until the effects of the substance have worn off.

Posttraumatic stress disorder is commonly misdiagnosed as some other mental disorder, resulting in inappropriate treatment of the condition. The clinician must consider posttraumatic stress disorder in patients who have pain disorder, substance abuse, other anxiety disorders, and mood disorders. In general, posttraumatic stress disorder can be distinguished from other mental disorders by interviewing the patient regarding previous traumatic experiences and by the nature of the current symptoms. Borderline personality disorder, dissociative disorders, factitious disorders, and malingering should also be considered. Borderline personality disorder can be difficult to distinguish from posttraumatic stress disorder. The two disorders

TABLE 11.6-1
DIAGNOSTIC CRITERIA FOR POSTTRAUMATIC STRESS DISORDER

A. The person has been exposed to a traumatic event in which both of the following were present:
   (1) the person experienced, witnessed, or was confronted with an event or events that involved actual or threatened death or serious injury, or a threat to the physical integrity of self or others
   (2) the person's response involved intense fear, helplessness, or horror. **Note:** In children, this may be expressed instead by disorganized or agitated behavior
B. The traumatic event is persistently reexperienced in one (or more) of the following ways:
   (1) recurrent and intrusive distressing recollection of the event, including images, thoughts, or perceptions. **Note:** In young children, repetitive play may occur in which themes or aspects of the trauma are expressed.
   (2) recurrent distressing dreams of the event. **Note:** In children, there may be frightening dreams without recognizable content.
   (3) acting or feeling as if the traumatic event were recurring (includes a sense of reliving the experience, illusions, hallucinations, and dissociative flashback episodes, including those that occur on awakening or when intoxicated). **Note:** In young children, trauma-specific reenactment may occur.
   (4) intense psychological distress at exposure to internal or external cues that symbolize or resemble an aspect of the traumatic event.
   (5) physiological reactivity on exposure to internal or external cues that symbolize or resemble an aspect of the traumatic event
C. Persistent avoidance of stimuli associated with the trauma and numbing of general responsiveness (not present before the trauma), as indicated by three (or more) of the following:
   (1) efforts to avoid thoughts, feelings, or conversions associated with the trauma
   (2) efforts to avoid activities, places, or people that arouse recollections of the trauma
   (3) inability to recall an important aspect of the trauma
   (4) markedly diminished interest or participation in significant activities
   (5) feeling of detachment or estrangement from others
   (6) restricted range of affect (e.g., unable to have loving feelings)
   (7) sense of a foreshortened future (e.g., does not expect to have a career, marriage, children, or a normal life span)
D. Persistent symptoms of increased arousal (not present before the trauma), as indicated by two (or more) of the following:
   (1) difficulty falling or staying asleep
   (2) irritability or outbursts of anger
   (3) difficulty concentrating
   (4) hypervigilance
   (5) exaggerated startle response
E. Duration of the disturbance (symptoms in criteria B, C, and D) is more than 1 month.
F. The disturbance causes clinically significant distress or impairment in social, occupational, or other important areas of functioning.

Specifiy if:
   Acute: if duration of symptoms is less than 3 months
   Chronic: if duration of symptoms is 3 months or more

Specify if:
   With Delayed Onset: if onset of symptoms is at least 6 months after the stressor

Table from DMS-IV, *Diagnostic and Statistical Manual of Mental Disorders*, ed 4. Copyright American Psychiatric Association, Washington, 1994. Used with permission.

may coexist or even may be causally related. Patients with dissociative disorders do not usually have the degree of avoidance behavior, the autonomic hyperarousal, or the history of trauma that patients with posttraumatic stress disorder report. Partly because of the publicity that posttraumatic stress disorder has received in the popular press, clinicians should also consider the possibility of a factitious disorder and malingering.

INTERVIEWING AND PSYCHOTHERAPEUTIC GUIDELINES

The diagnosis of posttraumatic stress disorder is missed if the clinician is not looking for it. Patients may present with signs of substance abuse, depression, generalized anxiety disorder, panic disorder, and dissociative disorders. Focus on reducing the patient's denial of the stress (if present) and on reviewing and processing the feelings brought on by reexperiencing the stress. Address any guilt and feelings of responsibility for the trauma.

Some patients are knowledgeable about posttraumatic stress disorder. The symptoms are difficult to measure objectively; consequently, they are often feigned by malingerers who are attempting to obtain medications or admission to a hospital. While weeding out the malingerers, do not miss the true cases. At least initially, accept the patient's symptoms as presented.

Attempt to gain the patient's trust, and engage the patient in talking about the experience in some detail. That approach applies especially to rape victims. It is also useful to engage the patient's family and friends, educate them about posttraumatic stress disorder, and encourage them to be supportive and understanding of the patient.

EVALUATION AND MANAGEMENT

Evaluate the patient for possible head injury and other physical traumas sustained if the traumatic stress involved physical injury. Physical and neurological examinations are mandatory. Further diagnostic testing, such as computed tomography (CT) or magnetic resonance imaging (MRI) and electroencephalogram (EEG), is indicated if the neurological examination findings are abnormal or if the patient has a history of neurological symptoms.

Psychotherapeutic approaches in posttraumatic stress disorder include behavior therapy, cognitive therapy, and hypnosis—all with an emphasis on short-term treatment.

DRUG TREATMENT

Start drug treatment only in the context of an ongoing therapeutic relationship, especially since substance abuse is common in posttraumatic stress disorder patients.

Antidepressant treatment of posttraumatic stress disorder remains controversial. Other drugs that have been used in the disorder include benzodiazepines, lithium (Eskalith), and β-blockers—for example, propranolol (Inderal), clonidine (Catapres), and carbamazepine (Tegretol). Those drugs are generally prescribed as part of an ongoing treatment plan, with the exception of the benzodiazepines—for example, estazolam (ProSom) 0.5 to 1 mg by mouth, clonazepam (Klonopin) 0.25 to 0.5 mg by mouth, or lorazepam (Ativan) 1 to 2 mg by mouth or intramuscularly (IM)—which may also be used in the office to treat the acute anxiety and the agitation that may accompany posttraumatic stress disorder.

11.7 Conversion Disorder

A diagnosis of conversion disorder implies that physical symptoms, particularly losses of physical functioning and alterations in physical functioning, are the result of some psychological conflict.

CLINICAL FEATURES AND DIAGNOSIS

Conversion symptoms are typically neurological and include paralysis, seizures, blindness, tunnel vision, aphonia, akinesia, and dyskinesia. The symptoms may achieve a primary gain by keeping a conflict unconscious or may achieve a secondary gain by causing some desired change in the environment. Patients with conversion disorder are not in conscious control of their symptoms, unlike malingering patients and those with factitious disorders.

The risk factors of any symptom in conversion disorder include true medical conditions, past conversion symptoms in the patient or the family, and histrionic personality traits. A lack of concern (*la belle indifférence*) about the symptom may be present. The onset is usually rapid and in response to some acute stress.

INTERVIEWING AND PSYCHOTHERAPEUTIC GUIDELINES

Conversion symptoms stem from psychological conflicts that are actually interpersonally based (for example, arm paralysis in a wife who wants to strike her husband). The person with whom the patient is in conflict may accompany the patient to the emergency room or the physician's office. Conduct separate interviews to determine the nature of the conflict. Providing a psychodynamic explanation for the symptoms may lead to its resolution (for example, "You don't want to see what he's doing to you.") Do not minimize the physical symptoms; declare that the symptoms are real for the patient. Begin to engage the patient in a psychotherapeutic process, focusing on working through the conflicts that led to the symptom.

EVALUATION AND MANAGEMENT

1. Rule out physical causes. In the case of a symptom of blindness, the signs suggesting a psychogenic origin include a failure to bump into objects, blinking or moving the head in response to the sudden appearance of a threatening object, and a loss inconsistent with neuroanatomy (for example, tunnel vision). Evaluate the patient for multiple sclerosis, systemic lupus erythematosus, and other neuro-

logical disorders. Hysterical blindness should not be confused with optic neuritis secondary to multiple sclerosis.

2. Consider the possibility of psychogenic symptoms superimposed on organically based symptoms. Patients with organic causes often have superimposed psychogenic syndromes.

3. Identify the patient's psychological stressors.

4. Evaluate the secondary gains, including attention from the family and the avoidance of work. If secondary gains are present, try to alter the environment, or use a behavioral approach.

5. Evaluate the patient for other psychiatric diagnoses, since a significant portion of conversion disorder patients have comorbid illnesses, such as somatization disorder, depression, personality disorders, and schizophrenia.

6. Hypnosis or an amobarbital (Amytal) interview may be used to relieve the patient's anxiety.

DRUG TREATMENT

An intravenous barbiturate or benzodiazepine may relieve the patient's anxiety and symptoms. However, the relief of symptoms with an anxiolytic does not necessarily rule out the presence of an underlying medical condition.

For a more detailed discussion of this topic, see F G Guggenheim, G R Smith: Somatoform Disorders, Chap 18, p 1251, in CTP/VI.

11.8 Depersonalization

Depersonalization is a disturbance in perception that involves a sense that one is unreal or somehow changed and is strange to oneself. Depersonalization, like derealization, can occur briefly to normal people under stress (for example, during physical or psychological trauma). Mild symptoms may occur in normal people when they are exposed to an unfamiliar environment.

CLINICAL FEATURES AND DIAGNOSIS

Patients with depersonalization may describe feeling as though they were detached from their own bodies, viewing their lives as though they were spectators. They may also feel mechanical or robotlike. The patients are aware that the symptoms are not reality, and they find the experience unpleasant.

Depersonalization that is severe enough to cause impairment and that occurs repeatedly, without other prominent symptoms, may fulfill the diagnostic criteria for depersonalization disorder (Table 11.8-1).

Depersonalization is also a symptom of a wide range of disorders including other dissociative disorders, schizophrenia, anxiety disorders (especially posttraumatic stress disorder), depression, and medical conditions. Depersonalization can also be caused by intoxication with cocaine, hallucinogens, cannabis, and other

TABLE 11.8-1.
DIAGNOSTIC CRITERIA FOR DEPERSONALIZATION DISORDER

A. Persistent or recurrent experiences of feeling detached from, and as if one is an outside observer of, one's mental processes or body (e.g., feeling like one is in a dream).
B. During the depersonalization experience, reality testing remains intact.
C. The depersonalization causes clinically significant distress or impairment in social, occupational, or other important areas of functioning.
D. The depersonalization experience does not occur exclusively during the course of another mental disorder, such as schizophrenia, panic disorder, acute stress disorder, or another dissociative disorder, and is not due to the direct physiological effects of a substance (e.g., a drug of abuse, a medication) or a general medical condition (e.g., temporal lobe epilepsy).

Table from DSM-IV, *Diagnostic and Statistical Manual of Mental Disorders*, ed 4. Copyright American Psychiatric Association, Washington, 1994. Used with permission.

substances and by withdrawal from alcohol and sedative-hypnotics. β-Blockers, anticholinergic drugs, and such medical conditions as epilepsy and endocrine disorders can also cause depersonalization.

INTERVIEWING AND PSYCHOTHERAPEUTIC GUIDELINES

The symptoms do not usually occur during the interview. However, a patient who is depersonalizing during the interview may be in a dreamlike state and only partially responsive to the environment. Be directive and help the patient cooperate with the interview and the examination. With some reassurance the symptom may stop, especially if the depersonalization is in response to anxiety. The goal of the interview is a definitive diagnosis. Organic disorders, depression, personality disorders, schizophrenia, and anxiety disorders must be ruled out before a diagnosis of depersonalization disorder is made. As a rule, consider the most severe diagnoses first (for example, organic disorders), and rule them out before considering other diagnoses.

EVALUATION AND MANAGEMENT

1. Consider possible causes based on the patient's history. First consider a history of substance use or withdrawal, then cognitive disorders and medical conditions. Schizophrenia usually presents with other associated symptoms, including thought disorder. A history of a recent severe trauma may indicate that the depersonalization is a normal reaction. A history of repeated episodes of depersonalization after a past trauma suggests posttraumatic stress disorder. A history of other dissociative symptoms suggests a dissociative disorder.
2. Prescribed medications, particularly steroids, can cause depersonalization symptoms.
3. On the mental status examination, look for symptoms of mood disorders, anxiety disorders, psychosis, and dissociative disorders.
4. Conduct a physical examination and a neurological examination. If the diagnosis remains unclear, order an organic workup, including urine toxicology screening, an electroencephalogram (EEG), and a computed tomography (CT) scan of the head.

DRUG TREATMENT

Drug treatment depends on the definitive diagnosis. If the depersonalization is a symptom of severe anxiety, use a short-acting benzodiazepine—for example, lorazepam (Ativan) 1 to 2 mg by mouth, oxazepam (Serax) 10 to 30 mg by mouth, estazolam (ProSom) 0.5 to 1 mg by mouth, or alprazolam (Xanax) 0.5 to 1 mg by mouth. In some cases a long-acting benzodiazepine may be used—for example, clorazepate (Tranxene) 7.5 to 15 mg by mouth, clonazepam (Klonopin) 0.25 to 0.5 mg by mouth, diazepam (Valium) 5 to 10 mg by mouth, or chlordiazepoxide (Librium) 10 to 25 mg by mouth. The symptoms may resolve after benzodiazepines are given.

For a more detailed discussion of this topic, see J Yager, M J Gitlin: Clinical Manifestations of Psychiatric Disorders, Chap 10, p 637; J C Nemiah: Dissociative Disorders, Chap 20, p 1281, in CTP/VI.

11.9 Derealization

Derealization is a disturbance in perception that involves a sense that one's environment is unreal or somehow changed and strange.

CLINICAL FEATURES AND DIAGNOSIS

Patients may describe feeling as though they were actors on a stage. Derealization is often associated with depersonalization. Both derealization and depersonalization can occur in normal people under severe stress; the disorders are considered final defense mechanisms protecting against overwhelming distress.

Derealization is also a symptom of a wide range of disorders—including schizophrenia, dissociative disorders, anxiety disorders (especially posttraumatic stress disorder), borderline personality disorder, depression, and organic mental disorders. Derealization can be caused by intoxication with cocaine or other psychostimulants, hallucinogens, or cannabis or by withdrawal from alcohol or sedative-hypnotics. β-Blockers, anticholinergic drugs, epilepsy, and endocrine disorders can also produce derealization.

INTERVIEWING AND PSYCHOTHERAPEUTIC GUIDELINES

The patient may be in a dreamlike state and only partially responsive to the environment. Be directive and help the patient cooperate with the interview and the examination. With some reassurance to the patient, the derealization may stop, thus allowing a comprehensive evaluation. The goal of the interview is a definitive diagnosis. Derealization is a nonspecific symptom and seldom occurs alone, without other symptoms.

EVALUATION AND MANAGEMENT

1. Consider possible causes. A history of substance use and withdrawal should be considered first, then organic mental disorders. Schizophrenia usually presents with other associated symptoms, including psychosis and thought disorder. A history of recent severe trauma may indicate that the derealization is a normal reaction. A history of repeated episodes after a past trauma suggests posttraumatic stress disorder.
2. Prescribed medications, particularly steroids, can cause derealization symptoms.
3. Rule out organic conditions with an electroencephalogram (EEG), urine toxicology screen, full medical evaluation, and endocrine workup (thyroid, pancreas, adrenal).
4. Look for symptoms of mood disorders, anxiety disorders, psychosis, and dissociative disorders.
5. The patient's behavior is usually either withdrawn or anxious and agitated.

DRUG TREATMENT

Drug treatment depends on the definitive diagnosis. If derealization is a symptom of severe anxiety, benzodiazepines may be used for a short time. For schizophrenia and other psychotic conditions, antipsychotics may be indicated.

For a more detailed discussion of this topic, see J Yager, M J Gitlin: Clinical Manifestations of Psychiatric Disorders, Chap 10, p 637; J C Nemiah: Dissociative Disorders, Chap 20, p 1281, in CTP/VI.

11.10 Fugue State

A *fugue state* is a prolonged dissociative period during which the patient performs complex activities, including unexpected travel and the assumption of a new identity. The episode usually lasts for hours to days but occasionally lasts for years. The new identity is apparently normal, and there is no obvious indication of a mental disorder. During the episode the patient is amnestic for the previous identity; after recovery, the patient is amnestic for the episode. Usually, the patient makes a complete recovery, and recurrences are uncommon.

CLINICAL FEATURES AND DIAGNOSIS

In the majority of cases, the new identity is incomplete, and the activities during the episode are only semipurposeful. The patient may avoid complex social interactions during the episode. In a minority of cases, a completely new personality is assumed. The new personality is usually more outgoing and friendly than the original personality.

Fugue states typically occur after a severe stress (such as a natural disaster), during wartime, or after a significant personal failure. Alcohol use may precipitate a fugue state. Patients with mood disorders and certain personality disorders (such as borderline, histrionic, and schizoid) are predisposed to dissociative fugue.

INTERVIEWING AND PSYCHOTHERAPEUTIC GUIDELINES

In general, the patient comes to clinical attention either when the episode is over and the patient has a memory gap or when someone who knew the patient previously brings the patient to clinical attention. Under either of those conditions, the patient is perplexed and bewildered by the situation and requires reassurance.

In the initial evaluation the objective is to engage the patient in an ongoing treatment plan. The goals are to explore the conflicts that led to the episode, to eliminate any persistent amnestic barriers, and to prevent recurrences.

EVALUATION AND MANAGEMENT

The differential diagnosis includes intoxication, temporal lobe epilepsy, dissociative amnesia, dissociative personality disorder (multiple personality disorder), factitious disorder, and malingering.

1. Urine drug screening and an electroencephalogram (EEG) help in the evaluation of possible drug intoxication or temporal lobe epilepsy.
2. Dissociative amnesia seldom involves travel or the assumption of a new identity.
3. In dissociative identity disorder (formerly known as multiple personality disorder), the old (also known as host) and new identities fluctuate.
4. Malingerers may avoid probing, detailed questions; may refuse to undergo laboratory tests; and are often difficult to identify. In general, do not assume that a patient is malingering unless strong evidence suggests it.

The clinician should identify the conflicts that led to the dissociation. Relaxation, hypnosis, and an interview facilitated by sedative-hypnotics—usually intravenous (IV) diazepam (Valium) or amobarbital (Amytal)—may help reduce the amnestic barriers (Table 11.10-1).

The most important objective of treatment is to break down the amnestic barriers and to restore the lost memory. Persistent lost memories can form the nidus for further amnesia and possible recurrence. Evaluate the patient for suicidality; some patients enter a fugue state when suicidal and again become suicidal when emerging from the fugue.

The clinician should refer the patient for psychotherapy to explore and to resolve the conflicts that led to the dissociation.

DRUG TREATMENT

Drug treatment is usually not needed, but severe anxiety may be treated with benzodiazepines.

TABLE 11.10-1
USING AMOBARBITAL DURING A PATIENT INTERVIEW

1. Have the patient recline.
2. Explain that the medication should make the patient relax and feel like talking.
3. Insert a narrow-bore scalp-vein needle into the forearm or hand.
4. Begin injecting a 5% solution of amobarbital (Amytal)—500 mg dissolved in 10 mL of sterile water—at a rate no faster than 1 mL/minute (50 mg/minute) to prevent sleep or sudden respiratory depression.
5. Interview:
   a. With a verbal patient, begin with neutral topics, gradually approaching areas of trauma, guilt, and possible repression.
   b. With a mute patient, continue to suggest that soon the patient will feel like talking. Prompting with known facts about the patient's life may also help.
6. Continue the infusion until the patient shows sustained rapid lateral nystagmus or drowsiness. Slight slurring of speech is common; the sedation threshold is usually reached at a dose between 150 mg (3 mL) and 350 mg (7 mL) but can be as little as 75 mg (1.5 mL) in an elderly patient or one with organic illness. Prompts to talk should have their strongest effect at this point.
7. To maintain the level of narcosis, continue the infusion at the rate of 0.5 to 1.0 mL every 5 minutes.
8. Conduct the interview as you would any other psychiatric interview, but with several caveats:
   a. Approach affect-laden or traumatic material gradually, and then work over it again and again to recover forgotten details, attendant feelings, and the patient's current reactions to them.
   b. In the mute or verbally inhibited patient, do not concentrate on traumatic topics (such as murderous rage toward someone) to prevent the development of panic after the interview.
9. Terminate the interview when enough material has been produced (about 30 minutes for a mute patient) or when the therapeutic goals have been reached (sometimes an hour or more). Have the patient recline for an additional 15 minutes until able to walk with close supervision.

Table from W R Dubin, K J Weiss: *Handbook of Psychiatric Emergencies,* p. 100. Springhouse, Springhouse, Pa., 1991. Adapted from J C Perry, D L Jacobs: Overview: Clinical applications of the Amytal interview in psychiatric emergency settings. Am J Psychiatry *139:* 552, 1982. Used with permission.

For a more detailed discussion of this topic, see J Yager, M J Gitlin: Clinical Manifestations of Psychiatric Disorders, Chap 10, p 637; J C Nemiah: Dissociative Disorders, Chap 20, p 1281, in CTP/VI.

11.11 Group Hysteria

Group hysteria is seen in a group of people who have experienced a significant stress, such as a personal or collective tragedy, and who present with various psychiatric symptoms of a similar nature.

CLINICAL FEATURES AND DIAGNOSIS

The common characteristics of the group suggest that the individual members have experienced a stress in a common way. They may be a family, the residents of a single building, coworkers, or the victims of a disaster. Usually, the cultural background of the group is uniform.

Usually, a few members of the group manifest symptoms, and the rest of the group follow; as the leaders' symptoms escalate, so do those of the rest of the group. The symptoms may include screaming, panic, fainting, agitation, and other symptoms of hysteria.

INTERVIEWING AND PSYCHOTHERAPEUTIC GUIDELINES

The group must be dispersed before an intervention can begin. Start with the persons who are leading in the manifestation of symptoms. Provide a reassuring environment that emphasizes that the situation is under control. Give each patient an opportunity to ventilate. Point out potential resources, such as families and social networks.

EVALUATION AND MANAGEMENT

1. To whatever extent is possible, isolate the individual members whose symptom manifestations are leading the group; encourage less emotional family members and paraprofessional staff members to calm the others.
2. Consider the culture of the group. Emotional reactions are encouraged in some cultures (for example, Latin American cultures) and discouraged in others (for example, Asian cultures). Devise a culturally appropriate plan.
3. Enlist the help of important people in the culture (for example, priests, neighborhood leaders) who may be the best equipped to dissipate the crisis appropriately.
4. Reassure the patients by providing an environment that shows that the situation is under control with the presence of enough staff members, rapid attention, and minimal unnecessary traffic in and out of the emergency area.
5. Give each patient a chance to discuss the stressful experience, to ventilate, and to describe the emotional process leading to the symptoms.
6. Encourage the patients to stay with extended family members who are not involved in the hysteria. Close friends and other social networks can also be used. Try to avoid immediately reassembling the group, which may lead to a recurrence of the group hysteria.

DRUG TREATMENT

Treat the severe agitation or anxiety with a brief course of short-acting benzodiazepines—for example, alprazolam (Xanax) 0.5 to 1 mg, lorazepam (Ativan) 1 to 2 mg, or oxazepam (Serax) 10 to 30 mg, all given by mouth every four hours as needed.

For a more detailed discussion of this topic, see N Wong: Group Psychotherapy, Combined Individual and Group Psychotherapy, and Psychodrama, Sec 31.4, p 1821, in CTP/VI.

12

Somatoform Disorders

12.1 Hypochondriasis

Hypochondriasis is an unreasonable concern about one's health and an unrealistic conviction that physical signs or symptoms are indicative of serious medical disease, despite reasonable assurance that such a disease is not present.

CLINICAL FEATURES AND DIAGNOSIS

The fear of disease is persistent, and itself leads to functional impairment. Several organ systems may be the focus of concern, or one system may predominate (Table 12.1-1).

About 10 to 15 percent of all patients seen in general medical practice have hypochondriasis. The peak incidence is in the fourth or fifth decade. Hypochondriasis may be more common in the relatives of patients with hypochondriasis than in the general population.

Hypochondriasis may be common in cultures that encourage somatization as an expression of psychic distress. Psychodynamically, hypochondriasis offers the patient a way to assume the sick role in avoidance of insurmountable problems or some overwhelming stress. The possible origins include (1) aggression toward others that is repressed and displaced into physical symptoms and (2) defense against guilt in which the physical symptoms are a deserved punishment for some sin. Psychosocially, the onset of symptoms often follows a major stressor.

The clinical features that indicate a good prognosis include the presence of depression or anxiety, a sudden onset, young age, a high socioeconomic status, the absence of organic disease, and the absence of a personality disorder. Hypochondria-

TABLE 12.1–1
DIAGNOSTIC CRITERIA FOR HYPOCHONDRIASIS

A. Preoccupation with fears of having, or the idea that one has, a serious disease based on the person's misinterpretation of bodily symptoms.
B. The preoccupation persists despite appropriate medical evaluation and reassurance.
C. The belief in Criterion A is not of delusional intensity (as in delusional disorder, somatic type) and is not restricted to a circumscribed concern about appearance (as in body dysmorphic disorder).
D. The preoccupation causes clinically significant distress or impairment in social, occupational, or other important areas of functioning.
E. The duration of the disturbance is at least 6 months.
F. The preoccupation is not better accounted for by generalized anxiety disorder, obsessive-compulsive disorder, panic disorder, a major depressive episode, separation anxiety, or another somatoform disorder.

Specify if:
   With poor insight: if, for most of the time during the current episode, the person does not recognize that the concern about having a serious illness is excessive or unreasonable

Table from DSM-IV, *Diagnostic and Statistical Manual of Mental Disorders*, ed 4. Copyright American Psychiatric Association, Washington, 1994. Use with permission.

cal patients are often resistant to psychiatric treatment; offering them treatment in a medical setting that emphasizes coping with chronic medical illnesses may improve their cooperation. The outcome is poor in about 25 percent of patients, and another two-thirds run a long-term fluctuating course.

INTERVIEWING AND PSYCHOTHERAPEUTIC GUIDELINES

Hypochondriacal patients may also have genuine medical conditions. Begin by assuming that all somatic complaints are due to medical causes, and proceed with an appropriate medical evaluation, including consultations if appropriate. Medical conditions with symptoms in multiple systems—such as acquired immune deficiency syndrome (AIDS), systemic lupus erythematosus, endocrinopathies, multiple sclerosis, myasthenia gravis, central nervous system (CNS) diseases, cancer, and syphilis—can be missed in a patient who appears to be hypochondriacal. Regular physical examinations and other noninvasive tests help reassure patients that the doctor is not ignoring their somatic complaints. Maintain an understanding attitude without reinforcing the patient's behavior.

Identify pervasive psychiatric disorders, such as depression and anxiety disorders, since the presence of such disorders suggests definitive treatments that can improve the prognosis.

EVALUATION AND MANAGEMENT

1. Rule out genuine medical conditions; even a known hypochondriac can get sick. However, avoid repetitive unnecessary medical testing.
2. Evaluate the patient for depressive and anxiety disorders, especially panic disorder. Also, examine the patient for somatic delusions, obsessions, and compulsions.
3. Group therapy may be the treatment of choice, especially in medical settings that emphasize coping skills. Groups also provide social contacts and support. Individual insight-oriented psychotherapy may also be effective.

DRUG TREATMENT

No specific drug treatment is indicated in cases of hypochondriasis. In the hypochondriacal anxious state the patient may benefit from an anxiolytic—for example, alprazolam (Xanax) 0.5 to 1 mg by mouth, oxazepam (Serax) 10 to 30 mg by mouth, or lorazepam (Ativan) 1 mg by mouth or intramuscularly (IM). If the course is episodic and similar to that of a depressive disorder, diagnose depression. A new onset of hypochondriasis in an elderly patient also suggests depression. Treatment with an antidepressant medication may relieve both the underlying depression and the hypochondriasis. In panic disorder, hypochondriasis may respond to benzodiazepines or antidepressants. If psychotic symptoms suggest a delusional disorder or schizophrenia, consider antipsychotics.

For a more detailed discussion of this topic, see F G Guggenheim, G R Smith: Somatoform Disorders, Chap 18, p 1251, in CTP/VI.

12.2 Pain

Pain is a complex symptom consisting of an unpleasant sensation underlying a potential physical disease and an associated emotional state. *Chronic pain* is pain that persists for more than six months. *Pain disorder* is pain in one or more sites that is not fully accounted for by a medical or neurological condition, and the symptoms of pain are associated with emotional distress and functional impairment; the disorder has a plausible causal relation with psychological factors.

CLINICAL FEATURES AND DIAGNOSIS

Pain is a subjective experience that cannot be objectively measured and that is greatly influenced by many factors other than the degree of physical disease or injury. Those factors include the patient's psychological makeup; the presence of depression, anxiety, or psychotic disorders; the reactions elicited in the family, health care providers, the employer, and the rest of the patient's environment; stressors; and the level of distraction by other stimuli. Pain may serve simultaneously as a symptom of stress and as a defense against stress.

A physiological classification of pain is given in Table 12.2-1.

TABLE 12.2-1
PHYSIOLOGICAL CLASSIFICATION OF PAIN

Type	Subtypes	Examples	Comments
Nociceptive	Somatic Visceral	Bone metastasis Intestinal obstruction	Caused by activation of pain-sensitive fibers; usually aching or pressure
Deafferentation	Peripheral Central Somatic Visceral Sympathetic-dependent Nonsympathetic-dependent	Causalgia Thalamic pain Causalgia Visceral pain in paraplegics Postherpetic pain Phantom pain	Caused by interruption of afferent pathways. Pathophysiology poorly understood, with most syndromes probably involving both peripheral and central nervous system changes. Usually dysesthetic, often burning and lancinating
Psychogenic	Somatization disorder Psychogenic pain Hypochondriasis Specific pain diagnoses, with organic contribution	Low back pain Atypical facial pain Chronic headache	Does not include factitious disorders—i.e., malingering and Munchausen syndrome

Table from *Merck Manual*, ed 15. Merck Sharp & Dohme Research Laboratories, Rahway, NJ, 1987. Used with permission.

TABLE 12.2–2
CHARACTERISTICS OF SOMATIC AND PSYCHOGENIC OR NEUROPATHIC PAIN

Somatic pain
Nociceptive stimulus usually evident
Usually well localized: visceral pain may be referred
Similar to other somatic pains in patient's experience
Relieved by anti-inflammatory or narcotic analgesics
Psychogenic or neuropathic pain
No obvious nociceptive stimulus
Often poorly localized
Unusual, dissimilar from somatic pain
Only partially relieved by narcotic analgesics

Table from E Braunwald, K Isselbacher, R G Petersdorf, J D Wilson, J B Martin, A S Fauci: *Harrison's Principles of Internal Medicine II, Companion Handbook*. McGraw-Hill, New York, 1988. Used with permission. Modified by R Maciewicz, J B Martin.

Differentiating somatic pain from psychogenic pain is often complex (Table 12.2-2). Somatic pain varies with time, the situational stress, the patient's emotional state, and the use of analgesics. A constant pain that is unaffected by any of these factors is often psychogenic. A sudden, dramatic presentation suggests histrionic and borderline personality disorders. If the course of the pain parallels that of depression, psychosis, or anxiety, those psychiatric diagnoses should be made and those conditions treated. If litigation is an issue, reliably evaluating how much of the pain is somatic and how much is psychogenic may not be possible. Malingering, factitious disorders, and drug-seeking behavior in substance abusers must always be ruled out.

INTERVIEWING AND PSYCHOTHERAPEUTIC GUIDELINES

Examine the effects that the pain has on the patient and the patient's environment. Have family members responded by increasing their care and nurturing? Has the primary physician responded by strengthened efforts to diagnose an unidentified medical condition? Does litigation depend on the patient's disability? Does the patient need to have pain to receive health care attention? Does the administration of analgesics depend on the patient's proving that pain is present, thus causing a battle between the patient and the nursing staff?

Whatever the quality of the complaint, assume that a somatic cause is present and perform a medical workup.

If the pain appears to be psychogenic, help the patient move past placing the responsibility on the physician to find the cause of the pain. Help the patient take some responsibility for coping with the pain through rehabilitation. Pain patients are sensitive to any implications that the pain is all in their heads, so the approach should be one of focusing on the pain as genuine and working out strategies to cope with the stress created by the pain.

EVALUATION AND MANAGEMENT

1. Perform a complete medical evaluation.
2. Obtain a detailed history of the pain, including the frequency and the duration of past episodes of the pain and the factors that exacerbate or relieve the pain.

3. Administer a complete mental status examination, and obtain a psychiatric history. Evaluate the patient for symptoms of depression, anxiety disorders, psychotic disorders, personality disorders, malingering, and drug-seeking behavior. Evaluate the patient for suicidality, since chronic pain increases the risk of suicide.

4. When medical and psychiatric causes have been ruled out, switch to a rehabilitation approach. Start by discussing the neurophysiological substrates of pain, and work toward explaining how those factors can cause stress, influence behavior, and lead to impairments in functioning.

5. Chronic pain programs are usually best suited for treating patients with chronic pain; they provide medical and psychiatric treatment, individual therapy, group therapy, and rehabilitation programs. Referral to chronic pain programs minimizes the treating physician's frustration and reduces direct conflicts with the patient.

6. Cognitive therapy is often useful. Conventional folk wisdom dictates, "If you think about your pain all the time, you'll make it worse." The cognitive approach expands on that concept. Use relaxation, visual imagery, and other techniques to distract the patient from the pain.

7. Individual psychotherapy is fraught with many obstacles but may be useful in some patients. A short-term problem-oriented supportive approach should focus on bolstering the patient's ego strengths and avoiding conflicts and anxiety.

8. Family therapy is often useful. The family almost always plays an important role in shaping the patient's behavior. Family therapy should focus on changing the pattern of responses to reinforce positive behavior and to ignore negative behavior.

9. Group therapy is helpful and places responsibility on the patient for the management of the pain. However, avoid creating situations in which group members compete to see who can be sicker or learn sick-role behaviors from each other.

10. Use physical therapy as needed.

11. Use increased sensory stimulation, such as massage, acupuncture, and transcutaneous nerve stimulation.

12. Use biofeedback and relaxation techniques.

13. Nerve blocks differentiate central sources of pain from peripheral sources of pain. Chemical or surgical ablation may follow. Table 12.2-3 lists procedures used in management of cancer pain.

14. Neurosurgery is a last resort, but it has helped some patients, although the relief from pain may also have been caused by the relief of severe depression or a change in personality.

15. Table 12.2-4 lists auxiliary methods of pain control.

DRUG TREATMENT

Base the drug treatment on as accurate a diagnosis as possible. Undertake drug treatment with the agents in Table 12.2-5 as part of a comprehensive, ongoing treatment plan; therefore, the medications should not be given in the emergency room or the primary care physician's office. Before beginning any drug treatment, decide unequivocally that drug treatment is clearly indicated. Avoid ambivalence

TABLE 12.2-3
PROCEDURES USED IN MANAGEMENT OF CANCER PAIN

| Site | Procedures | | |
	Anesthetic	Neurosurgical	Neuroaugmentative
Peripheral nerve	Temporary and neurolytic block	Neurectomy	Percutaneous electrical stimulation, acupuncture
Nerve root	Temporary and neurolytic block	Rhizotomy	—
Spinal cord	—	Dorsal root entry zone lesions, cordotomy, myelotomy	Dorsal column stimulation
Brainstem	—	Mesencephalic tractotomy	—
Thalamus	—	Thalamotomy	Deep brain stimulation
Cortex	—	Lobotomy, cingulotomy	—
Pituitary	Chemical hypophysectomy	Transsphenoidal hypophysectomy	—

Table from *Merck Manual*, ed 16, p 1417. Merck Sharp & Dohme Research Laboratories, Rahway, NJ 1992. Used with permission.

TABLE 12.2-4
AUXILIARY METHODS OF PAIN CONTROL

Approach	Procedure	Indication
Psychotherapy	Distraction Relaxation Hypnosis Biofeedback	Prominent depression or anxiety, muscle spasm, predictable pain
	Supportive and/or analytically oriented individual or group (including family) therapy	Abnormal behavior, secondary gain, coexistent psychopathology
Physiatrics	Physical or occupational therapy Prosthetics or orthotic devices	Incident pain, skeletal instability, disuse
Neuroaugmentative techniques	Transcutaneous electrical nerve stimulation. Counterirritation	Localized pain, neuropathic pain
Anesthesia	Trigger point injections	Myofascial pain

Table from *Merck Manual*, ed 16, p 1416. Merck Sharp & Dohme Research Laboratories, Rahway, NJ 1992. Used with permission.

in ordering pain medications to minimize undermedicating the patient or setting up situations in which the patient must struggle to receive medication.

In conditions with paroxysmal pain, such as trigeminal neuralgia, try such anticonvulsants as carbamazepine (Tegretol) first, and prescribe the anticonvulsant on a standing basis.

Tricyclic antidepressants are often helpful in chronic pain, regardless of whether they are being used to treat depression or insomnia. The dosage of antidepressant needed is often much less than that typically used for depression—for example, imipramine (Tofranil) or amitriptyline (Elavil), both given at 25 to 100 mg at bedtime.

TABLE 12.2–5
DRUGS USED TO RELIEVE PAIN

Nonnarcotic analgesics; equivalent doses and intervals

Generic name	Dose (mg)	Interval
Aspirin	750–1250	Every 3 hours
Phenacetin	750–1000	Every 3 hours
Acetaminophen	600–800	Every 3 hours
Phenylbutazone	200–400	Every 4 hours
Indomethacin	50–75	Every 4 hours
Ibuprofen	200–400	Every 4 hours
Naproxen	250–500	Every 4 hours

Narcotic analgesics compared with 10 mg morphine sulfate (MS)

Generic name	IM dose (mg)	Oral dose (mg)	Differences from MS
Oxymorphine	1	6	None
Hydromorphone	1.5	7.5	Shorter acting
Levorphanol	2	4	Good oral-IM potency
Heroin	4		Shorter acting
Methadone	10	20	Good oral-IM potency
Morphine	10	60	
Oxycodone	15	30	Shorter acting
Meperidine	75	300	None
Pentazocine	60	180	Agonist-antagonist
Codeine	130	200	More toxic

Anticonvulsants

Generic name	Oral dose (mg)	Interval
Phenytoin	100	Every 6–8 hours
Carbamazepine	200	Every 6 hours
Clonazepam	1	Every 6 hours

Antidepressants

Generic name	Oral dose (mg)	Range (mg/day)
Doxepin	200	75–400
Amitriptyline	150	75–300
Imipramine	200	75–400
Nortriptyline	100	40–150
Desipramine	150	75–300
Amoxapine	200	75–300
Trazodone	150	50–600

Table from R Maciewicz, J B Martin: Pain: Pathophysiology and management. In E Braunwald, K Issel-bacher, R G Petersdorf, J D Wilson, J B Martin, A S Fauci: *Harrison's Principles of Internal Medicine II.* McGraw-Hill, New York, 1988. Used with permission.

Nonnarcotic analgesics, such as aspirin and nonsteroidal anti-inflammatory drugs—for example, ibuprofen (Motrin)—are useful and should be given on a standing basis to achieve therapeutic blood levels.

Opioids are effective analgesics but produce rapid tolerance and dependence should be limited to short-term use. However, if the decision is made to use opioids, a sufficient dosage should be prescribed—that is, a dosage sufficient to cause analgesia. Some chronic pain patients become dependent on opioids and later require detoxification. Table 12.2-6 lists guidelines for management of opioid mainte-nance therapy.

Do not give placebos without the patient's agreement. Although placebo analgesic effects have been documented, a more effective treatment should not be withheld, and deception of the patient undermines trust in the physician.

For a more detailed discussion of this topic, see F G Guggenheim, G R Smith: Somatoform Disorders, Chap 18, p 1251; M S Lederberg, J C Holland: Psycho-Oncology, Sec 26.11, p 1570, in CTP/VI.

TABLE 12.2–6
GUIDELINES FOR MANAGEMENT OF OPIOID MAINTENANCE THERAPY IN PATIENTS WITH NONMALIGNANT PAIN*

Consent discussion required, specifically noting possibilities of side effects, minimal risk of addictive behaviors developing, and physical dependence of newborns in women who deliver while on therapy
Agreed-upon period of titration, aiming for at least partial relief of pain
After titration, agreed-upon monthly quantity of drug, with some leeway in daily dosage but return to maintenance dosage by the month's end
Monthly visits; careful documentation in the medical record of repeated assessment of continued efficacy and lack of evidence of opioid toxicity or signs of drug misuse or abuse
Return of function should continue to be major emphasis
Drug hoarding, diversion, or acquisition elsewhere should not be tolerated; if they occur, opioid dosage should be tapered and maintenance therapy stopped
Rapid escalation, or escalation without subsequent decrement, suggests need for hospitalization

*For use only after all nonopioid therapies are exhausted.
Table from *Merck Manual,* ed 16, p 1419. Merck Sharp & Dohme Research Laboratories, Rahway, NJ 1992. Used with permission.

12.3 Psychogenic Urinary Retention

Primary care physicians who treat patients with urinary retention must be aware that many factors may cause the condition. *Psychogenic urinary retention* is the transient inability to urinate because of emotional conflicts. Urinary retention may occur in social phobia (shy bladder), schizophrenia, and depression. Many psychotropic medications also cause urinary dysfunction, primarily because of their anticholinergic properties and particularly in overdoses. Psychogenic urinary retention may be accompanied by indifference, but urinary retention caused by toxicity is painful and requires urgent treatment.

CLINICAL FEATURES AND DIAGNOSIS

Psychogenic urinary retention is usually diagnosed by the process of exclusion. After all medical, neurological, and medication-induced causes have been ruled out a psychiatric referral is warranted. The emotional conflicts central to the diagnosis may be conscious or unconscious. If the conflicts are conscious, unfortunate experiences during socialization as a child may condition anxiety, fear of exposure, and shame on urination under certain (for circumstances example, in public places). The anxiety may grow and include a broad range of conditions. Avoidance becomes habitual. In those cases the patients are generally aware of the pattern of events that led to the difficulty in urinating.

If the patient's conflicts are unconscious, urinary retention is classified as a conversion disorder, formerly hysteria. The symptom is modeled on the patient's experience of others with urinary retention or the patient's own chance experience of difficulty in urinating. The disorder is precipitated by some internal threat outside the patient's conscious awareness and arises during extreme psychosocial stress. Conflicts about dependence, self-determination, and sexuality are common. Histrionic and dependent personality disorders contribute to the patient's vulnerability to conversion symptoms.

The onset is usually in adulthood, and women are affected more than men. Intermediate cases with varying degrees of conscious and unconscious motivation and insight also occur.

INTERVIEWING AND PSYCHOTHERAPEUTIC GUIDELINES

Patients with conscious anxiety readily describe the antecedents of their symptoms, and a straightforward history is sufficient for diagnosis. However, patients with unconscious conflicts and an established secondary gain do not respond well to the suggestion that the problem is psychogenic. Since the symptom serves a protective function and is a source of gratification, such patients resist uncovering the issues. Therefore, a subtle approach is suggested. Question the patients thoroughly about their histories, but do not directly focus on their toilet training or other emotionally charged issues. Devote particular attention to the stressful events that surrounded the onset of the urinary problems, but do not suggest a causative role.

Ascertain the patients' exposure and modeling by enquiring about family members with similar problems. That approach spares patients the threat of sudden confrontation with the source of their conflicts and allows the examiner to identify the problem without triggering increased defensiveness.

EVALUATION AND MANAGEMENT

1. The management of urinary retention includes intermittent catheterization. Most patients then resume spontaneous urination, although recurrences are common.
2. Urinary retention caused by schizophrenia or depression requires psychiatric treatment of the primary condition.
3. By the time of the consultation, self-catheterization may be established. Self-catheterization carries with it an attendant risk of infections, and it perpetuates the patient's emotional problems and maladaptive behavior. However, because of the importance of the symptom to the patient, unconscious resistance may interfere with evaluation and treatment. A psychiatric consultation or hospitalization may be necessary to ensure valid assessment and treatment compliance.
4. Successful treatment ultimately depends on resolving the underlying conflicts about dependence and on altering the patterns of reinforcement with behavior therapy. Problems with voiding tend to persist, and recurrences of urinary retention are common.

DRUG TREATMENT

Short-acting benzodiazepines may be useful for anxiety-based retention. Alprazolam (Xanax) 0.5 to 1 mg by mouth, oxazepam (Serax) 10 to 30 mg by mouth, estazolam (ProSom) 0.5 to 1 mg by mouth, or lorazepam (Ativan) 1 to 2 mg by mouth may induce urination within one hour. Anticholinergic-induced urinary retention may be treated with bethanechol (Urecholine) 2.5 to 5 mg subcutaneously.

For a more detailed discussion of this topic, see D H Barlow, M R Liebowitz: Specific Phobia and Social Phobia, Sec 17.2, p 1204; F G Guggenheim, G R Smith: Somatoform Disorders, Chap 18, p 1251, in CTP/VI.

12.4 Somatization Disorder

Somatization disorder is characterized by many somatic symptoms affecting multiple organ systems (for example, gastrointestinal and neurological) that cannot be explained adequately by physical and laboratory examinations. The disorder is chronic (with symptoms present for several years and beginning before age 30) and is associated with significant psychological distress, impairment in social and occupational functioning, and excessive medical help-seeking behavior. The disorder has also been called Briquet's syndrome.

CLINICAL FEATURES AND DIAGNOSIS

For the diagnosis, the onset of the symptoms must occur before age 30. During the course of the disorder, the patient must have complained of at least four pain symptoms: two gastrointestinal symptoms, one sexual symptom, and one pseudoneurological symptom, none of which physical or laboratory examinations completely explain.

Patients with the disorder have many somatic complaints and long, complicated medical histories. Nausea and vomiting (other than during pregnancy), difficulty in swallowing, pain in the arms and the legs, shortness of breath unrelated to exertion, amnesia, and complications of pregnancy and menstruation are among the most common symptoms. The belief that one has been sickly most of one's life is also common. Psychological distress and interpersonal problems are prominent; anxiety and depression are the most prevalent psychiatric conditions. Suicide threats are common, but actual suicide is rare (and often associated with substance abuse).

Somatization disorder is distinguished from other somatoform disorders because of the multiplicity of the complaints and the multiple organ systems (for example, gastrointestinal and neurological) affected. Hypochondriasis is characterized by the false belief that one has a specific disease, in contrast to somatization disorder, which is characterized by concern with many symptoms. The symptoms of conversion disorder are limited to one or two neurological symptoms, rather than the wide-ranging symptoms of somatization disorder. Pain disorder is limited to one or two complaints of pain symptoms.

The primary care physician must always rule out nonpsychiatric medical conditions that may explain the patient's symptoms. Several medical disorders often present with nonspecific, transient abnormalities in the same age group. Those medical disorders include multiple sclerosis, myasthenia gravis, systemic lupus erythematosus, acquired immune deficiency syndrome (AIDS), acute intermittent porphyria, hyperparathyroidism, hyperthyroidism, and chronic systemic infections. The onset of multiple somatic symptoms in patients over 40 should be presumed to be caused by a nonpsychiatric medical condition until an exhaustive medical workup has been completed.

Many mental disorders are considered in the differential diagnosis, which is made complicated by the observation that at least 50 percent of patients with somatization disorder have a coexisting mental disorder. Major depressive disorder, generalized anxiety disorder, and schizophrenia may all present with an initial complaint that focuses on somatic symptoms. In all those disorders, however, the symptoms of depression, anxiety, or psychosis eventually predominate over the somatic complaints.

INTERVIEWING AND PSYCHOTHERAPEUTIC GUIDELINES

A reasonable long-range primary care treatment strategy for somatization disorder is to increase the patient's awareness of the possibility that psychological factors are involved in the symptoms until the patient is willing to see a psychiatrist regularly.

Psychotherapy, both individual and group, decreases somatization disorder patients' personal health care expenditures by 50 percent, largely by decreasing their rates of hospitalization.

EVALUATION AND MANAGEMENT

1. Somatization disorder patients are best treated when they have a single identified physician as the primary caretaker. When more than one clinician is involved, the patient has increased opportunities to express somatic complaints.
2. The primary physician should see the patient during regularly scheduled visits, usually at monthly intervals. The visits should be relatively brief; although a partial physical examination should be conducted to respond to each new somatic complaint, additional laboratory and diagnostic procedures should generally be avoided.
3. Once somatization disorder has been diagnosed, the treating physician should listen to the somatic complaints as emotional expressions, rather than as medical complaints. However, patients with somatization disorder can also have bona fide physical illnesses; therefore, physicians must always use their judgment about what symptoms to work up and to what extent.

DRUG TREATMENT

Giving psychotropic medications whenever somatization disorder coexists with a mood or anxiety disorder is always a risk, but psychopharmacological treatment, as well as psychotherapeutic treatment, of the coexisting disorder is indicated. Medication must be monitored, because somatization disorder patients tend to use drugs erratically and unreliably. In patients without coexisting mental disorders, few available data indicate that pharmacological treatment is effective.

For a more detailed discussion of this topic, see F G Guggenheim, G R Smith: Somatoform Disorders, Chap 18, p 1251, in CTP/VI.

13

Factitious Disorders

13.1 Factitious Disorders

In *factitious disorders,* patients intentionally produce signs of medical or mental disorders and misrepresent their histories and symptoms. The only apparent objective of the behavior is to assume the role of a patient. For many persons, hospitalization itself is a primary objective and often a way of life. The disorders have a compulsive quality and are voluntary in that they are deliberate and purposeful.

CLINICAL FEATURES AND DIAGNOSIS

The psychiatric examination should emphasize securing information from any available friend, relative, or other informant, because interviews with outside sources often reveal the false nature of the patient's illness. Although time-consuming and tedious, verifying all the facts presented by the patient concerning prior hospitalizations and medical care is essential.

The differential diagnosis should include any disorder in which physical signs and symptoms are prominent, and the possibility of authentic or concomitant physical illness must always be explored. In somatoform disorders the symptoms are not voluntary. In hypochondriasis, patients do not want to undergo extensive tests or surgery. Malingerers have specific goals (for example, insurance payments, avoidance of jail term). Other disorders to consider are personality disorders (because of pathological lying), schizophrenia or other psychotic disorders (patients may have a somatic delusion), and substance use disorders.

Munchausen's Syndrome by Proxy

In *Munchausen's syndrome by proxy,* someone intentionally produces physical signs or symptoms in another person who is under the first person's care. The only apparent purpose of the behavior is for the caretaker to indirectly assume the sick role. The most common case of this disorder involves a mother who deceives medical personnel into believing that her child is ill. The deception may involve a false medical history, the contamination of laboratory samples, the alteration of records, or the induction of injury and illness in the child.

Self-Inflicted Dermatitis

Self-inflicted dermatitis (also called dermatitis artefacta and factitial dermatitis) is a disorder consisting of self-inflicted skin wounds. The patient may deny that the wounds are self-inflicted and complain of dermatological disease. However, the pattern of the lesions (linear or in a geometric shape) is pathognomonic of a factitious disorder. Self-inflicted dermatitis is more common in women than in men and is associated with borderline personality disorder. It also occurs in anxiety disorders, depression, and other personality disorders. It is rarely a symptom of a psychotic disorder.

INTERVIEWING AND PSYCHOTHERAPEUTIC GUIDELINES

Patients with factitious disorder are usually poorly motivated in psychotherapy; however, a working alliance with the physician is possible over time, and the patient may gain insights into the behavior. The patients are difficult to engage in an exploratory psychotherapy process and may insist that their symptoms are physical and, therefore, psychologically oriented treatment is useless.

Patients who feign psychiatric illness may have had a relative who was hospitalized with the illness they are simulating. Through identification, the patients hope to reunite with the relative in a magical way.

Patients with self-inflicted dermatitis have a need to have a dermatological condition; they may be attempting to achieve a secondary gain. After ruling out a true dermatological condition, try to identify the psychological needs that the symptom has been fabricated to satisfy. Do not lie or acknowledge that the injuries are from a genuine dermatological disorder. In addition, do not confront the patients directly and accuse them of malingering. Focus on the conflicts and the stresses that led to the behavior.

EVALUATION AND MANAGEMENT

1. Avoid unnecessary laboratory tests or medical procedures.
2. Rule out any psychiatric disorder in which physical signs and symptoms are prominent: somatoform disorders, hypochondriasis, malingering, personality disorders, schizophrenia or other psychotic disorders, and substance use disorders.
3. Rule out any authentic or concomitant organic disorders.
4. Patients should be confronted with the diagnosis of factitious disorder if appropriate. A data bank of patients with repeated hospitalizations for factitious disorder is available in some areas.

DRUG TREATMENT

Psychopharmacological therapy is useful with associated anxiety or depression.

For a more detailed discussion of this topic, see R M Jones: Factitious Disorders, Chap 19, p 1271, in CTP/VI.

13.2 Malingering

Malingering is the voluntary production of false or grossly exaggerated symptoms to achieve some clearly identifiable objective (for example, to win a lawsuit or to obtain controlled substances).

CLINICAL FEATURES AND DIAGNOSIS

The external motivations for malingering can be put into three categories: (1) to avoid responsibility, danger, or punishment; (2) to receive compensation, free room and board, or drugs; and (3) to retaliate after a loss. Malingering can be differentiated from factitious disorders in that the patient seeks a clearly definable objective (*secondary gain*) for the symptoms. In factitious disorders, the symptoms are intentionally produced to assume the sick role in the absence of other clearly defined objectives. With somatoform and conversion disorders, the symptoms are not produced intentionally.

Malingering is common, especially in such settings as prisons, the military, and industrial settings. Malingering may be more common in men than in women; it is often seen in adults with antisocial personality disorder and in children and adolescents with conduct disorder.

The first goal is to recognize malingering, so that unnecessary treatments are avoided. Malingering should be suspected in any patient who presents in a medicolegal situation, who has a marked discrepancy between the subjective complaints and the objective findings, who is noncompliant with diagnostic procedures or treatment, or who has antisocial personality disorder.

The symptoms are often vague, subjective, poorly localized, and impossible to measure objectively. Typical symptoms include pain in the head, the neck, the chest, or the back; dizziness; amnesia; loss of vision or sensation; fainting; seizures; and hallucinations and other psychotic symptoms. The patient often becomes angry if the doctor questions the symptoms. Malingerers may also cause self-inflicted injuries, may stage an injury or an accident to obtain compensation, and may tamper with data or records to support a false complaint. Malingerers may show *Vorbeireden,* in which they give approximate answers to questions when feigning psychiatric illness (for example, 2 + 2 = 5 or identifying a blue chair as red).

Sometimes, patients with true disease feign more severe symptoms than they actually have, which makes the proper identification difficult.

INTERVIEWING AND PSYCHOTHERAPEUTIC GUIDELINES

With suspected malingerers, it is important to maintain a neutral attitude and avoid being confrontational. Give the patients at least the same evaluation and respect given to any other patient. In fact, when malingering is suspected, the initial response should be to make a careful clinical evaluation to verify all suspicions and to rule out any genuine disease. Casual observation may reveal behavior inconsistent with the patients' complaints: for example, they may easily bend at the waist, despite complaints of severe back pain, or they may laugh and joke with other patients, despite somber complaints of depression during the interview.

EVALUATION AND MANAGEMENT

Malingerers do not want to be treated. The appropriate position for the primary care physician is initial clinical neutrality. If malingering is suspected, a careful differential investigation should be performed. If malingering seems the most likely diagnosis, then the patient should be tactfully confronted. However, the patient must not be abruptly shunned; the reasons underlying the deception should be elicited and possible pathways to the desired outcome explored. Any coexisting psychiatric disorders and medical conditions should be addressed. Only if the patient is utterly unwilling to interact with the physician under any terms other than manipulation should the possibility of a positive therapeutic outcome be abandoned.

DRUG TREATMENT

No drug treatment is indicated in this situation.

For a more detailed discussion of this topic, see M J Mills, M S Lipian: Malingering, Sec 28.2, p 1614, in CTP/VI.

14
Sexual Disorders and Sexual Abuse

14.1. Anorgasmia (Female Orgasmic Disorder)

Anorgasmia, also known as female orgasmic disorder, is the inability of the woman to achieve orgasm by masturbation or coitus. Women who can achieve orgasm with one of those methods are not necessarily categorized as anorgasmic, although some degree of sexual inhibition may be postulated.

CLINICAL FEATURES AND DIAGNOSIS

The diagnosis is made if there is a persistent or recurrent delay in, or absence of, orgasm following a normal sexual excitement phase. Women exhibit wide variability in the type or intensity of stimulation that triggers orgasm. The diagnosis of female orgasmic disorder should be based on the clinician's judgment that the woman's orgasmic capacity is less than expected for her age, sexual experience, and the adequacy of sexual stimulation she receives.

INTERVIEWING AND PSYCHOTHERAPEUTIC GUIDELINES

Women are usually comfortable discussing this topic with female doctors; however, male physicians who are sensitive and empathic can usually elicit the complaint. When present, the disturbance causes marked distress in most women, and interpersonal problems are usually part of the picture.

EVALUATION AND MANAGEMENT

1. Rule out the use of drugs of abuse and alcohol.
2. Medical conditions must be ruled out. Hypothyroidism, for example, can cause anorgasmia.
3. Psychiatric drugs are a reversible cause of anorgasmia (Table 14.1-1).
4. A hormonal pattern may contribute to responsiveness. Some women may experience anorgasmia only at a particular time in the menstrual cycle, but it is not clinically significant.
5. Alterations in testosterone, estrogen, prolactin, and thyroxin concentration have been implicated in female orgasmic disorder. Also, medications with antihistaminic or anticholinergic properties cause a decrease in vaginal lubrication. Some evidence indicates that dysfunctional women are less aware of their own physiological responses to arousal, such as vasocongestion, than are other women.

TABLE 14.1-1
PSYCHIATRIC DRUGS IMPLICATED IN FEMALE ORGASMIC DISORDER*

Amoxapine (Asendin)†
Clomipramine (Anafranil)‡
Fluoxetine (Prozac) ˘
Imipramine (Tofranil)
Nortriptyline (Pamelor) ˘
Phenelzine (Nardil)**
Thioridazine (Mellaril)
Tranylcypromine (Parnate)**
Trifluoperazine (Stelazine)

* The interrelation between female sexual dysfunctions and pharmacological agents has been less extensively evaluated than have male reactions. Oral contraceptives are reported to decrease libido in some women, and some drugs with anticholinergic side effects may impair arousal and orgasm. Benzodiazepines have been reported to decrease libido, but in some patients the diminution of anxiety caused by those drugs enhances sexual function.
   Both increases and decreases in libido have been reported with psychoactive agents. It is difficult to separate those effects from the underlying condition or from improvement of the condition. Sexual dysfunction associated with the use of a drug disappears when the drug is discontinued.
† Bethanechol (Urecholine) can reverse the effects of amoxapine-induced anorgasmia.
‡ Clomipramine is also reported to increase arousal and orgasmic potential.
˘ Cyproheptadine (Periactin) reverses fluoxetine- and nortriptyline-induced anorgasmia.
** MAOI-induced anorgasmia may be a temporary reaction to the medication that disappears even though administration of the drug is continued. Table by Virginia A. Sadock, MD.

PSYCHOTHERAPEUTIC TREATMENT

The physician can explore with the patient the many psychological factors associated with female orgasmic disorder: fears of impregnation, rejection by the sex partner, or damage to the vagina; hostility toward men; and feelings of guilt regarding sexual impulses. For some women, orgasm is equated with loss of control or with aggressive, destructive, or violent behavior; their fear of those impulses may be expressed through inhibition of excitement or orgasm. Cultural expectations and societal restrictions on women are also relevant. Nonorgasmic women may be otherwise symptom-free or may experience frustration in a variety of ways, including such pelvic complaints as lower abdominal pain, itching, and vaginal discharge, as well as increased tension, irritability, and fatigue. If a discussion of these issues brings no relief, the patient should be referred to a sex therapy center. (The most qualified centers are associated with medical schools or hospitals.) Other approaches—such as dual-sex therapy, in which the patient is treated with her partner or spouse, and other behavioral approaches, including masturbatory techniques—are also prescribed.

14.2. Hypersexuality

Hypersexuality usually refers to repeated sexual activity with different partners in the absence of ongoing relationships. Social evaluation of what is considered appropriate sexual behavior is highly dependent on culture. Therefore, hypersexuality must be defined in a social and cultural context; it is not based strictly on the quantity of sexual activity. A wide range of quantity of sexual activity can be considered normal. In homosexual patients it is more difficult to determine when a patient is hypersexual, since the range of socially acceptable sexual behavior may be wider in the gay community than among heterosexuals.

CLINICAL FEATURES AND DIAGNOSIS

Although the symptom of hypersexuality has been poorly studied, the vast majority of hypersexual patients suffer from psychological conditions rather than organic conditions. Mental disorders that may present with hypersexuality include personality disorders (such as borderline and histrionic personality disorders), mania, intoxication with such stimulant drugs as amphetamine and cocaine, and, less commonly, schizophrenia.

The terms "nymphomaniac" for women and "satyr" and "Don Juan" for men are commonly used for heterosexuals who repeatedly have sex with multiple partners, often compulsively. The theories about Don Juanism include unconscious homosexual desires defended against by repeated heterosexual contacts. Hypersexual women (nymphomaniacs) are often highly dependent and may have anorgasmia. They engage in sexual activities repeatedly because they fear a loss of love.

Hypersexuality may be a rare symptom of an organic disorder, such as epilepsy, especially temporal lobe epilepsy. Frontal lobe disease may present with hypersexuality as a form of disinhibited behavior.

INTERVIEWING AND PSYCHOTHERAPEUTIC GUIDELINES

Be nonjudgmental in interviewing the patient. In addition to a sexual history, the evaluation should include a full psychiatric history and a mental status examination.

EVALUATION AND MANAGEMENT

1. Perform a complete psychiatric evaluation and make a diagnosis.
2. Complete a sexual history, with emphasis on possible sexual disorders.
3. Evaluate the patient for possible exposure to human immunodeficiency virus (HIV) and other sexually transmitted diseases. Provide medical treatment if appropriate.
4. Consider giving a female patient a pregnancy test.
5. Is the hypersexual behavior placing the patient in potentially dangerous situations, especially if the patient is psychotic? Consider hospitalization in those cases.
6. When hospitalizing a hypersexual patient, consider a one-to-one watch to prevent destructive sexual interactions with other patients.

DRUG TREATMENT

No specific medication is used on an emergency basis for this condition. If the behavioral pattern is a manifestation of an underlying disorder, pharmacotherapy can be considered.

For a more detailed discussion of this topic, see J Yager, M J Gitlin: Clinical Manifestations of Psychiatric Disorders, Chap 10, p 637; R L Williams, I Karacan, C A Moore, M Hirshkowitz: Sleep Disorders, Chap 23, p 1373, in CTP/VI.

14.3. Impotence (Male Erectile Disorder)

Impotence is the inability to achieve penile erection. It is a common complaint of men seen by physicians and can produce considerable anxiety and suffering for the patient.

CLINICAL FEATURES AND DIAGNOSIS

The immediate objective in evaluating a complaint of impotence is making a specific diagnosis, determined by whether (1) the patient is truly impotent (unable to achieve a functional erection under any circumstances); (2) the patient is impotent because of a medical condition, a drug, or alcohol (Table 14.3-1 and Table 14.3-

TABLE 14.3-1
DISEASES IMPLICATED IN ERECTILE DYSFUNCTION

Infectious and parasitic diseases	Neurological disorders
Elephantiasis	Multiple sclerosis
Mumps	Transverse myelitis
	Parkinson's disease
Cardiovascular diseases	Temporal lobe epilepsy
Atherosclerotic disease	Traumatic or neoplastic spinal cord disease
Aortic aneurysm	Central nervous system tumors
Leriche's syndrome	Amyotropic lateral sclerosis
Cardiac failure	Peripheral neuropathies
	General paresis
Renal and urological disorders	Tabes dorsalis
Peyronie's disease	
Chronic renal failure	Pharmacological contributants (Table 14.3-3)
Hydrocele or varicocele	Alcohol and other addictive drugs (heroin,
	methadone, morphine, cocaine,
Hepatic disorders	amphetamines, and barbiturates)
Cirrhosis (usually associated with alcoholism)	Prescribed drugs (psychotropic drugs,
	antihypertensive drugs, estrogens, and
Pulmonary disorders	antiandrogens)
Respiratory failure	
	Poisoning
Genetics	Lead (plumbism)
Klinefelter's syndrome	Herbicides
Congenital penile vascular or structural	
abnormalities	Surgical procedures
	Perineal prostatectomy
Nutritional disorders	Abdominal-perineal colon resection
Malnutrition	Sympathectomy (frequently interferes with
Vitamin deficiencies	ejaculation)
	Aortoiliac surgery
Endocrine disorders	Radical cystectomy
Diabetes mellitus	Retroperitoneal lymphadenectomy
Dysfunction of the pituitary-adrenal-testis	
axis	Miscellaneous
Acromegaly	Radiation therapy
Addison's disease	Pelvic fracture
Chromophobe adenoma	Any severe systemic disease or debilitating
Adrenal neoplasias	condition
Myxedema	
Hyperthyroidism	

Table from V A Sadock: Normal human sexuality and sexual dysfunctions. In *Comprehensive Textbook of Psychiatry* ed 5, H I Kaplan, B J Sadock, editors, p 1045. Williams & Wilkins, Baltimore, 1989. Used with permission.

TABLE 14.3–2
PHARMACOLOGICAL AGENTS INPLICATED IN MALE SEXUAL DYSFUNCTION*

Drug	Impairs Erection	Impairs Ejaculation
Psychiatric drugs		
Tricyclic antidepressants†		
Imipramine (Tofranil)	+	+
Protriptyline (Vivactil)	+	+
Clomipramine (Anafranil)	+	+
Amitriptyline (Elavil)	+	+
Nortriptyline (Pamelor)		
Monoamine oxidase inhibitors		
Tranylcypromine (Parnate)	+	
Phenelzine (Nardil)	+	+
Other mood-active drugs		
Lithium (Eskalith)	+	
Amphetamines	+	+
Antipsychotics		
Fluphenazine (Prolixin)	+	
Thioridazine (Mellaril)	+	+
Mesoridazine (Serentil)	−	+
Perphenazine (Trilafon)	−	+
Trifluoperazine (Stelazine)	−	+
Reserpine (Serpasil)	+	+
Haloperidol (Haldol)	−	+
Antianxiety Drugs‡		
Chlordiazepoxide (Librium)	−	+
Antihypertensive drugs		
Clonidine (Catapres)	+	
Methyldopa (Aldomet)	+	+
Spironolactone (Aldactone)	+	−
Hydralazine (Apresoline)	+	−
Commonly abused drugs		
Alcohol	+	+
Barbituates	+	+
Cannabis	+	−
Cocaine	+	+
Heroin	+	+
Methadone	+	−
Morphine	+	+
Miscellaneous drugs		
Antiparkinsonian agents	+	+
Clofibrate (Atromid-S)	+	−
Digoxin (Lanoxin)	+	−
Glutethimide (Doriden)	+	+
Indomethacin (Indocin)	+	−
Phentolamine (Regitine)	−	+
Propranolol (Inderal)	+	−

*Both increases and decreases in libido have been reported with psychoactive agents. It is difficult to separate those effects from the underlying condition or from improvement of the condition. Sexual dysfunction associated with the use of a drug disappears when the drug is discontinued.
†The incidence of erectile dysfunction associated with the use of tricyclic antidepressants is low.
‡Benzodiazepines have been reported to decrease libido, but in some patients the diminution of anxiety caused by the drugs enhances sexual function.
Table from V A Sadock: Normal human sexuality and sexual dysfunctions. In *Comprehensive Textbook of Psychiatry*, ed 5, H I Kaplan, B J Sadock, editors, p 1045. Williams & Wilkins, Baltimore, 1989. Used with permission.

2); (3) the impotence is primary (the patient never had an erection sufficient for coitus) or secondary (the patient has had an erection sufficient for coitus in the past); (4) factors have contributed to secondary impotence; and (5) conditions make the impotence selective (for example, only with the man's wife but not with his girlfriend). After a few episodes of impotence, anticipatory anxiety about being

TABLE 14.3-3
DIAGNOSTIC CRITERIA FOR MALE ERECTILE DISORDER

A. Persistent or recurrent inability to attain, or to maintain until completion of the sexual activity, an adequate erection.
B. The disturbance causes marked distress or interpersonal difficulty.
C. The erectile dysfunction is not better accounted for by another Axis I disorder (other than a sexual dysfunction) and is not due exclusively to the direct physiological effects of a substance (e.g., a drug of abuse, a medication) or a general medical condition.

Specify type:
  Lifelong type
  Acquired type
Specify type:
  Generalized type
  Situational type
Specify:
  Due to psychological factors
  Due to combined factors

Table from DSM-IV, *Diagnostic and Statistical Manual of Mental Disorders*, ed 4. Copyright American Psychiatric Association, Washington, 1994. Used with permission.

impotent again inevitably contributes to continued impotence. The diagnostic criteria for impotence (male erectile disorder) are given in Table 14.3-3.

Primary impotence is uncommon (1 percent of men under age 35); secondary impotence is present in between 10 and 20 percent of all men. Prevalence increases with age, but, in the elderly, the availability of a sexual partner is more related to potency than is increasing age. General good health is also important.

INTERVIEWING AND PSYCHOTHERAPEUTIC GUIDELINES

Impotence is a sensitive topic for most men. Interview the patient alone; later, interview the identified partner alone. Ask the patient about drugs, medications, and alcohol use. Does the patient have erections in the morning, while masturbating, or with other partners? Many patients complaining of impotence do not have an organic cause. They should usually be referred for psychotherapy, including individual, couples, and sex therapy.

EVALUATION AND MANAGEMENT

1. Rule out the use of drugs and alcohol.
2. Obtain the patient's medical history. Could medical conditions (for example, diabetes mellitus) be the cause?
3. Determine the circumstances of the impotence—when, where, with whom, how frequent, how much effort was made. How anxious did the patient or the partner become?
4. If erections can ever be achieved (for example, in the morning, while masturbating, or with another partner), an organic cause is unlikely.
5. Sudden onset of erectile disorder is indicative of a psychological or pharmacological cause.
6. If drugs, alcohol, and medical conditions have been eliminated as possible causes, a sleep laboratory referral should be made to further evaluate the patient for

organic causes. Spontaneous erections occur during rapid eye movement (REM) sleep, and their tumescence can be measured. Some patients with mild organic impairments that cause impotence do have erections during REM sleep. Some depressed patients without organic impairment do not have erections during REM sleep.

7. If no erections occur during several nights in which electroencephalogram (EEG)-documented REM periods have occurred, refer the patient to a urologist. The next procedures to be done include an endocrine workup, penile doppler measurements of the blood flow, and nerve conduction studies.

8. Surgical placement of a penile prosthesis is a drastic course. Such prostheses are either semirigid or inflatable. Possible problems include infection, perforation, pain, and urinary retention. Often, the prostheses are not sexually satisfying for the partner.

9. Revascularization of the penis is an additional experimental treatment for impotence caused by vascular disease. Another proposed treatment is electrical stimulation of the penis.

DRUG TREATMENT

For impotence with an organic cause, invasive treatments can be considered, including the injection of vasoactive substances into the cavernosa of the penis. The drugs used include a combination of papaverine and phentolamine and a form of prostaglandin E (packaged as Caverject, which is injected into the corpora cavernosa to produce an erection). Priapism and venous sclerosis are rare complications. Other drugs that have been considered are vasoactive intestinal polypeptide, phenoxybenzamine (Dibenzyline), and gonadotropin-releasing hormone (which is inhaled). Yohimbine (Yocon) may sometimes be of use in treating psychotropic-drug-induced impotence.

For a more detailed discussion of this topic, see J Yager, M J Gitlin: Clinical Manifestations of Psychiatric Disorders, Chap 10, p 637; V A Sadock: Normal Human Sexuality and Sexual Dysfunctions, Sec 21.1a, p 1295; R L Williams, I Karacan, C A Moore, M Hirshkowitz: Sleep Disorders, Chap 23, p 1373, in CTP/VI.

14.4. Rape and Sexual Abuse

Rape is the forceful coercion of an unwilling victim to engage in a sexual act. Usually this act is sexual intercourse, although anal intercourse and fellatio can also constitute rape.

Rape is a life-threatening experience in which the victim has almost always been threatened with physical harm; like other acts of violence, it is a psychiatric emergency that requires immediate appropriate intervention. Left untreated, rape victims may suffer sequelae that persist for a lifetime.

Besides rape, other forms of sexual abuse include genital manipulation with foreign objects, infliction of pain, and forced sexual activity.

CLINICAL FEATURES AND DIAGNOSIS

Clinicians must have a high degree of suspicion for unreported rape, since about 50 percent of rapes are not reported. Patients' hesitation or anxiety while discussing their sexual histories should be a clue.

Rape is fundamentally an act of violent humiliation, rather than an act of sexual intimacy, and the basic interaction between rapist and victim is one of physical domination and submission. Some rapists are impotent during the rape; the victim's pain and suffering sexually arouse only a minority.

The overwhelming majority of rapists are male, and most victims are female. However, male rape does occur, often in penal institutions where men are detained. Women between the ages of 16 and 24 years are in the highest risk category, but female victims as young as 15 months and as old as 82 years have been raped. More than a third of all rapes are committed by rapists known to the victim, 7 percent by close relatives. A fifth of all rapes involve more than one rapist (gang rape).

Typical reactions in both rape and sexual abuse victims include shame, humiliation, anxiety, confusion, and outrage. Many victims wonder whether they are partly responsible and somehow invited the assault. In fact, victim behavior is less important in precipitating a rape than it is in precipitating a homicide or a robbery.

INTERVIEWING AND PSYCHOTHERAPEUTIC GUIDELINES

If possible, a female clinician should evaluate the patient, since the victim may find it easier to talk with a woman than with a man. The evaluation should take place in private. When rape or sexual abuse has not been acknowledged openly, be aware that many victims are hesitant to discuss the assault and avoid the topic. If the patient seems anxious when questioned about sexual history and avoids the discussion, do not validate the patient's avoidance by avoiding the topic. Recognize that the rape victim has undergone an unanticipated, life-threatening stress. It is legally and therapeutically important to take a detailed and complete history of the attack.

Rape and sexual abuse victims are often confused during the period after the assault. Be reassuring, supportive, and nonjudgmental. Educate the patient about the availability of medical and legal services and about rape crisis centers that provide multidisciplinary services.

EVALUATION AND MANAGEMENT

1. Offer appropriate medical, gynecological, and police services. Immediately treat the patient for the injuries sustained in the assault. If pregnancy is a possible consequence, consider giving progesterone or diethylstilbestrol by mouth for five days to prevent implantation. Provide treatment, including a course of antibiotics, for possible sexually transmitted diseases. Test for human immunodeficiency virus (HIV) at an appropriate time.

2. Offer crisis-intervention-oriented therapy. The objective is to minimize the psychological sequelae of the assault in the victim.
3. Refer the patient for ongoing psychotherapy, which should focus on reestablishing the patient's sense of control over the environment, reducing feelings of helplessness and dependence, and addressing and processing obsessional thoughts about the rape or abusive experience.
4. Refer the patient to group therapy for the victims of rape or sexual abuse. The groups are extremely helpful.
5. Encourage the patient to pursue the arrest and conviction of the rapist or sexual abuser. Reassure the patient that social support networks are available for the victims of rape and sexual abuse. Assess the availability of supportive friends and relatives.
6. Evaluate the patient for possible posttraumatic stress disorder. The disorder may not develop immediately, so educate the patient about the possible sequelae. Many rape and sexual abuse victims have symptoms that continue for years. The symptoms may include reliving the experience (flashbacks), preoccupation with the experience, feeling unable to make themselves clean, fear of being followed or of being alone, fear of returning to the site of the assault (often in the victim's home or neighborhood), nightmares, insomnia, and altered eating patterns. Such somatic symptoms as headaches, nausea and vomiting, and malaise are also common. In addition, the patient may avoid future sexual relationships or may experience such sexual symptoms as vaginismus.
7. Evaluate the patient for psychiatric conditions (for example, schizophrenia, substance dependence, and personality disorder) that may cause impaired judgment and place the patient in danger of rape or sexual abuse. If a psychiatric disorder is present, refer the patient for treatment of the underlying psychiatric disorder.

DRUG TREATMENT

Usually, no drug treatment is indicated. Some patients may experience overwhelming anxiety after the rape or sexual abuse. In those situations, short-term treatment with a benzodiazepine such as alprazolam (Xanax) 0.5 to 1 mg by mouth three times a day, lorazepam (Ativan) 1 to 2 mg by mouth three times a day, or oxazepam (Serax) 10 to 30 mg by mouth three times a day may be needed.

Insomnia can be treated with the medications listed above or with temazepam (Restoril) 15 to 30 mg by mouth at bedtime or flurazepam (Dalmane) 15 to 30 mg by mouth at bedtime.

For a more detailed discussion of this topic, see V A Sadock: Physical and Sexual Abuse of Adult, Sec 29.7, p 1729; B J Fauman: Other Psychiatric Emergencies, Sec 30.2, p 1752, in CTP/VI.

14.5. Incest

Incest is sexual activity (for example, fondling and coitus) with close blood relatives or family members (father-daughter, mother-son, siblings, stepparent-stepchild).

CLINICAL FEATURES AND DIAGNOSIS

Incest victims are usually female. The most commonly reported type of incest is father-daughter (75 percent of cases). Sibling incest is reported less often but may be just as common. Mother-son incest is the least common. The true prevalence of incest is unknown because of underreporting, but more than 10 percent of all women may have been victims of sexual abuse or incest. Families of low socioeconomic status may be less able to conceal incest than are families of higher status. Coitus occurs in about half of all incest cases. Homosexual incest (father-son and mother-daughter) is very rare; in those cases the father may not be otherwise homosexual and may be having sex with a daughter, as well as with a son.

In virtually all societies, parent-child incest is a taboo and indicates a breakdown of normal social and moral behavior. Socialized taboos against incest protect against the biological expression of recessive pathological genes. However, some societies sanction brother-sister marriages.

The clinical features associated with the initiators of incest include alcohol abuse, sociopathy, violence, overcrowding, increased physical proximity, rural isolation that prevents extrafamilial contacts, remarriage, intellectual deficiencies, and major mental disorders. Usually, the incestuous father is domineering, potentially violent, and feared, and the mother is passive or disabled and unable to interfere. Preexisting sexual discord often marks the parents' relationship.

In the typical father-daughter case of incest, the eldest daughter has been close to the father, who begins to approach her sexually at about age 10. Incest is usually identified when the child is 9 to 13 years old and after the sexual relationship has been going on for two to four years. The father becomes alternately and unpredictably parental and sexual with the daughter, leading to confusion about familial roles. The mother may at times be competitive and often refuses to believe the daughter's reports that her father has been approaching her sexually. The victim's mother may have abandoned the family in some way, often through illness. The siblings sense the special role that the victim has with the father, and they treat her as an outsider. The father, fearful that the incest will be revealed, interferes with his daughter's development of normal social relationships. Girls who have experienced incest have a higher than usual rate of adolescent pregnancy, suicide, and running away. If the victim runs away, the father may begin a sexual relationship with the next youngest daughter.

INTERVIEWING AND PSYCHOTHERAPEUTIC GUIDELINES

If incest is suspected, each family member should be interviewed alone, especially the abused child. Assure the child that he or she is safe and will be protected from possible retribution. The child should know that he or she can safely talk about the incest with professionals in a secure environment. Begin by approaching the topic indirectly. Ask about behaviors specifically, attempting to document precisely what happened. Usually, the parent denies the behavior. Relevant data should be elicited, including the level of privacy within the home, the nature of the parents' relationship, a parental childhood history of abuse, and embarrassment about the level of physical contact among family members.

Violence, depression, suicidality, somatic complaints, substance abuse, eating disorders, pregnancy, hypersexuality, personality disorders, and dissociative disorders may be related to incestuous experiences. Self-destructive behavior in a child may be a result of incest.

EVALUATION AND MANAGEMENT

1. The primary objective in incest cases is to reveal the fact that incest is occurring. Once the collusion, denial, and fear of other family members have been broken down, awareness and the fear of consequences usually prevent incest from recurring. Pay attention to suicide risk in all incest participants, particularly at the time of disclosure.
2. Examine the patient for bruising and trauma; check for venereal disease. Follow protocols similar to rape-evidence collection.
3. Involve legal child-protective agencies early to counteract the considerable pressure that will be exerted on the child to recant the story.
4. Evaluate the family members for primary psychiatric disorders that need to be treated. Evaluate siblings for possible victimization.
5. Individual psychotherapy is the preferred treatment for victims; it can be an avenue for the ventilation of anger.
6. Family therapy may help reconstruct a fractured family.
7. Group therapy is sometimes helpful for the survivors of incest who can discuss the topic openly in a group. Some groups specifically for female incest survivors help reduce the associated shame and stigma. Other groups are for the mothers of children who were incest victims. Often, the incest led to divorce, and the mothers have prominent feelings of rage and guilt.
8. Teach children clearly and simply that their genitals are their private parts and should not be touched by others, including family members.

DRUG TREATMENT

No specific drug treatment is indicated, although some underlying psychiatric disorders may require drug treatment later.

For a more detailed discussion of this topic, see J H Carter-Lourensz, G Johnson-Powell: Physical Abuse, Sexual Abuse, and Neglect of Child, Sec 47.3, p 2455, in CTP/VI.

14.6. Sexual Emergencies

Disorders of sexual function may bring patients to the office or to the emergency room. Impotence may occur for the first time in a previously well-functioning person and create overwhelming anxiety. Homosexual panic may happen unexpectedly with dire consequences (see Section 19.8). Other sexual disorders may so upset the patient's psychological equilibrium that the person involved feels compelled to seek immediate help.

Instead of the private office, some disorders present first to the medical emergency room, others to the psychiatric emergency room. In almost all cases, however, the physician finds signs and symptoms of mental illness of varying severity that need to be addressed. Some epileptic states, such as temporal lobe disorders, have been associated with sexual aberrations.

DIAGNOSIS AND CLINICAL FEATURES

Algolagnia

Algolagnia encompasses any form of sexual behavior associated with the giving or the receiving of pain.

In *sadism,* pain is inflicted on one person by another; in *masochism,* pain is received by the person or is self-inflicted. Unusual wounds—such as human bites, trunk lacerations (from whip lashings), bleeding of the nipples (in both sexes), and holes for metal rings in the labia of women or in the prepuce of men—are presumptive signs of sadomasochistic activities.

Anilingus

Anilingus involves the stimulation of the anus of one person by the mouth, the tongue, or the lips of another.

Foreign objects (for example, bottles and light bulbs) may be inserted into the anus. If they cannot be expelled, emergency evacuation is required.

Anal Intercourse

Anal intercourse occurs most often in homosexual men, but some heterosexual pairs also practice it. The woman may penetrate the man with a dildo that she either wears with a harness or inserts manually. Anal tears, fissures, and hemorrhoids may be sequelae of such activities. Chronic anal dilation is most often found in homosexual men who repeatedly experience anal penetration.

Aphrodisiacs

Aphrodisiacs are substances purported to excite sexual desire. Stimulants, sedatives, hallucinogens, and opioids may be used in an attempt to enhance sexual pleasure. Signs of intoxication or withdrawal from the substance may occur. Some substances (for example, capsaicin) may be rubbed on the genitalia and cause burns. Cantharides (Spanish fly) is toxic and causes hepatorenal damage.

Autoerotic Asphyxiation

Autoerotic asphyxiation involves masturbating while hanging oneself by the neck to heighten the erotic sensations and the intensity of the orgasm through mild hypoxia. Although those involved intend to release themselves from the noose after orgasm, an estimated 500 to 1,000 persons a year accidentally kill themselves by hanging. Most of those who indulge in the practice are male; transvestism is often associated with the habit, and the majority of deaths occur among adolescents. Autoerotic asphyxiation is usually associated with severe mental disorders such as schizophrenia and major mood disorders. The patient, if found alive, may be brought to the psychiatric emergency room and reported to be an attempted suicide.

Autoeroticism

Autoeroticism involves sexual arousal of oneself without the participation of another person (masturbation). At times, objects are used to enhance the experience. The objects include dildos inserted into the vagina, catheters or other objects inserted into the male or female urethra, and mechanical vibrators (with or without electrical sources), all of which can cause physical damage to the genitalia. Compulsive masturbation may produce penile or vaginal wounds and excoriations.

Bestiality

Bestiality is a sexual deviation in which a person engages in sexual relations with an animal. Both males and females may allow dogs or cats to lick their genitalia, which may cause urethritis, cystitis, or vaginitis. In rural areas, copulation with farm animals can produce vaginal infections and wounds in females and penile abrasions and infections in males.

Castration

Castration is mutilation of the penis or the testicles. Self-castration is carried out by severely ill psychotic persons and by transsexuals who have been denied male-to-female genital surgery and who hope to have a surgical procedure on an emergency basis.

Coprolalia

Coprolalia is the compulsive use of vulgar or obscene words. It is most often found in men who approach women in public places with lewd and graphic invitations to engage in sex acts of various kinds. Patients with Tourette's disorder may have coprolalia as an associated manifestation.

Coprophilia

In coprophilia, sexual pleasure is associated with feces. Men or women may eat feces (coprophagia) or play with feces (their own or their partners' feces). The practice may result in local infections of the mouth or the eyes and systemic infections (for example, hepatitis and parasitic infestation).

Diaphragm

A diaphragm is a dome-shaped contraceptive device, usually made of rubber, that obstructs the cervical os. On occasion, a woman is unable to remove her diaphragm, and she arrives at the medical emergency room or doctor's office with that complaint. Tampons may also unknowingly remain in the vagina for long periods, with resulting infections.

Dildo

A dildo is an artificial penis made of rubber, silicone, or latex used by both men and women. It may cause physical tears of the vaginal or anal areas or produce chronic anal dilation and encopresis.

Exhibitionism

Exhibitionism is a sexual disorder characterized by a compulsive need to expose one's body, particularly the genitals. It almost always occurs in men, who may be apprehended and brought to the emergency room for evaluation.

Frottage

Frottage is a sexual disorder in which men touch or rub their bodies against the breasts or buttocks of women in crowded places, such as subways. The perpetrator may be brought to the emergency room.

Koro

Koro is an acute anxiety reaction, most common in Asian men, characterized by the patient's fear that his penis is shrinking and may disappear into his abdomen, in which case he will die. It is a psychiatric emergency because it may result in suicide.

Priapism

Priapism is a persistent penile erection accompanied by severe pain. It may occur as a side effect of some psychotropic drugs, such as trazodone (Desyrel). It is a true medical emergency that requires the removal of blood from the engorged penile cavernosa by mechanical or surgical drainage. Without timely intervention, thrombosis and gangrene may develop.

Scopophilia

Also known as voyeurism, scopophilia is characterized by the compulsive desire to view sex organs or sex acts. Persons with the disorder are often apprehended as peeping Toms and brought for psychiatric evaluation.

Urolagnia

Urolagnia is a sexual disorder characterized by getting sexual pleasure from drinking urine or being urinated on. Skin, eye, or mouth infections may result.

INTERVIEWING AND PSYCHOTHERAPEUTIC GUIDELINES

If questions about sex are indicated, inquire in language that is familiar to the patient. Questions should be as specific as possible. A professional manner helps elicit truthful responses with a minimum of patient embarrassment and shame. Asking about sex practices is especially important to determine whether the patient is at risk for human immunodeficiency virus (HIV) infection and other sexually transmitted diseases.

EVALUATION AND MANAGEMENT

1. Treatment is geared first to the presenting complaint; physical injuries require immediate medical attention.
2. No specific therapy for the underlying sexual disorder is given on an emergency basis; however, diagnose the disorder, and recommend a treatment plan.
3. Most persons with sexually deviant behavior experience severe guilt and shame, and such patients can be motivated for psychiatric treatment. In addition, the primary care physician has the opportunity to provide reliable information to patients about sex, possibly for the first time.
4. Referral to a sex therapy clinic (one associated with a medical school is best) can be made for the definitive treatment of a wide range of sexual disorders.

DRUG TREATMENT

There is no effective drug treatment for these disorders. Anti-androgens have been used to diminish libido in men with various paraphilias with variable results. When anxiety is a major component, antianxiety agents may be of help. If there is an underlying psychosis, antipsychotic agents may be useful. Impulsive behavior may respond to serotonergic agents.

For a more detailed discussion of this topic, see J K Meyer: Paraphilias, Sec 21.2, p 1334; V A Sadock: Physical and Sexual Abuse of Adult, Sec 29.7, p 1729; B J Fauman: Other Psychiatric Emergencies, Sec 30.2, p 1752, in CTP/VI.

15
Eating Disorders

15.1. Anorexia Nervosa

Anorexia nervosa is an eating disorder characterized by a disturbed body image and severe self-imposed dietary limitations.

CLINICAL FEATURES AND DIAGNOSIS

Symptoms of anorexia nervosa include a body weight that is 15 percent below normal for the patient's age and height, an intense fear of being fat in spite of being underweight, a distorted body perception in which patients perceive themselves as fat although they are emaciated, and a loss of three or more consecutive menstrual periods because of starvation (Table 15.1-1).

The potentially fatal disorder usually begins between the ages of 13 and 20 and is 9 to 10 times more common in females than in males. The condition is thought to affect up to 1 percent of adolescent girls. Anorexia is more common in middle and upper socioeconomic groups than in low socioeconomic groups. Women who are pursuing careers that emphasize appearance are most vulnerable to the condition. Anorectic patients are often anxious, obsessive, and rigid. The disorder often begins in the context of a conflict about independence or sexuality. It may coexist with bulimia nervosa in cycles of rigid starvation followed by the loss of control, with eating binges causing guilt that leads to induced vomiting. Anorectic patients may also abuse diuretics or laxatives in an attempt to lose weight. Anorexia nervosa is

TABLE 15.1-1
DIAGNOSTIC CRITERIA FOR ANOREXIA NERVOSA

A. Refusal to maintain body weight at or above a minimally normal weight for age and height (e.g., weight loss leading to maintenance of body weight less than 85% of that expected; or failure to make expected weight gain during period of growth, leading to body weight less than 85% of that expected).
B. Intense fear of gaining weight or becoming fat, even though underweight.
C. Disturbance in the way in which one's body weight or shape is experienced, undue influence of body weight or shape on self-evaluation, or denial of the seriousness of the current low body weight.
D. In postmenarcheal females, amenorrhea, i.e., the absence of at least three consecutive menstrual cycles. (A woman is considered to have amenorrhea if her periods occur only following hormone, e.g., estrogen, administration.)

Specify type:
Restricting type: during the current episode of anorexia nervosa, the person has not regularly engaged in binge-eating or purging behavior (i.e., self-induced vomiting or the misuse of laxatives, diuretics, or enemas)
Binge-eating/purging type: during the current episode of anorexia nervosa, the person has regularly engaged in binge-eating or purging behavior (i.e., self-induced vomiting or the misuse of laxatives, diuretics, or enemas)

Table from DSM-IV, *Diagnostic and Statistical Manual of Mental Disorders*, ed 4. Copyright American Psychiatric Association, Washington, 1994. Used with permission.

thought to be related to depression, although antidepressant treatments are not always effective.

INTERVIEWING AND PSYCHOTHERAPEUTIC GUIDELINES

Anorectic patients may be uncooperative when brought in by their families for medical problems caused by starvation. Speak to the informants separately to get a history, since patients may deny or at least minimize the extent of their difficulties. Control is a major issue for anorectic patients, who are afraid that they will be forced to eat. Avoid any such power struggles, which are likely to be repetitions of family concerns. Concentrate on obtaining the patient's history while maintaining an empathic, supportive stance.

EVALUATION AND MANAGEMENT

1. Conduct a full medical evaluation. Some medical conditions (for example, cancer and gastrointestinal disorders) can present with severe weight loss, and those possibilities must be ruled out. Be particularly alert for nutritional deficiencies and metabolic diseases. Vomiting, diuretics, or laxatives can cause electrolyte imbalances.
2. Screen for substance abuse. Stimulant abuse can also produce weight loss, although the loss is typically not as much as that seen in anorexia nervosa. Check the patient's stool for phenolphthalein (for example, Ex-Lax) as evidence of laxative abuse.
3. Evaluate the patient for depression, as anorectic patients are often depressed.
4. Medical complications may necessitate forcible treatments such as intravenous fluids or nasogastric feedings. When there is a family crisis or a risk of suicide, hospitalization may be needed (Table 15.1-2).
5. Insight-oriented psychotherapy may not be useful. Cognitive approaches to change the patient's perceptions about body image and food are often helpful. Family therapy is strongly indicated.

TABLE 15.1-2
INDICATIONS FOR HOSPITALIZATION OF PATIENTS WITH EATING DISORDERS

Emergency
Weight loss >30% over 3 months
Severe metabolic disturbance (pulse <40 beats/minute, temperature <36°C, systolic blood pressure <70 mmHg, serum potassium <2.5 nmol/L despite oral potassium)
Severe depression or suicide risk
Psychosis
Diabetes mellitus in poor control
Failure of elective outpatient treatment
Elective
Family crisis
Complex differential diagnosis
Need to confront patient or family denial

Table from J R Hillard: Other emergencies. In *Manual of Clinical Emergency Psychiatry*, J R Hillard, editor, p 275. American Psychiatric Press, Washington, 1990. Adapted from D B Herzog: *Advances in Psychiatry: Focus on Eating Disorders.* Park Row, New York, 1987. Used with permission.

DRUG TREATMENT

Antidepressants are commonly used and may be of value. Cyproheptadine (Periactin) may be helpful because weight-gain is a side effect of the drug. Serotonergic antidepressants—such as fluoxetine (Prozac), sertraline (Zoloft), and paroxetine (Paxil)—may also be useful.

For a more detailed discussion of this topic, see P E Garfinkel: Eating Disorders, Chap 22, p 1361, in CTP/VI.

15.2 Bulimia Nervosa

Bulimia nervosa is an eating disorder characterized by episodic uncontrolled binge eating followed by self-induced vomiting or other purgative maneuvers designed to prevent weight gain.

CLINICAL FEATURES AND DIAGNOSIS

The diagnostic criteria for bulimia nervosa are listed in Table 15.2-1. The disorder is much more common in women than in men and usually begins in adolescence or early adulthood. The patient may engage in compulsive exercise and laxative abuse. Vomiting is a common feature and is usually induced by sticking a finger down the throat. Vomiting relieves postbinge bloating and allows the patient to binge without fear of gaining weight. The patient generally binges on sweet, soft, high-calorie foods, such as pastry and cakes. The patient may plan binging, although

TABLE 15.2-1
DIAGNOSTIC CRITERIA FOR BULIMIA NERVOSA

A. Recurrent episodes of binge eating. An episode of binge eating is characterized by both of the following:
 (1) eating, in a discrete period of time (e.g., within any 2-hour period), an amount of food that is definitely larger than most people would eat during a similar period of time and under similar circumstances
 (2) a sense of lack of control over eating during the episode (e.g., a feeling that one cannot stop eating or control what or how much one is eating)
B. Recurrent inappropriate compensatory behavior in order to prevent weight gain, such as self-induced vomiting; misuse of laxatives, diuretics, enemas, or other medications; fasting; or excessive exercise.
C. The binge eating and inappropriate compensatory behaviors both occur, on average, at least twice a week for 3 months.
D. Self-evaluation is unduly influenced by body shape and weight.
E. The disturbance does not occur exclusively during episodes of anorexia nervosa.

Specify type:
 Purging type: during the current episode of bulimia nervosa, the person has regularly engaged in self-induced vomiting or the misuse of laxatives, diuretics, or enemas
 Nonpurging type: during the current episode of bulimia nervosa, the person has used other inappropriate compensatory behaviors, such as fasting or excessive exercise, but has not regularly engaged in self-induced vomiting or the misuse of laxatives, diuretics, or enemas

Table from DSM-IV, *Diagnostic and Statistical Manual of Mental Disorders*, ed 4. Copyright American Psychiatric Association, Washington, 1994. Used with permission.

it may be done impulsively when the person is angry. Substance abuse, suicide attempts, shoplifting, depression, and emotional lability may be present.

Most bulimic patients are concerned about their sexual attractiveness, body image, and appearance to others. Unlike patients with anorexia nervosa, most bulimic patients are of normal weight. In contrast to patients with anorexia nervosa, most bulimic patients are sexually active and rarely amenorrheic or incapacitated. They are more disturbed by their eating disorder than are anorexics and are, therefore, more likely to seek help.

The prognosis for bulimia nervosa is better than for anorexia nervosa; however, bulimia can be chronic, with resulting medical complications, including dehydration, electrolyte imbalances leading to arrhythmias and sudden death, metabolic alkalosis, salivary gland enlargement, dental caries, esophagitis, esophageal tears, and gastric rupture.

The differential diagnosis includes seizure disorders, central nervous system (CNS) tumors, Kleine-Levin syndrome, and syndromes similar to Klüver-Bucy syndrome. Coexisting borderline personality disorder should be considered when assessing bulimic patients.

INTERVIEWING AND PSYCHOTHERAPEUTIC GUIDELINES

Assess the nature and the frequency of the binge-purge behavior without appearing judgmental or punitive. Patients may already feel guilty and ashamed. Encourage the patients to describe their behavior and associated feelings of anger, dysphoria, and loss of control. Try to interest them in ongoing treatment, so that an effective referral can be made. In addition, educate them about the medical consequences of binge-purge behavior while showing concern about their physical health.

EVALUATION AND MANAGEMENT

1. A complete medical evaluation is needed to detect possible electrolyte imbalances (particularly hypokalemia and hypochloremia), dehydration, and gastrointestinal damage. Screen for laxative abuse.
2. Order a complete psychiatric evaluation with attention to diagnosing comorbid depression, anorexia nervosa, substance abuse (for example, cocaine, alcohol, amphetamines, sedatives, and diet pills), and personality disorders.
3. Evaluate the patient for impulsivity and suicidality.
4. Consider hospitalizing patients with particularly poor impulse control, suicidality, or medical complications secondary to their eating disorders.
5. Refer the patient for cognitive-behavioral therapy, insight-oriented psychotherapy, or pharmacotherapy.
6. Consider admitting the patient to a specialized eating disorders unit if necessary.

DRUG TREATMENT

Antidepressants, including tetracyclics (imipramine [Tofranil]), serotonin-specific reuptake inhibitors (for example, fluoxetine [Prozac]), and monoamine oxidase inhibitors (MAOIs) are useful in treating bulimia. Those medications are used as part of a comprehensive treatment program. Particularly anxious or agitated patients can be given lorazepam (Ativan) 1 to 2 mg by mouth or intramuscularly.

For a more detailed discussion of this topic, see P E Garfinkel: Eating Disorders, Chap 22, p 1361, in CTP/VI.

16

Sleep Disorders

16.1. Insomnia

Insomnia is difficulty in falling asleep, difficulty in maintaining sleep, or insufficient sleep.

CLINICAL FEATURES AND DIAGNOSIS

Insomnia is a nonspecific symptom, rather than a specific disorder. Although it is the most common complaint presented to primary care physicians, insomnia usually does not receive an adequate workup. Typically, the complaint is rapidly treated with a hypnotic before sufficient medical and psychiatric evaluations have been made. Insomnia can be a symptom of many different psychiatric disorders, including depression, mania, anxiety disorders, psychotic disorders, substance abuse, and primary sleep disorders (Table 16.1-1). In the elderly, complaints of insomnia may be due to normal age-related changes in sleep architecture. The initial approach should be to describe the course and the severity of the insomnia and its relation to associated factors.

A complaint of insomnia is not clinically important unless there is associated impaired functioning (usually daytime sleepiness). People have individual differences in the amount of sleep they need, and some people are natural short sleepers, so a complaint of too few hours of sleep needs to be related to impaired daytime functioning to be significant. Furthermore, many patients who complain of insomnia, when monitored in a sleep laboratory, actually fall asleep rapidly.

INTERVIEWING AND PSYCHOTHERAPEUTIC GUIDELINES

Take the patient's history of substances taken, including alcohol, caffeine and other stimulants, sedative-hypnotics, and drugs of abuse, virtually all of which can cause insomnia. Prescribed medications, such as bronchodilators, can cause insomnia.

How long has the symptom been present, and what impairment has resulted? Is it related to some change in the environment? Does it occur only at home or only during the week?

Interview the bed partner about when the patient actually falls asleep. Ask the partner or the patient about related symptoms, such as snoring, gastroesophageal reflux, restless legs, and myoclonic jerks. Does the patient have nocturia due to excessive evening fluid intake or urinary tract disease?

Sleep hygiene is important. Is the room comfortable and quiet? Is the bed clean? Does the patient do distracting things in bed, such as watching television, eating, and reading? Do psychologically stimulating situations occur just before bedtime? Large meals, strenuous exercise, and more than one or two alcoholic beverages

TABLE 16.1-1
INSOMNIAS

Diagnosis	Signs and Symptoms	Comments	Treatment
Primary insomnia	Persistent insomnia without drug use or gross psychopathology. Repeated awakenings, anxious dreams, increased muscle activity, rapid pulse rates. Patient may sleep well when away from work, on vacation, or in a new sleep environment.	May be the result of any combination of chronic tension, anxiety, or negative conditioning to sleep environment. Usually diagnosed after eliminating all other possibilities.	Relaxation training, behavior modification, and inculcation of good sleep hygiene (regular bedtime, no stimulants before sleep, good sleep environment).
Insomnia related to anxiety or personality disorder	Persistent insomnia with a diagnosis of neurosis or personality disorder. EEG likely to reveal sleep fragmentation, with decreased slow-wave sleep (SWS) and, to a smaller extent, REM sleep.	Similar to the above, except that the psychiatric symptoms are more prominent. Often the insomnia parallels the severity of the psychiatric symptoms.	Sleep architecture improves with therapy of the underlying psychiatric symptoms. The treatments for primary insomnia may be helpful.
Insomnia related to depressive episode	With diagnosis of depression. Restless, unsatisfying sleep, multiple awakenings, sometimes shortened REM latency. Frequent insomnia in the early morning hours (terminal insomnia). Some depressed patients, particularly those with bipolar disorder or atypical depression, have hypersomnia. Reactive depressives usually have insomnia without shortened REM latency.	Insomnia is common among depressives, especially elderly depressives, who have little or no SWS.	Treatments for depression tend to correct sleep architecture.
Insomnia related to manic episode	Very little sleep (2 to 4 hours), with or without refreshing daytime naps. May not sleep until physically exhausted.	Frequently, the worried family complain of the patient's reduced sleep time.	Treatment for mania tends to correct sleep architecture.
Insomnia related to schizophrenia or other psychotic disorder	Severe increased sleep-onset latency (SOL) with poor sleep continuity. Patient may not sleep until exhausted.	Sleep may be out of phase with the usual circadian rhythms (inversion of the sleep-wake cycle).	Treatment of the psychosis with antipsychotics tends to correct sleep architecture.
Sedative hypnotic-, or anxiolytic-induced sleep disorder	On drug—decreased $3/_4$ REM, increased $1/_2$. Stage demarcations frequently blurred. After a few weeks of use, increased SOL, increased awakenings.	Results from tolerance to or withdrawal from drug. More common in elderly or very young. Withdrawal accompanied by restlessness, increased muscle tension, nausea.	Physician-supervised drug withdrawal. In abrupt withdrawal, complete sleep disruption is likely. Disturbed sleep may continue long after drug withdrawal. REM rebound is common in the withdrawal period.

Disorder	Description	Treatment
Amphetamine-induced, caffeine-induced, or cocaine-induced sleep disorder	On abrupt withdrawal—almost complete disruption of sleep. REM rebound (often nightmares). Increased SOL, decreased $3/4$ decreased REM. Disorders of hypersomnia may develop. The occasional crash is a classic symptom.	Physician-supervised drug withdrawal. In abrupt withdrawal, crashing (hypersomnia) is likely.
Breathing-related sleep disorder	Cessations of breathing lasting 10 seconds or more. Subsequent awakenings produce sleeplessness. Caffeine ingestion late in the day is a common cause. Patient should be checked after complete withdrawal for other sleep pathologies. More commonly associated with insomnia. Three types: Central sleep apnea syndrome—cessation of breathing effort. Obstructive sleep apnea syndrome—upper blockage of airflow in upper air passages; severe snoring; patients often obese. Central alveolar hypoventilation syndrome—hypoventilation without apneas or hypopneas; patients often obese.	Obstructive sleep apnea syndrome and central alveolar hypoventilation syndrome can be treated with weight loss or tracheostomy. A variety of drugs have been tried for central syndrome sleep apnea with little success. Hypnotic drugs can be detrimental to sleep apnea patients because of respiratory suppression.
Nocturnal myoclonus	Sleep-initiated periodic contractions in hip, leg, ankle, and foot, followed by partial or complete arousal. Episodes last 10 seconds or more. The EEG does not show seizure activity. Must be differentiated from seizures and from hypnic jerks—gross-motor jerks when falling asleep that are not pathological. Restless legs syndrome may accompany and is characterized by a deep creeping feeling in the legs and the feet.	No wholly satisfactory treatment. Benzodiazepines may relieve symptoms when taken at bedtime. Carbamazepine (Tegretol) for restless legs syndrome, but can depress bone marrow function. Opioids (e.g., oxycodone (Percodan)) at bedtime, but is addictive.
Alcohol-induced sleep disorder with onset during intoxication	Unsatisfying, unrefreshing sleep. Stages 3 and 4 completely absent in chronic alcoholism. REM disrupted and short. Strong REM suppression is the most common characteristic. There may be hypersomnia or terminal insomnia, with increased awakenings in the latter part of the night. Alcohol is frequently taken to hasten sleep onset, but it seriously disrupts REM, SWS, and sleep architecture.	Supervised withdrawal from alcohol.

Continued

TABLE 16.1-1—*continued*

Diagnosis	Signs and Symptoms	Comments	Treatment
Alcohol-induced sleep disorder with onset during withdrawal	Dramatically increased SOL, decreased $3/4$, REM rebound, frequent awakenings, restlessness.	Delirium and hallucinations characteristic of alcohol withdrawal may be present.	Sleep pattern normalizes somewhat in 10 to 14 days. However, sleep may be disturbed (increased awakenings, decreased $3/4$) for months to years in sober alcoholics.
Sleep disorder due to a general medical condition	Vary in type and severity. In general, increased SOL, increased awakenings, increased restlessness, and decreased $3/4$.	Particularly associated with insomnia are conditions with pain, pruritis, fever, dyspnea, and those requiring enforced sleep position (e.g., orthopedic problems).	Treat the underlying disorder if possible. Hypnotics can be helpful for acute illnesses when respiratory suppression is not contraindicated. Long-term use of hypnotics leads to habituation and tolerance and eventually may exacerbate insomnia.

Table adapted from I Karacan, R L Williams, C A Moore: Sleep disorders. In *Comprehensive Textbook of Psychiatry*, ed 5, H I Kaplan, B J Sadock, editors, p 1105. Williams & Wilkins, Baltimore, 1989. Used with permission.

should be avoided shortly before bedtime. Does the patient sleep late on weekends, only to be unable to fall asleep Sunday night? If so, that suggests a delayed sleep-wake cycle.

EVALUATION AND MANAGEMENT

1. Obtain a good medical history. Almost any medical condition associated with pain and discomfort (for example, arthritis) can produce insomnia. Some conditions (including neoplasms, vascular lesions, infections, and degenerative and traumatic conditions) are associated with insomnia even when pain and discomfort are not present. Endocrine and metabolic diseases frequently involve some sleep disturbance. The treatment for insomnia, whenever possible, is treatment of the underlying medical condition.
2. Instruct patients to wake up at the same time every day, no matter what time they went to sleep the night before. Although the patients will be sleepy the next day, they will fall asleep easily the next night. That is the best way to prevent delayed sleep-wake schedule disorder (characterized by sleeping late on the weekends).
3. A complete psychiatric evaluation may be necessary to diagnose depression, mania, anxiety disorders, and psychotic disorders if any are present. A definitive psychiatric diagnosis suggests a specific treatment.
4. If a definitive diagnosis is not obvious, ask the patient to complete a sleep diary over several weeks; this should include the time to bed, the time asleep, the time awake, naps, activity, and important events. This diary should then accompany the patient on a referral to a sleep disorders clinic.

DRUG TREATMENT

In general, if the insomnia is brief (less than three weeks), a trial of hypnotics may be appropriate. If the insomnia is chronic, avoid hypnotics and make a definitive diagnosis. Other contraindications for hypnotics include heavy snoring, other signs of sleep apnea, and possible dependence, tolerance, or abuse of sedative-hypnotics. If psychosis is present, consider prescribing an antipsychotic. Otherwise, benzodiazepines are usually the hypnotics of choice, because they have a wider therapeutic index, less enzyme induction, and lower dependence potential than do barbiturates. Zolpidem (Ambien) 5 to 10 mg has the advantage of being short-acting.

The choice of benzodiazepine depends on the route of metabolism and the elimination half-life. Treat initial insomnia without daytime anxiety with short-acting benzodiazepines—for example, triazolam (Halcion) 0.125 mg, temazepam (Restoril) 15 mg, and estazolam (ProSom) 1 mg. Middle insomnia or early-morning awakening may require a long-acting benzodiazepine, such as those used to treat insomnia with prominent daytime anxiety—for example, diazepam (Valium) 5 mg, flurazepam (Dalmane) 15 mg, and quazepam (Doral) 7.5 mg.

Start with the lowest dose and increase the dosage until it produces an effect. Most patients respond to any benzodiazepine if the dosage is increased sufficiently. When an effective dosage is reached, do not increase it further. Loss of efficacy at that dosage indicates tolerance and requires a drug washout. Inform patients that, after stopping the drug, they will have one to two weeks of rebound insomnia, which is not an indication for continued drug treatment.

The frequency of hypnotic use should be not more than three out of four nights, and the duration of use should not exceed several months.

For a more detailed discussion of this topic, see J Yager, M J Gitlin: Clinical Manifestations of Psychiatric Disorders, Chap 10, p 637; R L Williams, I Karacan, C A Moore, M Hirshkowitz: Sleep Disorders, Chap 23, p 1373, in CTP/VI.

16.2 Narcolepsy

Narcolepsy is characterized by the symptom tetrad of (1) excessive daytime somnolence, (2) cataplexy, (3) sleep paralysis, and (4) hypnagogic hallucinations.

CLINICAL FEATURES AND DIAGNOSIS

Excessive daytime somnolence is considered the primary symptom of narcolepsy. Many people are chronically sleepy because they do not get enough nocturnal sleep, but this symptom alone is not diagnostically significant for narcolepsy. Narcoleptic daytime somnolence is distinguished from fatigue by irresistible sleep attacks of short duration—that is, less than 15 minutes.

Other symptoms are also prominent in narcolepsy. *Cataplexy* is brief (seconds to minutes) episodes of muscle weakness or paralysis with no loss of consciousness. Laughter or anger often triggers it. Sleep paralysis is a temporary partial or complete paralysis that most commonly occurs on awakening. The patient is conscious but unable to move. Sleep paralysis generally lasts less than one minute. *Hypnagogic hallucinations* are dreamlike experiences during the transition from wakefulness to sleep.

Narcolepsy must be differentiated from (1) sleep apnea, (2) nocturnal movement disorders (myoclonus and restless legs syndrome), (3) the effects of drugs and alcohol, and (4) atypical depressive disorders.

INTERVIEWING AND PSYCHOTHERAPEUTIC GUIDELINES

The primary care physician should explain the disorder to the patient, especially the relation between sleep attacks and strong emotion. Memory problems may occur, and the patient needs reassurance that the disorder is treatable.

EVALUATION AND MANAGEMENT

1. A multiple sleep latency test, which is usually given at a sleep disorders clinic, is used as a diagnostic tool.
2. Advise the patient to have a regular bedtime and to take daytime naps.

3. Safety considerations, such as driving cautiously and avoiding sharp edges on furniture, are also advised.

DRUG TREATMENT

Tricyclics and monoamine oxidase inhibitors are used for rapid eye movement (REM)-related symptoms, mainly cataplexy.

Stimulants, such as 10 to 40 mg of dextroamphetamine (Dexedrine) and methylphenidate (Ritalin) 10 to 40 mg a day by mouth for daytime sleepiness are also used.

For a more detailed discussion of this topic, see R L Williams, I Karacan, C A Moore, M Hirshkowitz: Sleep Disorders, Chap 23, p 1373, in CTP/VI.

17

Impulse-Control Disorders

17.1 Intermittent Explosive Disorder

Intermittent explosive disorder is found in persons who have discrete episodes of loss of control of aggressive impulses, resulting in serious assaultive acts or the destruction of property.

CLINICAL FEATURES AND DIAGNOSIS

Sometimes the term "epileptoid personality" is used for the seizurelike quality of the aggressive episodes, which are not characteristic of the patient's usual behavior. Related symptoms and signs may include an aura, changes in the sensorium, increasing tension before the violent act, hypersensitivity to sound or light, amnesia, and nonspecific electroencephalographic (EEG) abnormalities.

Intermittent explosive disorder is more common in men than in women, and it usually begins before age 30. The men are often described as physically large but psychologically dependent, with threatened masculinity. The patient often witnessed parental violence in childhood. Usually, a history of family instability includes such problems as alcohol abuse, promiscuity, a poor work history, child abuse, and spouse abuse. The patient may have a history of pathological alcohol intoxication or disinhibition after taking other central nervous system (CNS) depressants.

The diagnostic criteria for intermittent explosive disorder are given in Table 17.1-1.

INTERVIEWING AND PSYCHOTHERAPEUTIC GUIDELINES

The patient is usually remorseful about the episode and should be approached with support and understanding. Focus on the explosive episodes as specific targets of treatment.

Psychotherapy with these patients is difficult, dangerous, and often unrewarding, as the therapist may have difficulties with countertransference and limit setting.

TABLE 17.1–1
DIAGNOSTIC CRITERIA FOR INTERMITTENT EXPLOSIVE DISORDER

A. Several discrete episodes of failure to resist aggressive impulses that result in serious assaultive acts or destruction of property.
B. The degree of aggressiveness expressed during the episodes is grossly out of proportion to any precipitating psychosocial stressors.
C. The aggressive episodes are not better accounted for by another mental disorder (e.g., antisocial personality disorder, borderline personality disorder, a psychotic disorder, a manic episode, conduct disorder, or attention-deficit/hyperactivity disorder) and are not due to the direct physiological effects of a substance (e.g., a drug of abuse, a medication) or a general medical condition (e.g., head trauma, Alzheimer's disease).

Table from DSM-IV, *Diagnostic and Statistical Manual of Mental Disorders*, ed 4. Copyright American Psychiatric Association, Washington, 1994. Used with permission.

Group psychotherapy may be of some help, as may family therapy, particularly when the explosive patient is an adolescent or a young adult.

EVALUATION AND MANAGEMENT

Rule out antisocial and borderline personality disorders, personality change due to a general medical condition, delirium, dementia, psychotic disorders, conduct disorder, mental retardation, and substance intoxication or withdrawal. In personality disorders, maladaptive behaviors are present between episodes. Psychotic symptoms and other mental status abnormalities usually easily differentiate psychotic disorders from intermittent explosive disorder. Conduct disorder shows a repeated pattern, rather than distinct episodes. Medical disorders that may resemble intermittent explosive disorder include brain tumor, epilepsy, and metabolic disorders. Intoxication with alcohol or sedative-hypnotics can lead to disinhibition and episodic violence. Intoxication with hallucinogens, cocaine, and other psychostimulants must also be considered.

DRUG TREATMENT

In the midst of an aggressive episode, the patient must be physically restrained. Administer an antipsychotic medication—for example, fluphenazine (Prolixin), trifluoperazine (Stelazine), thiothixene (Navane), or haloperidol (Haldol), all given at 5 mg by mouth or intramuscularly, repeated in 30 minutes if necessary.

There is no consensus about drug treatment. Anticonvulsants, antipsychotics, antidepressants, and lithium (Eskalith) have all been reported to be helpful. Benzodiazepines have also been used but may cause disinhibition through a paradoxical reaction. Propranolol (Inderal) has also been used.

For a more detailed discussion of this topic, see V K Burt: Impulse-Control Disorders Not Elsewhere Classified, Sec 24.1, p 1409, in CTP/VI.

17.2 Child, Elder, and Spouse Abuse

Child Abuse

Child abuse is defined as physical or psychological damage to a child under the age of 18 sustained because of neglect or maltreatment, usually by a parent, a parent surrogate, or a relative. The typical child abuser is a single, unemployed mother under age 30, although the abuser may also be another caretaker, such as the father, a babysitter, or a friend. Many victims of physical abuse are also abused sexually. About 500,000 new cases of physical and sexual abuse are reported each year, and 2,000 to 4,000 abused children die. An estimated 2 to 4 million children (out of 30 million children in the United States) have been abused. The most serious injuries have been reported in children under the age of 3 years.

Victims, family, and health care professionals tend to deny, underreport, and misdiagnose cases of abuse, especially in patients from upper socioeconomic groups. Physical and sexual abuse often occurs when the abuser is using drugs or alcohol. The perpetrators of abuse are likely to have personal histories of having witnessed abuse or have been abused themselves.

Abuse occurs most often in the context of volatile and dysfunctional interpersonal relationships, violent marital relationships, and heightened stress in the environment. The abused child is viewed in some way as different or special. The difference may involve such issues as mental retardation, high intelligence, hyperactivity, prematurity, serious illness, or physical or neurological abnormalities.

CLINICAL FEATURES AND DIAGNOSIS

Physical Abuse

Obvious cases of abuse may present with bruises, fractures, dislocations, burns, lacerations, focal neurological deficits, signs of intracranial bleeding, or abdominal injury. Malnutrition or dehydration may indicate food or water deprivation. Physical abuse is also called *battered child syndrome.*

Munchausen syndrome by proxy is a form of child abuse in which a caretaker (usually the child's mother) brings a child with a fabricated illness to medical attention. The caretaker may report nonexistent symptoms in the child (for example, reporting apneic episodes), alter laboratory tests (for example, putting blood in the child's urine sample), or induce illness by various methods (for example, administering a symptom-inducing medication). Children are then subjected to multiple unnecessary medical workups and treatments. The diagnosis should be suspected in cases involving children whose symptoms disappear when separated from their caretakers, who are often medically knowledgeable and overinvolved. The child usually presents as treatment-refractory or a diagnostic dilemma with ailments that include apnea, vomiting, failure to thrive, sepsis, and bleeding.

Sexual Abuse

Sexual abuse is difficult to diagnose reliably, since false allegations by parents occur, especially in child-custody cases. The physician should suspect sexual abuse of a child with evidence of genital injury or irritation, foreign bodies in the vagina or the rectum, excessive masturbation, venereal disease, or pregnancy.

Acute conditions may also present with a variety of symptoms and syndromes, from evidence of posttraumatic stress disorder to sleep disorders and somatic complaints. Regressive behaviors (thumb sucking, enuresis) often occur. Depression with suicidal ideation may be present.

Chronic conditions may involve a picture of hypersexuality on the child's part (preoccupation with sexual words and ideas, compulsive masturbation, seductive behavior), generalized low self-esteem, and a sense of isolation from peers and parents. Child victims are usually unable to give a reliable history.

The sexual abuser is usually male. The physician should consider whether an older sibling, cousin, uncle, or friend with whom the child has contact is a possible perpetrator. Sexual abuse can also occur in child-care centers.

Child victims can be of any age; even infants are abused. The use of children in (or the exposure of children to) pornography, talking about sex with young children, and allowing children to witness sex between adults are other forms of sexual abuse. Girls are sexually abused approximately twice as often as boys. Additional information about sexual abuse is found in Section 14.4.

Emotional Abuse

Grossly abnormal care can be the result of conscious cruelty, lack of parenting skills, or unwanted parenthood. There is an increased incidence of emotional abuse when the parent is mentally retarded. The most typical picture is a failure to thrive in a young child. The physician should look for hypokinesis, apathy, an unhappy facial expression, delayed responsiveness, malnutrition, and fearfulness.

See Table 17.2-1 for indicators of child abuse and neglect.

INTERVIEWING AND PSYCHOTHERAPEUTIC GUIDELINES

Interviews should be conducted in a manner that conveys respect and allows for the utmost privacy. When interviewing a child, do not suggest answers or press for accusatory responses. Several interviews may be necessary before a child feels safe enough to reveal specific information. Do not display strong emotions to the child, even if the abuse is personally abhorrent. Gently ask the child to describe what happened. Drawings and dolls can be helpful. Tell the parents that physicians are required by law to make a report to a child protective service when abuse is confirmed or even suspected. When the parents suspect that another adult has abused their child, reassure the parents that an honest, supportive, and direct approach with the child will lessen any further emotional trauma. Use open-ended questions with caretakers, such as, "How do you deal with the stress of being a parent?" and "How is Johnny punished when he is bad?" Interview the child and each parent alone and together. Note any change in behavior in each setting. Does the child become fearful in the presence of a parent? Does a parent appear threatening to the child? If any history of violence is presented, other questions can be gently directed toward other potential problem areas, such as drug and alcohol involvement, wife battering, and financial or legal problems.

EVALUATION AND MANAGEMENT

1. The physician who suspects child abuse is legally required to refer all such cases to the local child protection agency.
2. Always consider abuse in a child with any signs or symptoms listed in Table 17.2-1.
3. Almost a third of all abused children are under the age of 5 years and are unable to give a history. Children older than 5 years may feel too frightened,

TABLE 17.2–1
PHYSICAL AND BEHAVIORAL INDICATORS OF CHILD ABUSE AND NEGLECT

Type of Abuse	Physical Indicators	Behavioral Indicators

Physical abuse	Unexplained bruises and welts
	  on face, lips, mouth
	  on torso, back, buttocks, thighs
	  in various stages of healing
	  clustered, forming regular patterns like
	    articles used to inflict (e.g., electric
	    cord, belt buckle)
	  on several surface areas
	  regularly appear after absence,
	    weekend, or vacation
	Unexplained burns
	  cigar or cigarette burns, especially on
	    soles, palms, back, or buttocks
	  immersion burns (socklike, glovelike,
	    doughnut-shaped on buttocks or
	    genitalia)
	  patterned like electric burner, iron,
	    etc.
	  rope burns on arms, legs, neck, or torso
	  infected burns, indicating delay in
	    seeking treatment
	Unexplained fractures or dislocations
	  to skull, nose, or facial structure
	  in various stages of healing; multiple or
	    spinal fractures
	Unexplained lacerations
	  to mouth, lips, gums, eyes
	  to external genitalia in various stages
	    of healing
	Bald patches on scalp
		Feels deserving of punishment
		Wary of adult contacts
		Apprehensive when other children cry
		Behavioral extremes: aggressiveness or
		  withdrawal
		Frightened of parents
		Afraid to go home
		Reports injury by parents
		Vacant or frozen stare
		Lies very still while surveying surroundings
		Does not cry when approached by
		  examiner
		Responds to questions in monosyllables
		Inappropriate or precocious maturity
		Manipulative behavior to get attention
		Capable of only superficial relationships
		Indiscriminately seeks affection
		Poor self-concept

Physical
  neglect
	Underweight, poor growth pattern,
	  failure to thrive
	Consistent hunger, poor hygiene,
	  inappropriate dress
	Consistent lack of supervision, especially
	  in dangerous activities or long
	  periods
	Wasting of subcutaneous tissue
	Unattended physical problems or
	  medical needs
	Abandonment
	Abdominal distention
	Bald patches on the scalp
		Begging, stealing food
		Extended stays at school (early arrival
		  and late departure)
		Rare attendance at school
		Constant fatigue, listlessness, or falling
		  asleep in class
		Inappropriate seeking of affection
		Assuming adult responsibilities and
		  concerns
		Alcohol or drug abuse
		Delinquency (e.g., thefts)
		States there is no caretaker

Sexual abuse	Difficulty in walking or sitting
	Torn, stained, or bloody underclothing
	Pain, swelling, or itching in genital area
	Pain on urination
	Bruisers, bleeding, or lacerations in
	  external genitalia, vaginal or anal
	  areas
	Vaginal or penile discharge
	Venereal disease, especially in preteens
	Poor sphincter tone
	Pregnancy
		Unwilling to change for gym or
		  participate in physical education
		  class
		Withdrawal, fantasy, or infantile
		  behavior or knowledge
		Poor peer relationships
		Delinquent or runaway
		Reports sexual assault by
		  caretaker
		Change in performance in school

Emotional
  maltreatment
	Speech disorders
	Lag in physical development
	Failure to thrive
	Hyperactive or disruptive behavior
		Habit disorders (sucking, biting, rocking,
		  etc.)
		Conduct or learning disorders
		  (antisocial, destructive, etc.)
		Neurotic traits (sleep disorders, inhibition
		  of play, unusual fearfulness)
		Psychoneurotic reactions (hysteria,
		  obsession, compulsion, phobias,
		  hypochondria)
		Behavior extremes (compliant, passive;
		  aggressive, demanding)
		Overly adaptive behavior
		  (inappropriately adult, inappropriately
		  infantile)
		Developmental lags (mental,
		  emotional)
		Attempted suicide

Table from J W Lauer, I S Laurie, M K Salus, et al: *The Role of the Mental Health Professional in the Prevention and Treatment of Child Abuse and Neglect.* US Department of Health, Education and Welfare, National Center on Child Abuse and Neglect, Washington, 1979.

guilty, loyal, or anxious to give a reliable history. Take the history from the person bringing the child for medical attention. Obtain old records, if they are available, to identify a pattern of abuse.

4. Use the physical examination to obtain evidence of abuse or sexual trauma. Look for genital irritations, trauma, and discharges; also look for minor bruises, welts, fractures, lacerations, abrasions, abdominal injuries, and central nervous system injuries. Have a nurse present during the examination. Do not force the child to submit to an examination. In sex-abuse cases, check for sexually transmitted diseases. Hospitalize the victim if necessary.

5. Carefully document any evidence of abuse. Making a definitive diagnosis of abuse on one visit is sometimes impossible, so any documentation may be used in the future to identify a pattern. Complete a detailed physical examination, and obtain X-rays and a medical or surgical consultation, even if the patient is hesitant. Look for burns, head-injury fractures, and bruises. Photograph visible injuries.

6. Many centers have specific rape protocols that require the collection of specimens and physical evidence. Those protocols should be carefully followed.

7. In cases of suspected sexual abuse, obtain oral, anal, and vaginal cultures to rule out the presence of gonorrhea.

8. Identify and treat other psychiatric disorders, such as depression, anxiety, insomnia, and substance abuse.

9. Evaluate the dangerousness of returning the child to the home. Although separating a child from a parent is usually undesirable, the child must be removed and protected if the situation presents a persistent danger. That is a physician's legal responsibility. Children can be placed in foster homes or with relatives or friends. The possible abuser should not be confronted until the safety of the child has been assured by removing the child or the suspected abuser from the home. The arrival of the child victim in the emergency room may be a rare opportunity for intervention.

10. Report the case to an appropriate protective service agency (for example, Child Protective Services), which will initiate the legal process.

11. Intervention includes an evaluation of the abuser, the victim, and the family. Try to determine the duration and the pattern of abuse. Organize follow-up and monitoring plans that include the possibility of legal action to protect the victim.

12. Support groups may be helpful, especially for adolescent victims. Local and national programs can aid parents and children, such as the National Committee for the Prevention of Child Abuse.

13. Victims of child abuse often grow up to be child abusers themselves. Ask the parents about their personal histories of child abuse, and check for the presence of a mental disorder, especially substance abuse and alcohol dependence.

DRUG TREATMENT

Psychotropic medication is not used in the treatment of abused children. The psychiatric sequelae of abuse, such as depression or anxiety, may require appropriate medication; however, psychosocial approaches are preferred.

Elder Abuse

Elder abuse is the physical, sexual, or psychological mistreatment of elderly persons. Abuse is most likely to occur to men over age 75 who are bedridden or who have a chronic illness that requires constant nursing attention.

An estimated 1 million elders (out of 32 million elderly people in the United States) have been mistreated. The highest risk of abuse is by a family member (for example, a grown child who has no relief from caretaking activities). The typical abuser is a white, middle-class man between 40 and 60 years old who is under financial or mental stress.

CLINICAL FEATURES AND DIAGNOSIS

Physical Manifestations

The patient may show evidence of dehydration, malnutrition, bedsores, fecal impaction, dermatitides, lice infestation, bruises, welts, burns, punctures, hair pulling, or ammoniacal odor from urinary incontinence. Look for anogenital injuries as manifestations of sexual abuse.

Psychosocial Manifestations

On the mental status examination, look for confusion, psychomotor retardation or agitation, depression, suicidal ideas or attempts, anger or generalized apathy, and sleep disturbances (excessive sleep or insomnia).

Look for overt anger by a family member or a caretaker that is directed toward the patient and for inconsistencies between the histories given by a family member and the patient. Insistence by a family member that the patient be hospitalized or placed in a nursing home immediately or a refusal to have the physician see the patient alone should arouse suspicion of abuse.

INTERVIEWING AND PSYCHOTHERAPEUTIC GUIDELINES

Always interview the patient and the family members alone and together. Note any changes in behavior in each setting. Ask the patient: "Have you ever been hurt by a family member?" "Do they feed you?" "Do you get out of the house?" "Do you get a bath?" "Are you given any medicine?" Inquire about any observed physical signs: "How did you get that black-and-blue mark?"

EVALUATION AND MANAGEMENT

1. Report elder abuse to an appropriate health agency. Reporting is mandatory in most states (for example, California and New Jersey); it is voluntary in other states (for example, New York and Pennsylvania).
2. During the physical examination, look for fractured bones, contusions, and abrasions. Evidence of venereal disease and unusual genital infection suggest

sexual abuse. Attend to the patient's immediate medical needs. Hospitalize the patient if necessary. Photograph visible injuries.

3. Try to create a good working relationship with the elderly patient. If the patient is cognitively alert, the primary care physician should explain that the patient's claim of abuse is believed. Reassure the patient that help is available.

4. Develop a comprehensive, interdisciplinary plan—medical, psychological, and legal. If the patient is returned to the home, give the patient an emergency phone number and make a follow-up appointment.

5. Tell the family members that support services will be made available to help them provide care. Elder neglect (a form of abuse) may be unintentional. Family members may be overwhelmed by their responsibilities.

6. Plans depend on circumstances. The patient may be kept at home with a home worker and visiting nurse services or may be placed in a nursing home. Remember that most elderly abuse victims fear institutionalization more than the possibility of continued abuse.

7. Provide programs for abusers who may require psychiatric treatment. Support services are available locally and nationally (for example, National Coalition Against Domestic Violence).

DRUG TREATMENT

Medication in the elderly abused population should be used with extreme caution because confusion is often present and medication may mask physical or psychiatric signs and symptoms.

Patients with a clear sensorium who are extremely agitated may be sedated with a single small dose of diazepam (Valium) 2.5 mg by mouth.

Spouse Abuse

Spouse abuse is physical assault within the home (domestic violence) in which one spouse is repeatedly assaulted by the other. The victim is the wife in almost every case (battered wives) and is most commonly a woman under 35 years of age. Husband abuse occurs rarely and almost always in response to the wife's having been beaten or when a frail elderly man is married to a very young woman. Spouse abuse is reported in about 1.8 million households, but it is thought to be an underreported phenomenon. Between 2,000 and 5,000 deaths each year are attributed to spouse abuse.

The typical abuser is a man between 18 and 24 years who is unemployed and suffering from alcoholism, substance abuse, or some other mental disorder. He is often extremely possessive and jealous. The typical wife beater came from a violent home where he witnessed his mother's being beaten. His own father or mother may also have abused him as a child, and he may frequently abuse his own children. Most spouse abuse occurs repeatedly in a consistent pattern established early in a relationship. The abuse may increase in violence around the holidays. Violence often occurs when the husband sees his wife as less available than in the past because of her pregnancy, relationships with friends, going to school, or taking a job.

CLINICAL FEATURES AND DIAGNOSIS

Look for multiple injuries at various sites—contusions, lacerations, and abrasions, particularly around the face. Look for ecchymoses in the neck area, indicating a stranglehold.

Look for bruises over the chest, the breasts, the abdomen, and the pelvis that are not readily visible to observers, sometimes called bathing-suit-pattern injuries.

Pregnant women are often victims; look for injuries on the abdominal wall over the uterus.

A medical workup is essential, especially X-rays for fractures. Always consider head injuries, especially if the patient is confused or lethargic. Somatic symptoms—such as headaches, chronic pain, and gastrointestinal distress—are common. Depression, anxiety, insomnia, and suicidal gestures and attempts are also common.

INTERVIEWING AND PSYCHOTHERAPEUTIC GUIDELINES

The abused person often appears very guarded or depressed, and the abuser may appear nervous and possessive. Separate the victim from the abuser to get an accurate history, but remember that the victim may be too frightened to reveal the truth. The victim may initially describe problems in the marriage, issues of infidelity, or financial and legal problems without mentioning abuse. In fact, the victim may initially deny being abused. Be courteous and respectful of the patient, and show concern for her safety. Assure the patient that she is not to blame. Many women feel that they provoked the abuse—for example, by not making dinner. The patient may be frightened of her husband. Do not confront her or pressure her to lodge a complaint, but allow her to ventilate her anger. Explain that abuse is a common problem, that she is not alone, and that help is available.

The batterer may intimidate the patient, but the patient must be handled tactfully, as she may flee into denial and guilt if she feels that her husband is being confronted and exposed. Try to ask the patient if her husband has ever hit her. If he drinks, ask if he gets drunk and how he behaves if drunk. Does he curse or lose his temper? Is he jealous for any reason? Ask about her suicidal ideas and attempts; they are often seen in battered women.

EVALUATION AND MANAGEMENT

1. Admit the patient to a general hospital if there is a medical or surgical need or to a psychiatric hospital if the patient is actively suicidal. Make a diagnostic evaluation of any associated drug or alcohol abuse. Photograph the injuries for possible legal documentation, even if the patient does not wish to press charges at the time. Old hospital charts should be reviewed for evidence of prior abuse or trauma.
2. Refer the woman to a shelter if she is unwilling to return home.
3. Give her an emergency number to call if she feels threatened at any time after returning home or if she feels that her husband is menacing her.

4. Schedule a follow-up appointment, or refer the patient to a support group for battered wives—for example, National Woman Abuse Prevention Center.

DRUG TREATMENT

Extremely agitated patients may require sedation with a single dose of a benzodiazepine—for example, diazepam 2.5 to 5 mg intramuscularly (IM) or by mouth or lorazepam (Ativan) 1 to 2 mg IM or by mouth.

Psychiatric complications of spouse abuse, such as depression, may require antidepressant medication later as part of a comprehensive treatment plan.

For a more detailed discussion of this topic, see V A Sadock: Physical and Sexual Abuse of Adult, Sec 29.7, p 1729; J H Carter-Lourensz, G Johnson-Powell: Physical Abuse, Sexual Abuse, and Neglect of Child, Sec 47.3, p 2455; M Z Goldstein: Elder Abuse and Neglect, Sec 49.8d, p 2652, in CTP/VI.

17.2 Threats of Homicide or Assault

Threats of homicide or assaultive behavior are common in psychiatric settings. Since a statement of violent intent is a predictor of violence, determine which threatening patients are actually dangerous. This is a difficult decision to make, even for psychiatrists; however, some guidelines are outlined below.

CLINICAL FEATURES AND DIAGNOSIS

Factors that increase the likelihood of an assault include agitation, psychosis (especially paranoid delusions and command hallucinations), previous violence, recent stressors, intoxication with drugs or alcohol, withdrawal from alcohol or sedative-hypnotics, and organic disorders.

Some threats of assault (typically from borderline, antisocial, or histrionic personality disorder patients) are manipulative and without true intent. The evaluation of those patients can be difficult, but always err on the side of caution. Assume, at least initially, that all threats are potentially genuine. Threatening manipulative patients, on perceiving that they are not being taken seriously, may commit violent acts simply to prove that the clinician should have believed them.

INTERVIEWING AND PSYCHOTHERAPEUTIC GUIDELINES

Interaction should be firm, and limits should be clear. The patient must realize that any threats of homicide or assault are taken seriously and will elicit predictable responses from the authorities. A thorough search for weapons may be indicated. Perform a complete psychiatric evaluation, with special emphasis on obtaining a history of previous episodes of assault.

EVALUATION AND MANAGEMENT

1. Is a psychiatric illness responsible for the patient's threatening behavior? How specific are the patient's plans for violence? Does the patient have a specific intended victim? Has the patient obtained the means (for example, a weapon)? Does the patient have a specific reason for committing the violent act (for example, a domestic dispute, revenge against a rival drug dealer, or a response to command hallucinations)?
2. Has the patient committed violent acts in the past?
3. Has the patient been using drugs or alcohol? When was the last alcohol or drug ingestion?
4. Does the patient have a criminal record? If so, what are the specifics (for example, arrests, convictions, the nature of the crimes)?
5. Was the patient abused as a child? Did the patient have childhood conduct problems or the triad of bed-wetting, fire setting, and cruelty to animals?
6. The clinician has a duty to warn and protect the intended victim. If a specific intended victim is likely to be attacked, the clinician must notify that person, the police, or the family or friends of the intended victim who are likely to be able to intervene. In addition, the clinician must do anything reasonable to protect the intended victim. The duty to warn and to protect takes priority over the patient's confidentiality. Threats against the President of the United States must be reported to the Secret Service.
7. Hospitalization, medication, and restraint may be needed.

DRUG TREATMENT

Acutely agitated patients who are already being treated with antipsychotics or benzodiazepines should be given an additional dose of their medication. Violent, psychotic patients can be given haloperidol (Haldol) 2 to 5 mg by mouth or intramuscularly (IM), thiothixene (Navane) 2 to 5 mg by mouth or IM, fluphenazine (Prolixin) 2 to 5 mg by mouth or IM, or perphenazine (Trilafon) 8 mg by mouth or 5 mg IM. Patients who are intoxicated or in withdrawal from drugs or alcohol can be given lorazepam (Ativan) 1 to 2 mg by mouth or IM, estazolam (ProSom) 0.5 to 1 mg by mouth, or oxazepam (Serax) 10 to 30 mg by mouth. If the patient has delirium or dementia, give haloperidol 1 to 5 mg by mouth or IM.

For a more detailed discussion of this topic, see J R Lion: Aggression, Sec 3.4, p 310; K Tardiff: Adult Antisocial Behavior and Criminality, Sec 28.3, p 1622; B J Fauman: Other Psychiatric Emergencies, Sec 30.2, p 1752, in CTP/VI.

17.4 Violence

Violence is physical aggression inflicted by one person on another. When it is directed toward oneself, it is called self-mutilation (Section 10.5) or suicidal behavior (Section 10.6). Violence can be due to a wide range of psychiatric disorders, but it may also occur in normal people who cannot cope with life stresses in less severe ways. Violence and threats of violence are frequently encountered in psychiatric emergency settings and are frequent causes of psychiatric consultations. The physician and the staff members must know how to rapidly initiate a procedure for the prevention of escalating violence. The procedure may involve behavioral, pharmacological, and psychosocial interventions.

CLINICAL FEATURES AND DIAGNOSIS

The psychiatric conditions most commonly associated with violence include such psychotic disorders as schizophrenia and mania (particularly if the patient is paranoid or is experiencing command hallucinations), intoxication with alcohol and drugs, withdrawal from alcohol and sedative-hypnotics, catatonic excitement, agitated depression, personality disorders characterized by rage and poor impulse control (for example, borderline and antisocial personality disorders), and organic disorders (especially those with frontal and temporal lobe involvement). See Table 17.4-1 for diagnoses associated with violent behavior.

Other risk factors for violence include a statement of intent, a specific plan, the availability of the means of violence, male sex, young age (15 to 24 years), low socioeconomic status, poor social support system, history of violence, other antisocial acts, poor impulse control, history of suicide attempts, and recent stressors. A history of violence is the best predictor of violence. Additional important factors include a history of childhood victimization; childhood history of the triad of bedwetting, fire setting, and cruelty to animals; criminal record; military or police service; reckless driving; and family history of violence.

The first goal with the potentially violent patient is the prevention of immediate violence. The next objective is to make a diagnosis that will lead to a treatment plan, including measures to minimize the likelihood of subsequent violence.

TABLE 17.4-1
DIAGNOSES ASSOCIATED WITH VIOLENT BEHAVIOR

A. Psychotic disorders
  1. Schizophrenia (especially paranoid and catatonic)
  2. Mania
  3. Paranoid disorders
  4. Postpartum psychosis
B. Organic mental disorders
  1. Delirium
  2. Drug intoxication or withdrawal
C. Personality disorders
  1. Antisocial
  2. Paranoid and others with transient psychosis
D. Situational problems
  1. Domestic quarrels (spouse abuse)
  2. Child abuse
  3. Homosexual panic
E. Brain disorders
  1. Seizure disorders
  2. Structural defects (trauma, encephalitis)
  3. Mental retardation and minimal brain dysfunction
F. Dissociative states

Table from N Hanke: *Handbook of Emergency Psychiatry*, p 109. Collamore Press, Lexington, Mass, 1984. Used with permission.

INTERVIEWING AND PSYCHOTHERAPEUTIC GUIDELINES

Be supportive and nonthreatening to potentially violent patients. However, be firm, and present clear limits that can be enforced with physical restraint if necessary. Set limits by offering choices (for example, medication or restraints), not provocative directives ("Take this medicine now"). Tell the patients directly that violence is not acceptable. Reassure the patients that they are safe. Convey an attitude of calm and control. Offer the patients medication to help them relax.

EVALUATION AND MANAGEMENT

1. It is important for primary care physicians to protect themselves. Assume that violence is always a possibility. Never interview an armed patient. The patient should always surrender the weapon to a security guard. Know as much as possible about the patient before the interview. Never interview a potentially violent patient alone or in an office with the door closed. Interviewers should consider removing neckties, necklaces, and other articles of clothing or jewelry they are wearing that the patient can grab or pull. Stay within sight of other staff members. Do not give the patient access to areas where weapons may be available (for example, a crash cart or a treatment room). Do not sit close to a paranoid patient, who may feel threatened by the proximity. Keep at least an arm's length away from any potentially violent patient. Do not challenge or confront a psychotic patient. Always leave a route of rapid escape in case the patient attacks.
2. Be alert to the signs of impending violence; they include recent violent acts against people or property, clenched teeth and fists, verbal threats (menacing), weapons or objects potentially usable as weapons (for example, a fork, pens or pencils, a paperweight), psychomotor agitation (considered by many to be an important indicator), alcohol or drug intoxication, paranoid delusions, and command hallucinations.
3. Be sure that sufficient staff members are on hand to restrain the patient safely. Call for staff assistance before the patient's agitation has escalated. Often, a show of force through the presence of several able-bodied staff members is sufficient to prevent a violent act.
4. Physical restraint should be performed only by those who are trained to do so. For patients with suspected phencyclidine (PCP) intoxication, physical restraints (especially limb restraints) should be avoided, since self-injuries may occur. Usually, a benzodiazepine or an antipsychotic is given immediately after physical restraints are applied to provide a chemical restraint, but the drug choice depends on the diagnosis. Provide a nonstimulating environment.
5. Make a definitive diagnostic evaluation, including the patient's vital signs, physical examination, and psychiatric history. Evaluate the patient's suicide risk, and create a treatment plan that provides for the management of potential subsequent violence. Elevated vital signs may suggest withdrawal from alcohol or sedative-hypnotics.
6. Explore possible psychosocial interventions to reduce the risk of violence. If violence is related to a specific situation or person, try to separate the patient

from that situation or person. Try family interventions and other environmental manipulations. Would the patient still be potentially violent while living with other relatives?

7. Hospitalization may be necessary to detain the patient and to prevent violence. Constant observation may be necessary, even on a locked inpatient psychiatric ward.

8. If psychiatric treatment is not appropriate, involving the police and the legal system may be necessary.

9. Intended victims must be warned if there is a continued possibility of danger (for example, if the patient is not hospitalized).

DRUG TREATMENT

Drug treatment depends on the specific diagnosis. Benzodiazepines and antipsychotics are used most often for tranquilization. Fluphenazine (Prolixin), thiothixene (Navane), trifluoperazine (Stelazine), or haloperidol (Haldol), all given at 5 mg by mouth or intramuscularly (IM) or lorazepam (Ativan) 2 mg by mouth or IM may be tried initially. If the patient is already taking an antipsychotic, give more of the same drug. If the patient's agitation has not decreased in 20 to 30 minutes, repeat the dose. Avoid antipsychotics in patients at risk for seizures. Benzodiazepines may be ineffective in patients who are tolerant; these drugs may also cause disinhibition, which can potentially worsen the violence. For patients with epilepsy, first try an anticonvulsant—for example, carbamazepine (Tegretol)—and then a benzodiazepine. Chronically violent patients with organic disorders sometimes respond to β-blockers, such as propranolol (Inderal).

For a more detailed discussion of this topic, see J R Lion: Aggression, Sec 3.4, p 310; V K Burt: Impulse-Control Disorders Not Elsewhere Classified, Sec 24.1, p 1409; K Tardiff: Adult Antisocial Behavior and Criminality, Sec 28.3, p 1622; B J Fauman: Other Psychiatric Emergencies, Sec 30.2, p 1752, in CTP/VI.

18

Personality Disorders

18.1. Borderline Personality Disorder

Borderline personality disorder is characterized by a long-standing pattern of instability of mood, self-image, and interpersonal relationships. Borderline patients are frequent users of psychiatric emergency rooms and can present with a range of emergencies, most commonly suicidal ideation. The patients can consume a great deal of staff time and may be exasperating for mental health care providers, One defense mechanism those patients often use is splitting, in which the patient divides ambivalently regarded people into good people and bad people (for example, the therapist is good, and the emergency room or office staff members are bad).

The patients can often be difficult to manage and manipulative in their suicidal gestures, which are often made to gain attention or to express anger. However, there is always the risk that a suicidal gesture will inadvertently lead to a completed suicide. In the emergency room or office setting the goal is to devise a plan that resolves the crisis without sabotaging the long-term treatment objectives.

CLINICAL FEATURES AND DIAGNOSIS

The hallmarks of the disorder are instability and an almost constant state of crisis (Table 18.1-1). Under stress, borderline patients may have psychotic symptoms or major depression. They characteristically act out with manipulative, self-destructive acts or, less often, with rage directed toward others.

TABLE 18.1-1
DIAGNOSTIC CRITERIA FOR BORDERLINE PERSONALITY DISORDER

A pervasive pattern of instability of interpersonal relationships, self-image, and affects, and marked impulsivity beginning by early adulthood and present in a variety of contexts, as indicated by five (or more) of the following:

    (1) frantic efforts to avoid real or imagined abandonment. **Note:** Do not include suicidal or self-mutilating behavior covered in criterion 5.
    (2) a pattern of unstable and intense interpersonal relationships characterized by alternating between extremes of idealization and devaluation
    (3) identity disturbance: markedly and persistently unstable self-image or sense of self
    (4) impulsivity in at least two areas that are potentially self-damaging (e.g., spending, sex, substance abuse, reckless driving, binge eating). **Note:** Do not include suicidal or self-mutilating behavior covered in criterion 5.
    (5) recurrent suicidal behavior, gestures, or threats, or self-mutilating behavior
    (6) affective instability due to a marked reactivity of mood (e.g., intense episodic dysphoria, irritability, or anxiety usually lasting a few hours and only rarely more than a few days)
    (7) chronic feelings of emptiness
    (8) inappropriate, intense anger or difficulty controlling anger (e.g., frequent displays of temper, constant anger, recurrent physical fights)
    (9) transient, stress-related paranoid ideation or severe dissociative symptoms

Table from D8M-IV, *Diagnostic and Statistical Manual of Mental Disorders*, ed 4. Copyright American Psychiatric Association, Washington, 1994. Used with permission.

INTERVIEWING AND PSYCHOTHERAPEUTIC GUIDELINES

Borderline patients form an instant transference in which they may overvalue or devalue the primary care physician. Be empathic, but maintain enough objectivity to make therapeutic decisions in the patient's best interests. Set limits for acceptable and unacceptable behavior in the physician's office. Do not join in when the patient attempts to split the staff.

EVALUATION AND MANAGEMENT

1. Assess the patient's dangerousness. The most common emergency in borderline patients is a suicidal gesture, commonly by slashing the wrists or taking a drug overdose. Evaluate the potential lethality of the patient's behavior. Was the self-destructive act a genuine suicide attempt with an intent to die or a gesture used as a cry for help without an intent to die? If the gesture is repeated, could it lead to an accidental suicide? Is the behavior a well-developed coping mechanism, with multiple similar gestures in the past, or is it new? If the patient is not admitted to the hospital, what other options are available for the patient? Can crisis intervention relieve an acute stress, or will a release simply return the patient to the same environment that led to the attempt, perhaps making the patient feel more hopeless than before?

2. Was the gesture designed to gain attention and an attempted rescue by others? If so, has that goal been achieved? Who responded? Was the response the desired one? Was the gesture designed to discharge a dysphoric affect? If so, has that affect been discharged, at least in the short term? Was the gesture designed to obtain hospitalization? If so, how does hospitalization now fit into the patient's longitudinal course? Frequent brief hospitalizations may not be desirable and may reinforce hospital dependence. Was the gesture designed to obtain control over a situation? If so, has that been achieved?

3. Evaluate the patient's related symptoms, such as drug and alcohol abuse, sexual promiscuity, binging and purging, fighting, and other signs of poor impulse control.

4. What is the patient's current treatment? Contact the patient's therapist, if possible, and organize a plan for the patient that places the resolution of the immediate emergency in the context of the patient's ongoing treatment. Try to avoid hospitalization unless that is the therapist's plan (Table 18.1-2). Patients may present in an emergency because of some conflict encountered in the ongoing psychotherapy.

5. Unless there is an indication for hospital admission, attempt to resolve the crisis without hospitalization. Manipulate the environment to reduce the stress, perhaps by recruiting the assistance of friends and relatives. Give the patient the opportunity to ventilate and discharge some hostile affect. Consider a family session for crisis intervention. Try to develop some rapport with the patient. Reassure the patient, as reasonably as possible, that someone does care.

6. Consider a wide range of psychotherapeutic and psychopharmacological approaches, ranging from insight-oriented psychotherapy to antidepressants, anti-

TABLE 18.1–2
**USE OF HOSPITALIZATION FOR PATIENTS WITH BORDERLINE PERSONALITY DISORDER OR
OTHER SEVERE PERSONALITY DISORDERS**

Indications for admission
- The patient's ongoing therapist wants the patient admitted as part of an ongoing treatment plan or for reevaluation.
- Suicidal gestures are escalating.
- Secondary major depression or substance abuse requires admission.
- Psychotic reaction that does not respond to emergency interventions (structured environment and/or antipsychotic medication) occurs.
- Severe losses or other stresses occur.

Contraindications to admission*
- Repeating a treatment that has already failed
- Using the hospital because nothing else works
- Attempting to make major characterologic change
- Attempting to try a new medication in the absence of any positive indication for its success
- Trying to convince patients to change their living situations
- Treating the patient's unwillingness to follow treatment plans
- Sheltering malingerers or patients facing legal charges

* Table adapted from I D Glick, H Klar, P Broff: When should chronic patients be hospitalized? Hosp Community Psychiatry 35: 934, 1984. Table from J R Hillard: Personality disorders. In *Manual of Clinical Emergency Psychiatry,* J R Hillard, editor, p 268. American Psychiatric Press, Washington, 1990. Used with permission.

psychotics, benzodiazepines, lithium (Eskalith), and other drugs. Behavior therapy, family therapy, and group therapy may also be useful.

DRUG TREATMENT

Agitation or anxiety may be reduced with benzodiazepines, although the risk of abuse and dependence is great. Initiating a benzodiazepine should be considered only as part of a complete plan (for example, to avoid hospitalization) and should be continued only during an acute episode. Benzodiazepines may cause disinhibition. For nonpsychotic patients, the risks of benzodiazepines are usually less severe than the risks of antipsychotic side effects, especially tardive dyskinesia. Borderline patients are subject to psychotic symptoms in response to stress. Brief treatment with antipsychotics can be considered for those minipsychotic episodes. If depression is also present, serotonergic agents, such as paroxetine (Paxil), fluoxetine (Prozac), and sertraline (Zoloft), may be helpful.

For a more detailed discussion of this topic, see J G Gunderson, K A Phillips: Personality Disorders, Chap 25, p 1425, in CTP/VI.

18.2. Other Personality Disorders

Other personality disorders include paranoid, schizoid, schizotypal, antisocial, histrionic, narcissistic, avoidant, and dependent types. These personality disorders are generally not associated with the emergency situations that may occur with borderline personality disorder; however, patients exhibiting these personality disorders or similar personality traits create difficulties for the primary care physician.

Chapter 1 discusses the management of several personality types during the diagnostic interview.

For a more detailed discussion of this topic, see J G Gunderson, K A Phillips: Personality Disorders, Chap 25, p 1425, in CTP/VI.

19

Other Conditions That May Be a Focus of Clinical Attention

19.1. Akinesia (Decreased Motor Activity)

Akinesia is markedly decreased motor activity, including diminished facial expressiveness and eye blinking.

CLINICAL FEATURES AND DIAGNOSIS

Akinesia may be a side effect of antipsychotic medication or a symptom of catatonia, schizophrenia, depression, or an organic disorder. When it is a side effect of medication, it may be mistaken as a psychiatric symptom—for example, psychomotor retardation in depression or withdrawn behavior in schizophrenia.

INTERVIEWING AND PSYCHOTHERAPEUTIC GUIDELINES

Because the akinetic patient's responses will be slow or nonexistent, being a tolerant interviewer will be rewarded. The patient may be well aware of what the interviewer is saying and doing; therefore, any actions should be explained. Collateral informants may be particularly useful.

EVALUATION AND MANAGEMENT

1. Obtain the patient's vital signs. Fever may indicate neuroleptic malignant syndrome or another medical disorder.
2. Obtain the patient's history of antipsychotic treatment.
3. Examine the patient for waxy flexibility. If it is present, consider catatonia as a possible diagnosis (see Section 6.4). Catatonia may be a sign of a mental disorder, but antipsychotics may also induce it, especially in patients with organic disorders.
4. If catatonia is present, consider referring the patient to a psychiatrist for a drug-facilitated interview with amobarbital (Amytal) or diazepam (Valium). Sedative-hypnotics may reduce anxiety and allow the catatonic patient to talk. If catatonia is related to an organic disorder, cognition may worsen with the sedative-hypnotic. Although sedative-hypnotics may further sedate an akinetic patient, they are useful for diagnostic purposes.
5. Akinesia secondary to depot antipsychotics (fluphenazine [Prolixin] and haloperidol [Haldol]) may be particularly severe and clinically indistinguishable from catatonia. Such a severe presentation is most likely if the depot medication is given too often or at too high a dosage. Some weeks of administering the depot

medication at a lower dosage may be needed before improvement is seen. Obtain psychiatric consultation in severe cases.

DRUG TREATMENT

A decreased antipsychotic dosage may relieve the akinesia. If a decreased dosage is not possible, a different antipsychotic may be indicated. The addition of an anticholinergic medication (for example, benztropine [Cogentin] 2 mg by mouth, intramuscularly, or intravenously) may also be helpful.

For a more detailed discussion of this topic, see J Yager, M J Gitlin: Clinical Manifestations of Clinical Disorders, Chap 10, p 637; S G Siris, M R Lavin: Schizoaffective Disorder, Schizophreniform Disorder, and Brief Psychotic Disorder, Sec 15.1, p 1019; D P Van Kammen, S R Marder: Dopamine Receptor Antagonists, Sec 32.15, p 1987, in CTP/VI.

19.2. Anger

Anger is an emotion, ranging from irritability to rage, that all people experience. Usually, anger is in reaction to an unpleasant or threatening stimulus.

CLINICAL FEATURES AND DIAGNOSIS

Most often, the diagnosis of anger is obvious and self-evident. Sometimes, anger is masked and presents as depression, apathy, or agitation.

INTERVIEWING AND PSYCHOTHERAPEUTIC GUIDELINES

Repeatedly reassure the patient that the situation is under control and that any concerns will be listened to empathically and noncritically. Try to determine if the patient is psychotic. Do not try to convince a delusional patient that the delusion is false.

Determine if the patient is depressed or experiencing grief. In the first six months after a significant loss, a grieving person may experience and express tremendous resentment about the loss. A depressed patient may also present with a primary picture of irritability, frustration, and apparent anger when, in fact, the primary underlying problem is depression.

If patients are intoxicated with drugs or alcohol or both, they can become emotionally disinhibited and angry. In addition, demented patients often experience confusion, disorientation, frustration, and disinhibition, which can lead to angry outbursts.

If the patient is not psychotic, depressed, grieving, demented, or using substances, try to explore the reasons for the anger, and allow the patient to express the emotions felt.

EVALUATION AND MANAGEMENT

1. The primary objective is to prevent the escalation of the patient's anger to violence or other maladaptive acts. Often, if the patient can express anger verbally in a safe setting, it may significantly relieve the affect.
2. Be sure that sufficient staff members are present to restrain the patient if the anger escalates to violence.
3. Isolate the patient from the object of the anger. For example, if the patient is angry at his or her family, have the family wait in another room.

DRUG TREATMENT

If the patient's anger is escalating and violence or other maladaptive behavior seems imminent, medicate the patient. Patients with severe anger problems— especially those who may be violent—should always be referred for a psychiatric evaluation.

If the patient is already taking a tranquilizer (a benzodiazepine or an antipsychotic), increase the dosage of that drug unless the patient is elderly or demented or is abusing substances. In those cases, benzodiazepines in particular may produce a paradoxical effect, which can lead to increased agitation and anger.

For patients not already taking a tranquilizer, benzodiazepines and antipsychotics are effective. Start with benzodiazepines (for example, lorazepam [Ativan] 1 to 2 mg by mouth or intramuscularly [IM]), since they have fewer side effects than do antipsychotics. If several doses of a benzodiazepine are ineffective, use an antipsychotic (for example, haloperidol [Haldol] 2 to 5 mg by mouth or IM or chlorpromazine [Thorazine] 25 to 100 mg by mouth or 10 to 25 mg IM).

For a more detailed discussion of this topic, see Lion, J R: Aggression, Sec 3.4, p 310, in CTP/VI.

19.3. Anniversary Reaction

An *anniversary reaction* is a set of behaviors, symptoms, or dreams that occur on the anniversary of a significant past event.

CLINICAL FEATURES AND DIAGNOSIS

Patients with recurrent depression often become depressed at the same time of year as in previous episodes. Patients who have suffered a significant medical illness (for example, myocardial infarction) may present with symptoms of the illness on the anniversary of the first episode. Family members of a patient who died of an acute illness may have symptoms of their relative's illness on the anniversary of the death.

INTERVIEWING AND PSYCHOTHERAPEUTIC GUIDELINES

Reassurance and a calm exploration of the chronology of the reaction are needed. Explain to the patient that anniversary reactions are likely to recur for several years and that feelings about the event should be expressed.

EVALUATION AND MANAGEMENT

1. Determine the temporal pattern of the symptoms.
2. Identify the events that precipitated the episode. In anniversary reactions of an acute medical illness, a variety of stimuli may be present; often, family members are helpful in identifying the precipitants.
3. If the reaction is determined to be a recurrence of mental illness, explore the possible causes with the patient, and refer the patient to a psychiatrist for psychotherapy. In many cases, however, ventilation of feelings in the office may be sufficient, with no other treatment necessary.

DRUG TREATMENT

Drug treatment is generally not indicated unless a severe reaction, such as major depression, psychosis, or extreme agitation, is present.

For a more detailed discussion of this topic, see H S Akiskal: Mood Disorders: Clinical Features, Sec 16.6, p 1123; S Zisook: Death, Dying, and Bereavement, Sec 29.6, p 1713, in CTP/VI.

19.4. Disaster Survivors

Disaster survivors are people who have survived a sudden, unexpected, overwhelming stress that is greater than that normally expected in life. Typical stresses include earthquakes, floods, fires, plane crashes, mud slides, and building collapses. Concentration camp internment, famine, and radiation contamination are also extraordinary stresses.

CLINICAL FEATURES AND DIAGNOSIS

The common emotions in disasters include fear, panic, anger, frustration, numbness, confusion, helplessness, and guilt. The psychiatric syndromes that patients may present include posttraumatic stress disorder, other anxiety disorders, and depression. Some victims experience brief depersonalization or derealization. Psychiatric syndromes may be identified in those who are physically injured, those who escaped physical injury, family members of the victims, and rescue workers.

INTERVIEWING AND PSYCHOTHERAPEUTIC GUIDELINES

Be empathic and supportive. Make the patients as comfortable as possible. Reassure them with whatever facts are available, and minimize the spread of rumors. If the facts may be overwhelming for a patient, delay telling the facts, but do not intentionally tell a patient something that is not true. Emotional reactions to the stress vary considerably, so be prepared to handle a wide range of emotional states. Work with the victims to mobilize support and a plan of action. Remind the victims of their past successful coping skills.

Obtain a detailed account of the victims' experiences. Was the event unexpected, anticipated, or a repetition of a similar experience? Past histories can be useful in understanding the patients' present maladaptive reactions.

EVALUATION AND MANAGEMENT

1. Treat any acute medical problems.
2. Provide some psychological relief. Cognitive approaches may be useful. The survivors' feelings of guilt may respond to such interventions as, "What could anyone else have done in that situation?" Reassure the survivors that guilt, frustration, and hopelessness are normal reactions to the level of stress experienced and that those feelings will pass with time. Recruiting survivors to help other victims may relieve hopelessness.
3. Encourage the patients to talk about their feelings and how they experienced the disaster. Uninjured survivors and family members of dead victims may feel guilty about not being hurt when their friends and family members have died. Rescue workers may have similar feelings, plus anger and frustration.
4. Group therapy with victims, families, and rescue workers may be helpful, especially in relieving the feelings of helplessness and loneliness.
5. Referral to a psychiatrist may be necessary if symptoms continue unabated.

DRUG TREATMENT

Medications are usually not needed, although severe anxiety may be relieved with a brief course of short-acting benzodiazepines—for example, oxazepam (Serax) 15 to 30 mg, alprazolam (Xanax) 0.5 to 1 mg, lorazepam (Ativan) 1 to 2 mg, or estazolam (ProSom) 0.5 to 1 mg, all given by mouth three times a day. In some cases a long-acting benzodiazepine may be used—for example, diazepam (Valium) 5 to 10 mg by mouth two times a day, chlordiazepoxide (Librium) 10 to 25 mg by mouth three times a day, clorazepate (Tranxene) 2.5 to 5 mg by mouth three times a day, or clonazepam (Klonopin) 0.25 to 0.50 mg by mouth two times a day. Insomnia can be treated with flurazepam (Dalmane) 15 to 30 mg by mouth as needed, quazepam (Doral) 7.5 to 15 mg by mouth as needed, temazepam (Restoril) 15 to 30 mg by mouth as needed, or triazolam (Halcion) 0.125 to 0.25 mg by mouth as needed.

For a more detailed discussion of this topic, see A J Fyer, S Mannuzza, J D Coplan: Panic Disorders and Agoraphobia, Sec 17.1, p 1191; J R T Davidson: Posttraumatic Stress Disorder and Acute Stress Disorder, Sec 17.4, p 1227; N Wong: Group Psychotherapy, Combined Individual and Group Psychotherapy, and Psychodrama, Sec 31.4, p 1821.

19.5. Dyskinesia (Abnormal Movement)

Dyskinesia is any disturbance of movement.

CLINICAL FEATURES AND DIAGNOSIS

In psychiatry the most commonly seen dyskinesias are the acute and chronic movement disorders caused by antipsychotic drugs. In addition, patients taking maintenance antipsychotic agents may experience withdrawal dyskinesia if and when the antipsychotic dosage is reduced. Dyskinesias in patients receiving antipsychotic medications are common. Acute extrapyramidal side effects—including parkinsonism, dystonia, and akathisia—can be caused by any antipsychotic, except perhaps clozapine (Clozaril), and are most common in patients receiving high-potency antipsychotics. See Chapter 23 for more information on antipsychotic-induced movement disorders.

A wide range of neurological conditions can also present with abnormal movements. The disorders with established genetic transmission include Huntington's chorea, Wilson's disease, Tourette's disorder, Lesch-Nyhan syndrome, and essential tremor; other disorders include Parkinson's disease, dystonia musculorum deformans, and many other syndromes related to either focal insults (for example, cerebrovascular diseases) or diffuse insults (for example, anoxia, hepatic failure, hypocalcemia, and hypothyroidism) to the basal ganglia. Connective tissue diseases, such as systemic lupus erythematosus, can cause dyskinesia. In women, dyskinesias may occur in pregnancy or as a side effect of oral contraceptives. 1-Methyl-4-phenyl-1,2,3,6-tetrahydropyridine (MPTP), a synthetic opioid drug of abuse, can destroy substantia nigra neurons and cause Parkinson's disease. In general, dyskinesias are not present during sleep.

INTERVIEWING AND PSYCHOTHERAPEUTIC GUIDELINES

The interviewing style depends largely on the acuteness and the severity of the complaint. A patient with an acute antipsychotic-induced dystonia is in extreme distress and should be reassured that the condition can be treated. Less acute conditions should be carefully evaluated, looking for neurological causes.

EVALUATION AND MANAGEMENT

1. Determine whether antipsychotic medication is a possible cause of the dyskinesia. If the patient is taking an antipsychotic, consider acute extrapyramidal side

effects, withdrawal dyskinesia, and tardive dyskinesia. If the patient has taken antipsychotics in the past, consider tardive dyskinesia. Dyskinesia may have multiple causes in one patient.

2. Consider other drugs that may cause dyskinesias, possibly psychostimulants or L-dopa (lerodopa [Larodopa]). Also consider head injury or exposure to toxins (for example, MPTP and carbon monoxide).

3. Consider the age of the patient. In the elderly, look for cerebrovascular diseases, Parkinson's disease, and tumors; in children, look for perinatal injury, kernicterus, juvenile Huntington's chorea, Sydenham's chorea (after rheumatic fever), Lesch-Nyhan syndrome, Tourette's disorder, athetosis, and myoclonus caused by subacute sclerosing panencephalitis.

4. Look for genetic disorders in the patient's family history.

5. Refer the patient for a neurological examination.

6. Conduct a full medical workup, including complete blood count (CBC), thyroid function tests, Venereal Disease Research Laboratory (VDRL) test, chemistry panel tests, erythrocyte sedimentation rate (ESR), urinalysis, urine toxicology screen, blood drug levels, electroencephalogram (EEG), and a computed tomographic (CT) scan or a magnetic resonance imaging (MRI) scan of the head. A lumbar puncture and further brain imaging may also be indicated.

DRUG TREATMENT

Treatment depends on making a definitive diagnosis. Some conditions are responsive to pharmacological manipulations of the cholinergic or dopaminergic systems. Tardive dyskinesia requires careful planning of any antipsychotic exposure. Although they cause the patient discomfort, dystonia and parkinsonism can usually be rapidly managed with anticholinergic agents, such as benztropine (Cogentin) 1 to 2 mg by mouth or intramuscularly. Acute dystonia usually responds to 50 mg of diphenhydramine (Benadryl) given intravenously (IV). Akathisia is less responsive to anticholinergic medications, but other drugs, such as benzodiazepines and β-blockers, may be helpful.

For a more detailed discussion of this topic, see J A Grebb: Medication-Induced Movement Disorders, Sec 32.2, p 1909; G L Hanna: Tic Disorders, Chap 41, p 2325, in CTP/VI.

19.6. Dysprosody (Flat Speech)

Dysprosody is the loss of the normal ability to vary the intonation of speech to express emotions.

CLINICAL FEATURES AND DIAGNOSIS

Speech is flat, monotonous, and without inflection. Dysprosody is seldom a specific complaint. It is seen in cases of brain dysfunction, particularly in the elderly. Dysprosody may be similar to the monotonous speech of depressed patients and schizophrenic patients with negative symptoms.

INTERVIEWING AND PSYCHOTHERAPEUTIC GUIDELINES

Do not focus on the dysprosody. Attempt to determine the underlying cause of the disorder by taking a psychiatric history and conducting a mental status examination. Pay particular attention to the presence of dementia by conducting a cognitive examination and performing a medical workup.

EVALUATION AND MANAGEMENT

1. Besides dementia, depression and schizophrenia must be ruled out. Patients with substance use disorder—particularly sedatives or hypnotics—may also show dysprosody. Some persons with articulation or speech disorders may have a flat intonation of speech. Dysprosody may be an early sign of Parkinson's disease.
2. Treat the underlying disorder. Speech therapy is of value for articulation or speech disorders if present.

DRUG TREATMENT

Underlying psychiatric disorders are treated with the appropriate medication (for example, antipsychotic agents for schizophrenia). Depression will respond to standard antidepressants. As the underlying condition improves, dysprosody diminishes.

For a more detailed discussion of this topic, see G D Strauss: The Psychiatric Interview, History, and Mental Status Examination, Sec 9.1, p 521; R W Butler, P Satz: Personality Assessment of Adults and Children, Sec 9.4, p 544, in CTP/VI.

19.7. Hypertensive Crisis

Hypertensive crisis is a potentially life-threatening emergency that occurs when patients taking monoamine oxidase inhibitors (MAOIs) eat food containing tyramine or take contraindicated drugs, such as sympathomimetic agents. The primary care physician should give patients careful instructions on diet and drug interaction before prescribing MAOIs (Table 19.7-1).

CLINICAL FEATURES AND DIAGNOSIS

The symptoms of hypertensive crisis include severe occipital headache, stiff neck, sweating, nausea, and vomiting.

TABLE 19.7-1
INSTRUCTIONS FOR PATIENTS TAKING MONOAMINE OXIDASE INHIBITORS (MAOIs)

Background Information
Foods rich in tyramine and some related amines have been known to cause serious side effects and hypertensive responses in patients taking MAOIs. Tyramine is an amino acid found in many protein substances and is produced by fermentation, aging, spoiling, or pickling. The enzyme MAO found in the liver normally inactivates tyramine. In the presence of an MAOI, tyramine is not deactivated by MAO and is allowed to circulate and indirectly cause the release of norepinephrine from nerve endings. This may lead to detrimental side effects, especially hypertensive responses.

Summary of Guidelines to Follow While Taking an MAOI
1. The foods in the high-tyramine category should be completely avoided. If you consume small quantities of foods in this category without symptoms, do not assume that you can repeat this. These foods vary greatly in tyramine content and their ability to cause a severe reaction. You may have a reaction the second time.
2. You are allowed foods with moderate to low tyramine content (categories 2 and 3). These foods should be eaten in moderation. Try to avoid eating combinations of foods in these categories because of the possible additive effects of tyramine.
3. Avoid aged, spoiled, improperly refrigerated, or frozen foods. Do not eat tuna fish that has been in the refrigerator for 2 or 3 days. Eat only fresh food or freshly prepared frozen or canned foods. Beware of many foods that derive their flavor from aging, smoking, or pickling. Also note that cooking of degraded protein does not alter the tyramine content of these foods.
4. Avoid any foods that have previously caused adverse side effects.
5. Cheeses have been responsible for the greatest number of reported hypertensive responses. Observe that many foods contain cheese as an ingredient, such as cheese crackers, pizza, and cheese bread.
6. There are certain prescription and nonprescription medicines that should be avoided. See list of MAOI Drug Incompatibilities (Table 19.7-2) Be certain to tell your physician, dentist, or pharmacist that you are taking an MAOI.
7. Call your physician immediately or go to your nearest emergency medical facility if you should suffer from the following symptoms: a throbbing, explosive headache of sudden onset associated with flushing, visual disturbances, nausea or vomiting. Major muscle jerks, confusion, or excitement may also occur, and in the case of a reaction with another drug, sometimes without a severe headache.

Table from D L Murphy, T Sunderland, R M Cohen; Monoamine oxidase-inhibiting antidepressants: A clinical update. Psychiatr Clin North Am 7:549, 1984. Used with permission.

Interactions of MAOIs with sympathomimetic agents and other specific drugs are potentially fatal (Table 19.7-2). MAOIs combined with meperidine (Demerol) or dextromethorphan (Dexedrine and many over-the-counter cough medications) can produce restlessness, dizziness, tremor, sweating, muscle twitching, seizures, and severe hyperpyrexia—in some cases eventually leading to shock and death. The concomitant use of serotonin-specific reuptake inhibitors (SSRIs) (for example, fluoxetine [Prozac], paroxetine [Paxil], and sertraline [Zoloft]) and MAOIs can produce rigidity, fever, confusion, and death. MAOIs cannot be used until the SSRIs have been discontinued for at least five weeks.

Tricyclic antidepressants have been safely and effectively combined with MAOIs in closely monitored patients. The best rule is to use low dosages of both drugs, increase them slowly, and monitor the patients closely.

Patients should continue a tyramine-free diet for at least two weeks after the MAOI has been discontinued (Table 19.7-3).

The most common side effects of MAOIs are unrelated to diet and drug interactions; the side effects include orthostatic hypotension, weight gain, edema, insomnia, and sexual dysfunction. Both orthostatic hypotension and hypertensive crisis can present with fainting or unconsciousness.

TABLE 19.27–2
MAOI DRUG INCOMPATIBILITIES

Generally Contraindicated Hazardous Potentiations*	
Stimulants	Weight-reducing or antiappetite drugs; amphetamines, cocaine
Decongestants	Sinus, hay fever, and cold tablets; nasal sprays or drops; asthma tablets or inhalants, cough preparations (or any products containing ephedrine, phenylephedrine, or phenylpropanolamine)
Antihypertensives	Methyldopa, guanethidine, reserpine
Tricyclics	Imipramine, desipramine, clomipramine
MAOIs	Tranylcypromine, after other MAOIs
Sympathomimetics	Dopamine, Metaraminol
Amine precursors	L-dopa, L-tryptophan
Narcotics	Meperidine (Demerol)
Some Potentiation Possible	
Narcotics	Morphine, codeine
Sedatives	Alcohol, barbiturates, benzodiazepines
Local anesthetics containing vasoconstrictors	
Sympathomimetics	Ephedrine, norepinephrine, isoproterenol
General anesthetics	

*Under certain circumstances, some of these drugs may be used together with MAOIs in specialized treatment approaches and with additional precautions. For example; TCAs and L-tryptophan have been used with MAOIs in antidepressant regimens. Also of note, other agents from these drug classes are safely used (for example, the antihypertensive agent chlorothiazide) as only mild potentiation occurs. Table from D L Murphy, T Sunderland, R M Cohen: Monoamine oxidase-inhibiting antidepressants: A clinical update. Psychiatr Clin North Am 7: 549, 1984. Used with permission.

TABLE 19.7–3
MAOI DIETARY RESTRICTIONS

High Tyramine Content—Not Permitted	
Aged, matured cheeses (unpasteurized)	Cheddar, Camembert, Stilton, bleu, Swiss
Smoked or pickled meats, fish, or poultry	Herring, sausage, corned beef
Aged putrefying meats, fish, and poultry	Chicken or beef liver, paté, game
Yeast or meat extracts	Bovril, marmite, brewer's yeast (beware of drinks, soups, and stews made with those products)
Red wines	Chianti, burgundy, sherry, vermouth
Italian broad beans	Fava beans
Moderate Tyramine Content—Limited Amounts Allowed	
Meat extracts	Bouillion, consomme
Pasteurized light and pale beers	
Ripe avocado	
Low Tyramine Content—Permissible	
Distilled spirits (in moderation)	Vodka, gin, rye, scotch
Cheese	Cottage cheese, cream cheese
Chocolate- and caffeine-containing beverages	
Fruits	Figs, raisins, grapes, pineapple, oranges
Soy sauce	
Yogurt, sour cream (made by reputable manufacturers)	

Table from D L Murphy, T Sunderland, R M Cohen: Monoamine oxidase-inhibiting antidepressants: A clinical update. Psychiatr Clin North Am 7: 549, 1984. Used with permission.

INTERVIEWING AND PSYCHOTHERAPEUTIC GUIDELINES

Keep the interview brief, and focus on identifying the type and the amount of any tyramine-containing foods eaten and contraindicated medications taken. Patients with potentially dangerous conditions should be referred for possible intensive care unit (ICU) admission. Medications taken in an overdose attempt present a much greater risk than do inadvertent toxic combinations.

EVALUATION AND MANAGEMENT

1. Check the patient's vital signs. Rule out orthostatic hypotension caused by the MAOI itself. Hypotension may also be related to the rate of the MAOI dosage increase. Headaches may have many different causes, so do not assume that a patient taking an MAOI is in a hypertensive crisis until the patient's blood pressure has been taken, even if the headache is severe.
2. Identify the quantity of the tyramine-containing food or contraindicated medication taken.
3. Provide ICU monitoring and supportive treatment of the patient's vital functions as needed.
4. Evaluate the patient for suicidality.

DRUG TREATMENT

Give phentolamine (Regitine) 5 mg intravenously (IV) repeated as needed or phenoxybenzamine (Dibenzyline) 100 mg IV drip over an hour (both are α-adrenergic receptor blockers). An alternative drug is diazoxide (Hyperstat) 300 mg IV, which relaxes the arteriolar smooth muscles. Nifedipine (Procardia) can be used by having the patient bite into a 10 mg capsule before swallowing its contents with water. Chlorpromazine (Thorazine) 50 to 100 mg by mouth also has prominent hypotensive effects and can be used to lower the patient's blood pressure. Some psychiatrists prescribe chlorpromazine to their patients taking MAOIs and advise them to carry the pills with them in case they experience a hypertensive crisis.

For a more detailed discussion of this topic, see W Katon, M D Sullivan, M R Clark: Cardiovascular Disorders, Sec 26.4, p 1491; S L Dubovsky: Electroconvulsive Therapy, Sec 32.28, p 2129, in CTP/VI.

19.8. Homosexual Panic

Homosexual panic does not occur in people who are comfortable with issues related to homosexuality. Instead, it typically occurs in persons with strong homophobic traits who have an experience that suggests someone of the same gender is sexually interested in them. This triggers unrecognized feelings or fears of homosexuality, causing the patient to mount a massive defense, which produces a panic state characterized by anxiety, fear, agitation, and possibly violence and paranoid delusions.

CLINICAL FEATURES AND DIAGNOSIS

The population with the highest rate of homosexual panic are adolescent boys and young men in school dormitories, military barracks, or penal institutions.

The precipitant of homosexual panic may be a sexual conversation with a friend or, more commonly, physical contact, such as bathing together, fondling, sleeping together, or wrestling. In those situations a patient's unacceptable homoerotic fantasies may be aroused and then projected onto the other person involved in the encounter, precipitating a strong reaction in the patient. Homosexual panic may also occur when a person is solicited to engage in a homosexual act against his or her will.

Homosexual panic may be associated with underlying psychiatric conditions, such as mood disorders or schizophrenia. In severe cases the patient can be violent. Patients may have ideas of reference or paranoid delusions in which they believe that others accuse them of homosexuality.

INTERVIEWING AND PSYCHOTHERAPEUTIC GUIDELINES

Be supportive and reassuring. Give the patient an opportunity to ventilate emotionally and process what has occurred. A clinician of the patient's gender should not be overly friendly to avoid any possibility that the patient will misperceive it as sexual interest.

EVALUATION AND MANAGEMENT

1. Arrange for a clinician of the opposite sex to evaluate the patient if possible.
2. Evaluate the patient for possible paranoid delusions. Homosexual panic may represent the beginning of a paranoid disorder or schizophrenia.
3. Obtain the patient's drug history. Could the homosexual panic have been exacerbated by alcohol or sedative-hypnotic withdrawal or by cocaine or other stimulant intoxication?
4. Minimize the physical examination unless it is clinically necessary. The patient can easily misinterpret the physical examination as a sexual assault. Defer the rectal, pelvic, and genital examinations if possible. Hospitalization is usually indicated for patients who are violent or acutely psychotic.
5. Refer the patient for psychotherapy.

DRUG TREATMENT

For severe anxiety, a benzodiazepine may be needed—for example, alprazolam (Xanax) 0.5 to 1 mg by mouth or lorazepam (Ativan) 1 to 2 mg by mouth. If the patient is psychotic, antipsychotics may be indicated—for example, thiothixene (Navane), trifluoperazine (Stelazine), fluphenazine (Prolixin), or haloperidol (Haldol), all given at 5 mg by mouth for a short term. If possible, avoid giving medication by injection, which can be perceived as a sexual assault.

For a more detailed discussion of this topic, see B J Fauman: Other Psychiatric Emergencies, Sec 30.2, p 1752, in CTP/VI.

19.9. Hospitalization

Whether a patient requires psychiatric hospitalization is one of the most important decisions the primary care physician makes. The clinician should be familiar with the available alternatives to hospitalization, such as outpatient clinics, day programs, crisis-intervention programs, and psychosocial modification of the patient's environment.

Patients may be hospitalized in several ways. Since state laws vary, physicians should be familiar with their local regulations. In general, patients should be hospitalized voluntarily; however, dangerous or suicidal patients may require involuntary admission, a difficult process that a psychiatrist must carry out.

In adolescents, hospitalization is usually indicated to manage the acute onset of a psychosis and in cases where the psychiatric symptoms seriously disrupt the patients' functioning in school or at home and sufficiently disturb the patients and their families.

Informal Hospitalization

Admission and discharge may be requested orally, and the patient may leave at any time, even against medical advice. Most medical and surgical patients are admitted informally.

Voluntary Hospitalization

Voluntary hospitalization requires a written application for both admission and discharge. After the patient requests a discharge, the physician may convert a voluntary hospitalization to involuntary hospitalization.

Involuntary Hospitalization

Involuntary hospitalization severely limits the patient's autonomy and rights. It does not require the patient's consent and is often used for patients who are dangerous to themselves or others. Involuntary hospitalization requires certification by two physicians; the certificate may last up to 60 days and can be renewed. A court may order it in response to a petition by a hospital or the patient's family.

Emergency Hospitalization

Emergency hospitalization (temporary or one-physician commitment) is a convenient form of involuntary commitment that requires certification by only one physician; the certificate lasts up to 15 days. A second physician must examine the patient within 48 hours to confirm the need for emergency admission. After 15 days, the patient must be discharged, converted to involuntary status, or converted to voluntary status.

Short-Term Involuntary Protective Order

Patients with life-threatening medical illnesses who refuse treatment and who have mental disorders that prevent them from making decisions about their medical care can be involuntarily hospitalized for medical care by order of a judge. Patients who are dangerous to themselves or others must always be hospitalized or otherwise detained to prevent the occurrence of a dangerous act. Other indications for hospitalization include a need for treatment that is not available in other settings, or a lack of ability to care for oneself.

INTERVIEWING AND PSYCHOTHERAPEUTIC GUIDELINES

If patients are expected to be uncooperative with hospitalization, have sufficient staff members present before informing them. Explain to patients clearly what their rights are and what the procedures are for being discharged. Voluntary patients and parents requesting voluntary admission of a minor may incorrectly believe that they are permitted to be discharged immediately after they request it. Explain that they must request discharge in writing and that the physician has an option to convert them to involuntary status.

EVALUATION AND MANAGEMENT

1. Is the patient dangerous (for example, suicidal or homicidal)? Suicidal patients must be admitted to prevent a suicide attempt if outpatient care is not feasible. Some suicidal patients may continue to be actively suicidal even in the hospital and may require constant or one-to-one observation. Homicidal patients may also be admitted, but a mental illness and an indication for treatment should be present. Some homicidal persons are appropriately referred to the police if no treatable mental illness is detected. If a homicidal patient is not admitted or otherwise detained, the clinician has a duty to warn and protect the intended victim.
2. Does the patient have a mental illness and does the mental illness warrant inpatient treatment? Would manipulation of the environment, referral to outpatient treatment, medication, crisis intervention, or family therapy reduce the need for hospitalization?
3. Does the patient have a first-episode psychosis? First-episode psychoses generally require inpatient evaluation and treatment.
4. Is hospitalization the appropriate treatment? Some patients, including those with borderline personality disorder, may become dependent on the hospital and regress when admitted. During crises they may require admission, but hospitaliza-

tion should be avoided if possible. Instead, devising a long-term treatment plan in cooperation with the outpatient therapist is preferable.

5. Does the patient have sufficient supports if not hospitalized? The supports may include family, friends, the community, a church, and mental health providers.
6. How will the patient perceive not being hospitalized? If a patient has requested hospitalization, will not admitting the patient result in feelings of neglect and abandonment? Will a minor suicide gesture escalate to a dangerous attempt?
7. How will hospitalization affect the patient's work or school functioning? Hospitalization that creates absence from work or school may cause more problems.
8. Are family, friends, and hospital records available as sources of history? Clinicians are often faced with the difficult decision of whether to hospitalize with only limited data. Collateral sources of history can provide information crucial to making the most appropriate decision.
9. Is the patient medically ill? The physician must be careful not to hospitalize patients on a psychiatry unit if they have medical problems that cannot be managed adequately. In some cases the medical or surgical problem may be responsible for the psychiatric presentation. Some patients may require admission to a medical or surgical unit, with follow up by the psychiatric consultation service.

DRUG TREATMENT

If the patient is violent, an antipsychotic or antianxiety agent may be used. In most situations medication can be withheld until the patient has been admitted and has been more thoroughly evaluated as an inpatient.

For a more detailed discussion of this topic, see B J Fauman: Other Psychiatric Emergencies, Sec 30.2, p 1752; L J Kiser, J D Heston, D B Pruitt: Partial Hospitalization, Sec 46.4, p 2428; M J Stuber: Children's Reaction to Illness, Hospitalization, and Surgery, Sec 47.4, p 2469, in CTP/VI.

19.10. Impending Death of Psychogenic Origin

Medically healthy people can die from overwhelming psychic stress. One proposed mechanism is that severe anxiety leads to massive central nervous system (CNS) autonomic discharges, which cause ventricular fibrillation. Another proposed mechanism is that the severe stress causes a shutdown of the hypothalamic-pituitary-adrenal axis, leading to shock and changes in the immune system. A patient who has suffered a major loss may become so hopeless that the will to live is lost.

CLINICAL FEATURES AND DIAGNOSIS

In voodoo cultures the effectiveness of a death curse is related to whether the intended victim believes in the power of the curse. The belief that one will die because of a curse may be enough to cause voodoo death. Patients may be dehydrated or in a state of starvation. Arrhythmias may be present.

INTERVIEWING AND PSYCHOTHERAPEUTIC GUIDELINES

Rapidly intervene with cognitive approaches. Involve the patient's family, or use other culturally appropriate interventions. Attempt to relieve or remove the stressor. Persons with cardiac arrhythmias should be advised to prepare themselves in advance for stressful situations and to anticipate anxiety-provoking events.

EVALUATION AND MANAGEMENT

When voodoo is involved, try to call on another person who is believed to have psychic powers to break the death curse. Patients with cardiac arrhythmias should be seen by the cardiologist in the emergency room. If impending death is not related to voodoo, try to identify other stressful life events.

DRUG TREATMENT

No specific drug treatment is indicated, but severe anxiety may be treated with benzodiazepines.

Patients with known cardiac disease may benefit from agents that raise the electrical threshold of the heart or prevent a rapid heart rate. A cardiologist should be consulted.

For a more detailed discussion of this topic, see J E Mezzich, K-M Lin: Acute and Transient Psychotic Disorders and Culture-Bound Syndromes, Sec 15.3, p 1049; F G Guggenheim, G R Smith: Somatoform Disorders, Chap 18, p 1251, in CTP/VI.

19.11. Jaundice

Jaundice (also called icterus) is a yellow pigmentation of the skin caused by deposits of bilirubin. Although it is a rare drug side effect, primary care physicians may see patients with jaundice associated with antipsychotic treatment.

CLINICAL FEATURES AND DIAGNOSIS

Jaundice may be detected as yellowing of the sclera or as darkening of the urine. In patients who are taking chlorpromazine (Thorazine), another phenothiazine, or a cyclic antidepressant, obstructive jaundice may be an allergic reaction to the drug.

Some phenothiazines reported to cause jaundice include chlorpromazine, thioridazine (Mellaril), prochlorperazine (Compazine), and fluphenazine (Prolixin). Nonphenothiazine antipsychotics, such as haloperidol (Haldol), have not been associated with jaundice.

Jaundice develops during the first month of drug treatment and is often preceded by a flulike syndrome. The liver is not inflamed, and liver function tests indicate a cholestatic type of jaundice (increased direct-indirect bilirubin ratio, increased alkaline phosphatase, and absence of prominent elevation of serum glutamic-oxaloacetic transaminase [SGOT] and serum glutamic-pyruvic transaminase [SGPT]). The syndrome usually resolves after several weeks, but it can in rare cases have a long-term course.

INTERVIEWING AND PSYCHOTHERAPEUTIC GUIDELINES

Reassure the patient that the symptom is probably a drug side effect, that it will resolve within a few weeks, and that a complete return to normal is expected.

EVALUATION AND MANAGEMENT

1. Consider other causes of jaundice, such as hepatitis. Perform a physical examination, including the liver. Obtain blood tests, including a complete blood count (CBC), and liver function tests. The CBC often shows eosinophilia in chlorpromazine-induced jaundice.
2. Check the result of the baseline liver function tests if they are available.
3. Discontinue the drug causing jaundice. Patients with jaundice should avoid alcohol.

DRUG TREATMENT

If the patient still requires medication for a psychiatric condition, consider changing to a different drug. Nonphenothiazine antipsychotic may be substituted for phenothiazines. Jaundice requires no specific treatment.

For a more detailed discussion of this topic, see M A Schuckit: Alcohol-Related Disorders, Sec 13.2, p.775; A A Lipton, R Cancro: Schizophrenia: Clinical Features, Sec 14.7, p 968, in CTP/VI.

19.12. Leukopenia and Agranulocytosis

Both leukopenia and agranulocytosis are characterized by a decreased number of white blood cells (WBC) in the peripheral blood. *Leukopenia* is defined as fewer than 3,500 WBC per cubic millimeter, with a granulocyte count of fewer than 1,500 per cubic millimeter (granulocytopenia). *Agranulocytosis* is defined as fewer than 500 granulocytes per cubic millimeter.

CLINICAL FEATURES AND DIAGNOSIS

Leukopenia is a relatively common and benign side effect of drugs, but agranulocytosis is potentially fatal, as the patient is vulnerable to bacterial infection. Patients taking psychotropic drugs in whom leukopenia develops should be monitored closely by the primary care physician for continued decrease in the WBC count that can lead to agranulocytosis.

Drugs that can cause leukopenia and agranulocytosis include antipsychotics, tricyclic antidepressants, and carbamazepine (Tegretol). The usually clinically benign pattern of many patients taking those drugs is to have an initial WBC drop to between 3,500 and 5,000 followed by WBC fluctuation.

Drug-induced leukopenia and agranulocytosis usually resolve after the causative drug has been discontinued. The key objective is to identify the problem early, before infections overcome the patient. Often, patients with agranulocytosis present with high fever and are severely ill with pharyngitis and oral or perianal ulcerations. In those patients the offending drug must be discontinued.

Phenothiazines

Between 5 and 15 percent of patients treated with phenothiazines experience leukopenia, which is usually benign but requires monitoring. About 1 of every 1,000 patients taking phenothiazines have agranulocytosis. The risk is greatest for the elderly and for women. Phenothiazine-induced agranulocytosis usually occurs in the first three to five weeks of treatment, and 90 percent of cases occur in the first eight weeks.

Clozapine

Agranulocytosis induced by clozapine (Clozaril) is not related to the dosage or to the patient's age. It is rare in the first four weeks of treatment and is most likely to occur between the 5th and the 25th week of treatment. Therefore, a four-week trial of clozapine presents only a minimal risk of agranulocytosis. Only patients who are improving should be continued into the period of increased risk. Patients taking clozapine should have their WBC measured weekly, even if they have no leukopenia.

INTERVIEWING AND PSYCHOTHERAPEUTIC GUIDELINES

Patients with possible leukopenia or agranulocytosis must understand that those conditions are potentially dangerous side effects of their medications. Encourage them to seek medical attention and to have a complete blood count (CBC) for even minor infections, such as a cold. Do not allow the patients to minimize the significance of the problem. Engage the patient's family members, if necessary, to ensure cooperation with medical follow-up.

EVALUATION AND MANAGEMENT

1. If the WBC falls below 3,500, follow the WBC with a differential white blood cell count three times a week.
2. Monitor the patient closely for signs of infection. Check the CBC in any antipsychotic-treated patient who has a fever or a sore throat during the first eight weeks of treatment (the period when the effect usually occurs with phenothiazines).

3. In cases of leukopenia, immediately discontinue clozapine and other drugs. Usually, leukopenia does not progress to agranulocytosis.
4. Refer to a hematologist. Bone marrow biopsy may help if the cause of the agranulocytosis is unclear or if it continues after the offending drug has been discontinued.
5. If the WBC falls below 1,000 or if the granulocytes count falls below 500, protect the patient from infection in reverse isolation.

DRUG TREATMENT

Use antibiotics to treat the infections as indicated by culture and sensitivity results. Institute other supportive treatment as necessary. If drug treatment is absolutely necessary for behavioral control, use a short-acting benzodiazepine—for example, lorazepam (Ativan) 1 to 2 mg by mouth or intramuscularly (IM), oxazepam (Serax) 10 to 30 mg by mouth, or alprazolam (Xanax) 0.5 to 1 mg by mouth, all given every four hours as needed.

For a more detailed discussion of this topic, see A A Lipton, R Cancro: Schizophrenia: Clinical Features, Sec 14.7, p 968, in CTP/VI.

19.13. Nocturia

Nocturia is excessive urination at night.

CLINICAL FEATURES AND DIAGNOSIS

Nocturia can be caused by any medical condition in which urinary output exceeds bladder capacity and by some psychiatric and neurological conditions. Any medical condition that can cause polyuria can cause nocturia, including diabetes mellitus, diabetes insipidus (including lithium-induced nephrogenic diabetes insipidus), primary polydipsia (excessive water drinking), drugs (for example, diuretics), and many types of renal disease. Polyuria that is not due to excessive water intake implies impaired renal-concentrating ability. Seizure disorders can cause nighttime incontinence.

INTERVIEWING AND PSYCHOTHERAPEUTIC GUIDELINES

The two most important clinical objectives are to identify the possible presence of renal disease and to determine if primary polydipsia is the cause of the polyuria. Patients who voluntarily drink excessive amounts of water daily may be difficult to differentiate from patients with diabetes insipidus. The primary care physician should explain to the patient that this condition is treatable.

EVALUATION AND MANAGEMENT

1. Laboratory tests should be ordered, including routine urinalysis, urine osmolality, blood chemistries, complete blood count, serum osmolality, thyroid function tests, electrocardiogram, and electroencephalogram.
2. The drugs the patient is taking should be identified. Lithium (Eskalith), phenytoin (Dilantin), and propoxyphene (Darvon) can cause nephrogenic diabetes insipidus.
3. Order a complete psychiatric evaluation of patients in whom a clear medical cause is not identified. Primary polydipsia may be a sign of a psychotic disorder (for example, certain schizophrenic patients suffer from water intoxication), obsessive-compulsive disorder, or an organic disorder.
4. The patient should be advised to stop drinking anything four hours before bedtime if nocturia is due to excessive nocturnal fluid intake.

DRUG TREATMENT

No specific drug treatment exists. Some patients benefit from imipramine (Tofranil) 50 to 100 mg at bedtime because of its anticholinergic side effects.

For a more detailed discussion of this topic, see E D Caine, H Grossman, J M Lyness: Delirium, Dementia, and Amnestic and Other Cognitive Disorders and Mental Disorders Due to a General Medical Condition, Chap 12, p 705; Substance-Related Disorders, Chap 13, pp 755–887, in CTP/VI.

19.14. Photosensitivity

Photosensitivity is characterized by easy and sometimes severe sunburning that occurs as a side effect of antipsychotic medication (dopamine receptor antagonists, most commonly phenothiazines). It is reportedly most common with low-potency antipsychotics, although high-potency antipsychotics have also been implicated.

CLINICAL FEATURES AND DIAGNOSIS

The proper medical term is "cutaneous photosensitivity," which is subdivided into phototoxic reactions and photoallergic reactions. Phenothiazine-induced photo-sensitivity is phototoxic and can occur after only several minutes of exposure to bright, direct sunlight; it does not require previous exposure to the sun (as is necessary for photoallergic reactions). Maculopapular, urticarial, edematous, and petechial lesions can develop with sufficient skin concentration of the drug and appropriate wavelengths of ultraviolet light (290 to 400 nm).

A gray-blue hyperpigmentation in patients taking a phenothiazine can develop in areas often exposed to sunlight. That skin hyperpigmentation is sometimes associated with eye changes, described as brown granular deposits in the anterior lens and posterior cornea, that do not impair vision. Those eye changes are usually found only in patients who have taken high dosages of chlorpromazine (Thorazine) for many years. The eye changes are unrelated to the retinitis pigmentosa that can be caused by high dosages of thioridazine (Mellaril) (see Section 19.15) and that can lead to blindness. Dosages of thioridazine of more than 800 mg a day should be avoided.

INTERVIEWING AND PSYCHOTHERAPEUTIC GUIDELINES

The primary care physician should educate patients that the skin effects are an interaction of the antipsychotic medication and exposure to sunlight. Patients should be advised to avoid the sun if they are taking these drugs.

EVALUATION AND MANAGEMENT

1. Other possible causes of erythema (contact dermatitis, for example) should be considered.
2. The patient's exposure to the sun should be minimized.
3. Treat sunburn if present.
4. It is important to consult a dermatologist if symptoms do not clear.
5. If possible, change to a nonphenothiazine antipsychotic drug.

DRUG TREATMENT

Sunscreens with a high sun protection factor (SPF) should be used. Local dermatological treatment and systemic analgesics or anti-inflammatory drugs may increase the patient's comfort. However, the phenothiazine-induced photosensitivity reaction may not be prostaglandin-mediated, so anti-inflammatory drugs that inhibit prostaglandin synthesis—for example, indomethacin (Indocin)—may not be effective in reducing the erythema.

For a more detailed discussion of this topic, see F G Guggenheim, G R Smith: Somatoform Disorders, Chap 18, p 1251; B J Fauman: Other Psychiatric Emergencies, Sec 30.2, p 1752, in CTP/VI.

19.15. Pigmentary Retinopathy

Pigmentary retinopathy is characterized by retinal infiltrations. It is similar to retinitis pigmentosa and can be caused by the long-term use of thioridazine (Mellaril) at dosages of 1,600 mg a day or higher.

CLINICAL FEATURES AND DIAGNOSIS

An ophthalmological examination reveals retinal pigmentation and visual impairment in a patient who has been taking thioridazine for a long time.

Thioridazine can conjugate with the melanin of the pigment layer of the retina, resulting in degeneration of the outer layers of the retina and leading to impaired vision or even blindness. The condition may not resolve even after the drug is discontinued. Patients who have been taking thioridazine at dosages greater than 800 mg a day should be evaluated by an ophthalmologist. Complaints of impaired vision in patients taking thioridazine must be thoroughly evaluated.

INTERVIEWING AND PSYCHOTHERAPEUTIC GUIDELINES

Educating the patient is the priority. Make the patient aware that pigmentary retinopathy is a potential side effect of thioridazine and is dose-related. Most patients with the problem have either chronic psychotic disorders (for example, schizophrenia and schizoaffective disorder) or chronic behavioral problems (for example, agitation associated with dementia of the Alzheimer's type and other organic disorders).

The primary care physician should emphasize the clinical benefits of thioridazine, and discuss possible alternatives, such as other antipsychotics. The patient should be informed that all antipsychotics have some side effects in addition to their desired clinical effects.

EVALUATION AND MANAGEMENT

1. Request an ophthalmology consultation.
2. Early pigmentary retinopathy can be best detected by using small colored objects to test the patient's central visual field.

DRUG TREATMENT

Thioridazine should be discontinued or the dosage lowered. If antipsychotics are still needed, consider changing to an antipsychotic of a different class. In general, thioridazine should not be used at dosages greater than 800 mg a day.

For a more detailed discussion of this topic, see F G Guggenheim, G R Smith: Somatoform Disorders, Chap 18, p 1251, in CTP/VI.

19.16. Pregnancy

Pregnancy is the condition that exists from conception until the birth of the baby.

CLINICAL FEATURES AND DIAGNOSIS

The diagnosis can be obtained from the patient's history and physical examination. In early or doubtful cases, the diagnosis can be confirmed or ruled out by urine and blood pregnancy tests. The blood test—human chorionic gonadotropin (HCG)—is more sensitive than the urine test, but it is also more expensive and takes longer.

Pregnancy is always a significant stress to both the prospective mother and her family. Many factors can increase the stressfulness of the situation, including pregnancy as the result of rape or incest, teenage pregnancy, pregnancy in families with insufficient resources, alcohol or drug dependence in the expectant mother, pregnancy in the context of marital conflict, and other adverse environmental conditions.

INTERVIEWING AND PSYCHOTHERAPEUTIC GUIDELINES

Reactions to the pregnancy can vary, depending on the circumstances and the psychological makeup of the patient and her family members. Cultural factors have great influence on reactions to pregnancy and should be considered during evaluation. It should be determined whether the patient's family members and her friends from the same culture feel that her thoughts and behavior are abnormal. The physician's cultural beliefs, values, or judgments should not be imposed on the patient, whose reactions should be explored and understood.

EVALUATION AND MANAGEMENT

1. In teenage pregnancy the patient may want an abortion while the patient's parents do not. In general, crisis-intervention approaches should be used to try to negotiate an agreement between the patient and her parents. When no agreement is possible, most states consider the teenager capable of making her own informed decision and do not allow the parents to prevent the abortion.
2. In pregnancy caused by rape or incest, abortion is frequently recommended. Victims of rape and incest require psychiatric evaluation and treatment.
3. Heavy alcohol use during pregnancy has been associated with low birth weight (although cigarette smoking confounds that finding) and fetal alcohol syndrome. The safe level of alcohol consumption during pregnancy is not known, so alcohol should be avoided completely during pregnancy.
4. The use of illicit drugs during pregnancy has a wide range of deleterious effects on the fetus and the newborn. Those effects include dependence on and withdrawal from opioids, sedative-hypnotics, and cocaine. Opioid withdrawal in pregnancy can lead to a miscarriage. If opioid withdrawal is planned during pregnancy, it is safest during the second trimester. Methadone and probably other opioids used during pregnancy have been associated with intellectual development problems in the child. Cocaine use may cause spontaneous abortion during early pregnancy and premature labor during late pregnancy.
5. False pregnancy (also called pseudocyesis and hysterical pregnancy) is the presence of the physical symptoms of pregnancy—including abdominal distention, the cessation of the menses, nausea, breast enlargement and hyperpigmentation, and sometimes even labor—in a patient who is not pregnant. The patient believes that she is pregnant. Sometimes, a negative pregnancy test convinces the woman, but often the patient is seriously ill and requires extensive treatment, primarily psychotherapy that explores the psychological need to be pregnant.
6. Most obstetricians permit sexual intercourse during pregnancy until the last four or five weeks antepartum.

DRUG TREATMENT

Drug treatment should be avoided unless the patient is clearly psychotic, unmanageable, and a danger to herself, her baby, or others. In those cases a high-potency antipsychotic—for example, fluphenazine (Prolixin) or haloperidol (Haldol), both given at 0.5 to 2 mg by mouth or intramuscularly (IM) as needed—may be used.

The approach to take with medications is to compare the risk to the fetus of giving the medication with the risk to the mother of not giving the medication. In general, medications should not be given during pregnancy, since they can be teratogenic or cause other toxic effects to the fetus or the newborn by passing across the placenta or into the breast milk. The two most teratogenic drugs in the psychopharmacopeia are lithium and anticonvulsants. Lithium administration during pregnancy is associated with a high incidence of birth abnormalities, including Ebstein's malformation, a serious abnormality in cardiac development. Other psychoactive drugs (antidepressants, antipsychotics, and anxiolytics), although less clearly associated with birth defects, should also be avoided during pregnancy if possible.

For a more detailed discussion of this topic, see S L Berga, B L Parry: Psychiatry and Reproductive Medicine, Sec 29.4, p 1693, in CTP/VI.

19.17. Restraints

The physical restraint of patients may be necessary to prevent violence.

CLINICAL FEATURES AND DIAGNOSIS

Impending violence requires immediate intervention. Patients who are agitated, threatening violence, so severely disorganized that there is a risk of injury, or attempting to injure themselves must be restrained if they are not amenable to verbal intervention.

Physical restraint is important, useful, and often necessary. Although the experience can be humiliating, frustrating, and confusing for the patient, the stress is only temporary. The consequences of uncontained violence may be irreversible. Many patients feel more in control after they have been restrained and know that clear limits to their behavior are imposed.

INTERVIEWING AND PSYCHOTHERAPEUTIC GUIDELINES

The patient should always be offered a chance to stop the behavior that is leading to potential restraint. The patient should be authoritatively directed to stop the behavior. It is important to provide a quiet space alone (under visual observation) where the patient can try to calm down. It should be repeatedly explained that the continued behavior will lead to physical restraint. The patient should be offered an opportunity to take medication that may avoid the necessity of physical restraint. However, there should be no negotiation with the patient. Specific behaviors that

TABLE 19.17–1
USE OF RESTRAINTS

1. Preferably five or a minimum of four persons should be used to restrain the patient. Leather restraints are the safest and the surest type of restraints.
2. Explain to the patient why he or she is going into restraints.
3. A staff member should always be visible and reassuring the patient who is being restrained to help alleviate the patient's fear of helplessness, impotence, and loss of control.
4. Patients should be restrained with legs spread-eagled and one arm restrained to one side and the other arm restrained over the patient's head.
5. Restraints should be placed so that intravenous fluids can be given if necessary.
6. The patient's head is raised slightly to decrease the patient's feelings of vulnerability and to reduce the possibility of aspiration.
7. The restraints should be checked periodically for safety and comfort.
8. After the patient is in restraints, the clinician begins treatment, using verbal intervention.
9. Even in restraints, a majority of patients still take antipsychotic medication in concentrated form.
10. After the patient is under control, one restraint at a time should be removed at five-minute intervals until the patient has only two restraints on. Both of the remaining restraints should be removed at the same time, because it is inadvisable to keep a patient in only one restraint.
11. Always thoroughly document the reason for the restraints, the course of treatment, and the patient's response to treatment while in restraints.

Table data from W R Dubin, K J Weiss: Emergency psychiatry. In *Psychiatry*, vol 2, R Michaels, J O Cavenar, H K H Brodie, A M Cooper, S B Guze, L L Judd, G L Klerman, A J Skolnit, editors, p 9. Lippincott, Philadelphia, 1987. Used with permission.

warrant physical restraint should be identified, and, if they continue, restraint should proceed. The patient should not feel that there is any doubt regarding what interventions are necessary.

EVALUATION AND MANAGEMENT

1. Physical restraint should be left to those who are specifically trained to do it. Applying physical restraints is among the most hazardous of activities in mental health care. Improper restraint can lead to the injury of a staff member or the patient and even to patient death.
2. A sufficient number of staff members should be available to safely restrain the patient. If physical restraint is a possibility, sufficient staff members should be called in early. Having an excess number of staff members waiting in the area is better than to have insufficient staff members at the moment that restraint is required. Sometimes, simply the presence of several staff members and the perception that restraint is inevitable produce a change in the patient's behavior.
3. A chemical restraint should be offered before carrying out physical restraint.
4. In choosing a restraint, using a type with which the staff members have been trained and are familiar is important. The improper use of restraints can lead to injury. Restraint of only one limb should be avoided, since thrashing can cause a sprain or a fracture in the patient (Table 19.17-1).
5. Once the patient is restrained, medication should be offered again if the patient has not yet complied. Patients who remain agitated in restraints should be medicated until they are calm.
6. The patient's vital signs must be monitored every half hour while the patient is in restraints.
7. Reevaluate the need for restraints by an objective assessment of the patient's behavior as frequently as possible, preferably every 15 to 30 minutes.
8. Document the reasons for placing the patient in restraints.

DRUG TREATMENT

The vast majority of patients who require physical restraint benefit from medication that can provide chemical restraint and may reduce the need for physical restraint. It is probably more distressing to the patient to be physically subdued than to receive an injection. The three classes of drugs used most often are antipsychotics, benzodiazepines, and barbiturates. All can provide rapid behavioral control.

The choice of drug is based on what medication (if any) the patient is already taking, the drug's undesirable side effects, the patient's concomitant medical problems and other contraindications, and the availability of parenteral preparations for intramuscular (IM) administration. Drug dependence is a relative contraindication for benzodiazepines and barbiturates, since the dosages of those drugs required for dependent patients may be high and their use may lead to continued abuse. The presence of psychosis supports the use of antipsychotics, although the desired effect is immediate tranquilization, rather than a true antipsychotic effect, which takes days to weeks.

Most restrained patients comply with the oral administration of a liquid medication, but an IM injection is usually effective more rapidly.

If a patient is taking an antipsychotic drug, an additional dose of that drug should be given—for example, haloperidol (Haldol) 5 mg IM or 10 mg by mouth, perphenazine (Trilafon) 5 mg IM or 8 mg by mouth, or chlorpromazine (Thorazine) 10 to 25 mg IM or 50 to 100 mg by mouth. If the patient is taking an antipsychotic drug for which there is no parenteral form available—for example, thioridazine (Mellaril)—use the most similar available drug, such as chlorpromazine.

Benzodiazepines and barbiturates are alternatives to antipsychotics. Since most of the drugs are equally effective, the choice is often based on what is the most rapidly and conveniently available parenteral form. Commonly used drugs include lorazepam (Ativan) 1 to 2 mg IM or by mouth and amobarbital (Amytal) 250 mg IM or by mouth. Benzodiazepines are also used with patients taking antipsychotics as a short-term antipsychotic augmentation to avoid escalating the antipsychotic dose simply to provide behavioral control.

For a more detailed discussion of this topic, see K Tardiff: Adult Antisocial Behavior and Criminality, Sec 28.3, p 1622; B J Fauman: Other Psychiatric Emergencies, Sec 30.2, p 1752; T G Gutheil: Legal Issues in Psychiatry, Sec 52.1, p 2747, in CTP/VI.

19.18. Seclusion

Seclusion is the isolation of a patient in an environment of low stimulation. Seclusion may or may not include locking the door of the room.

CLINICAL FEATURES AND DIAGNOSIS

The indications for seclusion are similar to those for restraints but are less severe. The indications include potential assault, self-injurious behavior, and disorganization to the point of risking self-harm. Seclusion, quiet time, or time out is often an effective alternative to physical restraints and injection with a tranquilizing medication. Many agitated patients, if removed from a stimulating environment that may be provocative, can regain behavioral control of themselves. The isolation provides an opportunity for self-reflection in a low-stimulation environment.

Seclusion rooms must be as safe as possible. Remove any potentially dangerous objects from both the patient and the room, and keep the patient under observation.

INTERVIEWING AND PSYCHOTHERAPEUTIC GUIDELINES

In restraint, limits are externally imposed on patients; in contrast, the objective of seclusion is to give patients the opportunity to regain composure themselves.

Before secluding a patient, the behavior that may lead to seclusion should be as specifically as possible described, providing the patient an opportunity to stop the behavior and avoid being secluded. It is necessary that the patient feels they have any ally who is helping prevent seclusion, but it should be indicated that, if the behavior continues, seclusion is inevitable.

If the dangerous behavior does continue, repeated fair warnings should be given that seclusion may be necessary. The patient should be told that seclusion will be required for a limited time until the behavior has ceased.

It is important to be firm, set clear limits, and prevent escalation of the dangerous behavior. If appropriate, medication should be offered that may improve the patient's behavioral control and avoid the need for seclusion or restraints.

EVALUATION AND MANAGEMENT

1. Behaviors that may lead to seclusion or restraints should be identified.
2. The patient should be informed clearly that the behaviors must stop; otherwise, seclusion will be necessary.
3. Enough staff members should be available to enforce seclusion if needed.
4. If the dangerous or disruptive behavior continues, insist that the patient go into the quiet room, possibly with the door open or unlocked. If necessary, the patient may be physically forced into the seclusion room, and the door may be locked.
5. Any items from the patient that could be used to injure self or others (for example, sharp objects) should be removed.
6. The patient should be checked at least every 15 minutes and given regular and predictable opportunities to show behavioral control to obtain release from seclusion. The patient should be encouraged to comply.
7. If agitation or violence persists while the patient is in seclusion (for example, head banging, punching walls, kicking the door), physical restraints or chemical restraint with an injection of tranquilizing medication may be necessary.
8. It is important to document clearly and justify the use of seclusion in the medical record.

DRUG TREATMENT

Seclusion may or may not be used in conjunction with pharmacological agents. If drugs are used, the patient must be checked frequently (at least every 15 minutes) for adverse drug effects.

For a more detailed discussion of this topic, see K Tardiff: Adult Antisocial Behavior and Criminality, Sec 28.3, p 1622; T G Gutheil: Legal Issues in Psychiatry, Sec 52.1, p 2747, in CTP/VI.

19.19. Serotonin Syndrome

Serotonin syndrome is a potentially fatal toxic reaction that occurs when monoamine oxidase inhibitors (MAOIs) are coadministered with serotonergic psychotropic agents such as clomipramine (Anafranil), fluoxetine (Prozac), and tryptophan. It may also be seen with overdoses of MAOIs.

CLINICAL FEATURES AND DIAGNOSIS

The diagnosis of serotonin syndrome is based on a history of the ingestion of the offending drug combinations and the production of the characteristic signs and symptoms, including hyperthermia, diaphoresis, excitement, rigidity, hyperreflexia, hypotension, headache, tremor, confusion, coma, and death.

The risk of the reaction's occurring in combination with MAOIs is thought to be related to the non-MAOIs' degree of serotonergicity. Therefore, clomipramine and tryptophan are at high risk of causing the syndrome in combination with MAOIs. Serotonin-specific reuptake inhibitors also cause serotonin syndrome in combination with MAOIs.

Reactions can occur even if MAOIs are started several weeks after discontinuing serotonergic agents.

Patients have recovered spontaneously on discontinuation of the psychotropics involved; however, serious medical complications—including disseminated intravascular coagulation, rhabdomyolysis, and death—have occurred.

Tyramine reactions and neuroleptic malignant syndrome should be considered in the differential diagnosis. A history of antipsychotic drug intake and no history of serotonergic drug intake should indicate neuroleptic malignant syndrome, rather than serotonin syndrome.

INTERVIEWING AND PSYCHOTHERAPEUTIC GUIDELINES

The patients require prompt medical treatment. Therefore, keep the interview brief and medically oriented. Obtain a history of the patient's ingestion of the agents that can produce the syndrome. Reassure the patient that recovery is likely within days to weeks.

EVALUATION AND MANAGEMENT

1. Obtain the patient's vital signs.
2. Perform a full medical workup.
3. Discontinue the offending agents.
4. Give the patient supportive and symptomatic medical care.

DRUG TREATMENT

No specific drug treatment is indicated. Medical complications should be treated symptomatically. Avoid offending drug combinations. Intravenous dantrolene (Dantrium) or oral cyproheptadine (Periactin) may be useful in treating serotonin syndrome due to the combination of MAOIs and serotonergic agents.

For a more detailed discussion of this topic, see J A Grebb: Medication-Induced Movement Disorders, Sec 32.2, p 1909, in CTP/VI.

19.20. Terminal Illness

Terminal illness is not simply a biological event leading to death; it involves a complex psychological process of adaptation that varies among individual patients and cultures. Reactions to having a terminal illness may be measured or extreme. Common reactions to a serious, potentially fatal diagnosis include numbness, frank disbelief, and diffuse anger. Healthy responses, reflecting some degree of acceptance, include sadness and fear. The most worrisome initial manifestation is the lack of an emotional response.

CLINICAL FEATURES AND DIAGNOSIS

In general, people die as they have lived. Frank psychopathology in reaction to having a terminal illness is relatively rare. Most adults have developed the psychic apparatus necessary to cope with the stress of dying.

Cognitive equilibrium is maintained by subdividing the process of dying into components, putting things into a favorable perspective, and temporarily minimizing the consequences. Denial is used constructively in that phase. Catastrophic fantasies may be reassessed and better intermediate situations discovered by seeking information, adopting a concrete problem-solving approach, and finding meaningful, realistic, alternative short-term goals.

Affective equilibrium is maintained by suppressing the emotions, ventilating, seeking the support of others, and, eventually, accepting reality. The natural consequence of the process is bereavement. Insomnia, appetite disturbances, anxiety, and a depressed mood are common at some points in the process.

Although psychiatric symptoms are present, a psychiatric diagnosis is not reached unless the patient shows both distress and impairments in function. The patient should be assessed for suicidal ideation, and a thorough psychiatric evaluation should be conducted.

INTERVIEWING AND PSYCHOTHERAPEUTIC GUIDELINES

The primary care physician should show respect for the patient's mind and spirit and care for the patient's body. The patient should be allowed to be the executive decision maker. Educating the patient eases the decision-making process. Most decisions can be anticipated and options presented in advance, while the patient is in the best frame of mind.

At some point, the patient's family should be involved, giving them emotional and physical support is important.

The primary care physician should avoid making the patient's important decisions. Some states now provide a process by which patients may document their treatment wishes and may designate an alternate decision maker.

EVALUATION AND MANAGEMENT

1. Patients should be provided with accurate and appropriate data.
2. Allow patients to ventilate their fears and reassure them that they will not be abandoned.
3. Patients' priorities should be ascertained, deferring to the patients' definitions of quality of life.
4. It is necessary that patients be helped to maintain hope.
5. At some point, the transition should be made from a primary objective of curing to caring. Palliation may be more appropriate than aggressive treatment.
6. Overly zealous treatment should be avoided, especially if the treatment conflicts with patients' or the family's wishes.
7. As death nears, and with it the specter of failure, the tendency of health care providers to withdraw should be avoided.

DRUG TREATMENT

The terminally ill must always be kept free from disabling pain; the liberal use of narcotic preparations is strongly encouraged. The phase of coping with a catastrophic condition is one of the few clear indications for sedatives. Family members, particularly spouses, may also be severely affected, and, given the importance of family members in supporting the patient, hypnotics may be appropriate. Dependence liability is low in that population. The short-acting benzodiazepines are probably best: lorazepam (Ativan) 0.5 to 1 mg by mouth one to three times a day and at bedtime, alprazolam (Xanax) 0.5 to 1 mg by mouth two times a day and at bedtime, or oxazepam (Serax) 10 to 30 mg by mouth two times a day and at bedtime. Using these medications in the early days or weeks can reduce the fear of loss of control while the patient and the family regroup.

For a more detailed discussion of this topic, see S Zisook: Death, Dying, and Bereavement, Sec 29.6, p 1713, in CTP/VI.

19.21. Tremor

Tremor is an involuntary oscillating movement of parts of the body (for example, the limbs or the head) that results from alternating contractions of opposing muscle groups.

CLINICAL FEATURES AND DIAGNOSIS

Fine tremors that occur at rest are typical of anxiety, fatigue, and toxic and metabolic disorders. Coarse tremors are seen in Parkinson's disease and cerebellar disease. Tremors may also be classified by the phase of movement. A static tremor is present when the limb is at complete rest, as in Parkinson's disease. An action tremor may be of the postural type, present while sustaining any posture and throughout movement, or the intention type, absent while sustaining any posture and during early movement but worsening when a target is approached.

The differential diagnosis of tremor is wide and includes a physiological variety, benign essential or familial tremor, and senile tremor. Other causes include anxiety, hyperthyroidism, caffeine, hallucinogens, stimulants, cocaine, opioid withdrawal, alcohol withdrawal, benzodiazepine withdrawal, and many psychotropic medications. Sedatives and alcohol may be used for anxiety and essential tremor, so those conditions may suddenly appear to be much worse during abstinence. Occasionally, a persistent movement disorder may be attributable to hallucinogen abuse in the distant past.

Lithium (Eskalith) can produce an action tremor of 7 to 16 cycles per second that is similar in appearance to essential tremor. Wilson's disease typically first manifests with tremor before progressing to athetoid movements. Cerebellar lesions caused by tumors, vascular and degenerative diseases, and multiple sclerosis result in intention tremors.

INTERVIEWING AND PSYCHOTHERAPEUTIC GUIDELINES

A medically oriented interview should be conducted, paying close attention to the patient's medication history. The patient should be reassured that treatment is often effective.

EVALUATION AND MANAGEMENT

1. Management begins with a thorough medical and psychiatric workup to resolve the differential diagnostic issues.
2. A neurological consultation may be needed.

DRUG TREATMENT

Drug treatment of tremor depends on the cause. Tremor caused by benzodiazepine withdrawal may require no specific treatment if the benzodiazepine was used in therapeutic dosages for weeks to months. If the drug was used in very high dosages for months or sometimes in therapeutic amounts for a period of years, seizures may result when it is withdrawn, and detoxification may be indicated. Drugs with a long half-life are less likely to be associated with an abstinence syndrome than drugs with a short half-life.

Tremor alone caused by alcohol withdrawal does not require alcohol detoxification, but a rapid pulse and other signs of withdrawal suggest an increased level of concern. Prophylactic thiamine and folate are always appropriate treatments.

Pseudoparkinsonism caused by antipsychotics is easily managed, if severe, with benztropine (Cogentin) 1 to 2 mg intramuscularly (IM). Oral administration of benztropine is almost as rapid as IM administration. Maintenance treatment with 1 to 6 mg a day in divided doses should then be continued. An alternative is diphenhydramine (Benadryl) 50 mg, which has the advantage of sedation.

Historically, sedatives have been used to treat tremor, but they have been replaced by the more effective, less abusable β-blockers, which may be used either intermittently for performance anxiety or continuously for essential tremor. Atenolol (Tenormin) 50 mg orally is often sufficient for episodic anxiety; atenolol 50 mg twice daily may be given if necessary. Lithium-induced tremor can be treated with β-blockers or with a reduction of the lithium dosage.

For a more detailed discussion of this topic, see J Yager, M H Gitlin: Clinical Manifestations of Psychiatric Disorders, Chap 10, p 637; E D Caine, H Grossman, J M Lyness: Delirium, Dementia, and Amnestic and Other Cognitive Disorders and Mental Disorders Due to a General Medical Condition, Chap 12, p 705; J A Grebb: Medication-Induced Movement Disorder, Sec 32.2, p 1909; J W Jefferson, J H Greist: Lithium, Sec 32.16, p 2022, in CTP/VI.

Area C

Treatment and Management

20
Basic Principles of Psychopharmacology

Our current understanding of the normal and disordered brain makes the drug treatment of psychiatric disorders a somewhat empirical practice. Nevertheless, many biological therapies have proved to be highly effective and constitute the treatment of choice for certain psychopathological conditions. As such, biological therapies form a key part of the armamentarium for the treatment of psychiatric disorders.

Drug therapy and other biological treatments of psychiatric disorders may be defined as an attempt to modify or correct pathological behaviors, thoughts, or moods by chemical or other physical means. The ability to correlate physical brain states to functional neural manifestations (behaviors, thoughts, and moods) is at the frontier of biological knowledge: it is both highly complex and imperfectly understood. What is well-known is that the various parameters of normal and abnormal behavior (for example, perception, affect, and cognition) may be profoundly affected by physical changes in the central nervous system (for example, cerebrovascular disorders, epilepsy, legal and illicit drugs).

Because the pharmacotherapy of psychiatric disorders is one of the most rapidly evolving areas in clinical medicine, any practitioner, especially the primary care physician, who prescribes such drugs must remain current with the research literature. The key areas for regular update are the emergence of new agents (for example, risperidone [Risperdal], tacrine [Cognex], and venlafaxine [Effexor]), the demonstration of new indications for existing agents (for example, naltrexone [ReVia], divalproex [Depakote]), the clinical usefulness of plasma concentrations, and the identification and treatment of drug-related adverse events.

The practice of pharmacotherapy in psychiatry should not be oversimplified to a one diagnosis-one pill approach. Drug selection, prescription, administration, psychodynamic meaning to the patient, and family and environmental influences all impinge on the practice of pharmacotherapy. Some patients may view a drug as a panacea, and other patients may see medication as an assault. The nursing staff and relatives, as well as the patient, must be instructed regarding the reasons, the expected benefits, the risks, and (sometimes) the theoretical basis of pharmacotherapy. Yet another critical factor to the success of drug treatment is the theoretical biases of the treating psychiatrist: every pharmacotherapeutic decision is a function of his or her theoretical beliefs about such treatments.

Drugs must be used in effective dosages for sufficient periods, as determined by previous clinical investigations and personal experience. Subtherapeutic doses and incomplete trials should not be given to a patient simply because the psychiatrist is excessively concerned about the development of adverse effects. The prescription of drugs for psychiatric disorders must be made by a qualified practitioner and requires continuous clinical observation of treatment response and the emergence of adverse effects. The dosage of the drug should be adjusted accordingly, and appropriate treatments for emergent adverse effects must be instituted as quickly as possible.

Chapter 21 lists the psychotherapeutic drugs according to the generic name, the trade name, and pharmacological category and lists the major drugs used in the various psychiatric disorders.

HISTORY

Biological therapies such as electroconvulsive therapy (ECT) (pioneered by Ugo Cerletti and Lucio Bini), insulin coma therapy (developed by Manfred Sakel), and psychosurgery (introduced by António Egas Moniz) all began in the first third of the 20th century and heralded the biological revolution in psychiatry. In 1917 Julius von Wagner-Jauregg introduced malaria toxin to treat syphilis and is the only psychiatrist to have won a Nobel prize.

In the second half of the 20th century, chemotherapy as a treatment for mental illness became a major field of research and practice. Almost immediately after the introduction of chlorpromazine (Thorazine) in the early 1950s, psychotherapeutic drugs became a mainstay of psychiatric treatment, particularly for the seriously mentally ill patient.

In 1949 the Australian psychiatrist John Cade described the treatment of manic excitement with lithium. While conducting animal experiments, Cade had somewhat incidentally noted that lithium carbonate made the animals lethargic, thus prompting him to administer the drug to several agitated psychiatric patients.

In 1950 Charpentier synthesized chlorpromazine (an aliphatic phenothiazine antipsychotic) in an attempt to develop an antihistaminergic drug that would serve as an adjuvant in anesthesia. H. Laborit reported the ability of the drug to induce an "artificial hibernation." Reports by Paraire and Sigwald, John Delay and Pierre Deniker, and Heinz Lehmann and Hanrahan described the effectiveness of chlorpromazine in treating severe agitation and psychosis. Chlorpromazine was quickly introduced into American psychiatry, and many similarly effective drugs have since been synthesized, including haloperidol (Haldol) (a butyrophenone antipsychotic) in 1958 by Paul Janssen.

Imipramine (Tofranil) (a tricyclic antidepressant) is structurally related to the phenothiazine antipsychotics. While carrying out clinical research on chlorpromazinelike drugs, Thomas Kuhn found that imipramine, although not very effective in reducing agitation, did seem to reduce depression in some patients. The introduction of monoamine oxidase inhibitors (MAOIs) to treat depression evolved from the observation that the antituberculosis agent iproniazid had mood-elevating effects in some patients. In 1958 Nathan Kline was one of the first investigators to report the efficacy of MAOI treatment in depressed psychiatric patients.

By 1960, with the introduction of chlordiazepoxide (Librium) (a benzodiazepine antianxiety agent synthesized by Richard Sternbach at the Roche laboratories in the late 1950s), the psychiatric drug armamentarium had grown to include antipsychotics, tricyclics, MAOIs, antidepressants, an antimanic agent (lithium [Eskalith]), and antianxiety agents (the new benzodiazepines in addition to the older drugs, such as the barbiturates). The next 30 years were devoted primarily to clinical studies demonstrating the efficacy of those drugs and to the development of related compounds in each category. The efficacy of each class of drugs for treating specific psychiatric syndromes and for explaining their pharmacodynamic effects provided the impetus to develop the various neurotransmitter hypotheses of mental disorders (for example, the dopamine hypothesis of schizophrenia, the monoamine hypothesis of mood disorders).

Since 1960 the major additions to the psychotherapeutic drugs have been the anticonvulsants, particularly carbamazepine (Tegretol) and valproate, which are effective in treating some patients with bipolar disorder. Buspirone (BuSpar), a nonbenzodiazepine anxiolytic, was introduced for clinical use in America in 1986. Several serotonin-specific reuptake inhibitors—for example, fluoxetine (Prozac)—and the serotonergic-specific tricyclic drug clomipramine (Anafranil) are effective in the treatment of depression and some anxiety disorders, including obsessive-compulsive disorder. The most recently introduced drugs include a dopamine receptor antagonist that may be associated with few neurological adverse effects (risperidone), the first drug for the treatment of cognitive decline in dementia of the Alzheimer's type (tacrine), and two new antidepressants, venlafaxine and nefazodone (Serzone), that may eventually be shown to have some therapeutic advantage over currently available drugs. The burgeoning knowledge of basic neuroscience and neuropharmacology is expected to lead to the development of many new psychotherapeutic drugs during the next decade.

PHARMACOLOGICAL ACTIONS

Pharmacokinetic interactions describe how the body handles a drug; pharmacodynamic interactions describe the effects of a drug on the body. In a parallel fashion pharmacokinetic drug interactions refer to plasma concentrations of drugs, and the pharmacodynamic drug interactions refer to receptor activities of drugs.

Pharmacokinetics

The principal divisions of pharmacokinetics are drug absorption, distribution, metabolism, and excretion.

Absorption.   A psychotherapeutic drug must first reach the blood on its way to the brain, unless it is directly administered into the cerebrospinal fluid or the brain. Orally administered drugs must dissolve in the fluid of the gastrointestinal (GI) tract before the body can absorb them. Drug tablets can be designed to disintegrate either quickly or slowly; the absorption depends on the drug's concentration and lipid solubility and the GI tract's local pH, motility, and surface area. Depending on the drug's pK and the GI tract's pH, the drug may be present in an ionized form that limits its lipid solubility. If the pharmacokinetic absorption factors are favorable, the drug may reach therapeutic blood concentrations more quickly if it is administered intramuscularly. If a drug is coupled with an appropriate carrier molecule, intramuscular administration can sustain the drug's release over a long period. Some antipsychotic drugs are available in depot forms that allow the drug to be administered only once every one to four weeks. Although intravenous administration is the quickest route to achieve therapeutic blood concentrations, it also carries the highest risk of sudden and life-threatening adverse effects.

Distribution.   Drugs can be freely dissolved in the blood plasma, bound to dissolved plasma proteins (primarily albumin), or dissolved within the blood cells. If a drug is bound too tightly to plasma proteins, it may have to be metabolized and excreted before it can leave the bloodstream, thus greatly reducing the amount of active drug reaching the brain. The lithium ion is an example of a water-soluble drug that is not bound to plasma proteins. The distribution of a drug to the brain is determined by the blood-brain barrier, the brain's regional blood flow, and the drug's affinity with its receptors in the brain. Both high blood flow and affinity favor the distribution of the drug to the brain. Drugs may also reach the brain after passively diffusing into the cerebrospinal fluid from the bloodstream. The volume of distribution is a measure of the apparent space in the body available to contain the drug. The volume of distribution can also vary with the patient's age, sex, and disease state.

Metabolism and Excretion.   The processes of metabolism and excretion metabolism are often called "biotransformation." The four major metabolic routes for drugs are oxidation, reduction, hydrolysis, and conjugation. Although the usual result of metabolism is to produce inactive metabolites that are more readily excreted than is the parent compound, many examples of active metabolites are produced from psychoactive drugs. The liver is the principal site of metabolism, and bile, feces, and urine are the major routes of excretion. Psychoactive drugs are also excreted in sweat, saliva, tears, and milk; therefore, mothers who are taking psychotherapeutic drugs should not breast-feed their children. Disease states or coadministered drugs that affect the ability of the liver or the kidneys to metabolize and eliminate drugs can both raise and lower the blood concentrations of a psychoactive drug.

Four important concepts regarding metabolism and excretion are time of peak plasma concentration, half-life, first pass effect, and clearance. The time between the administration of a drug and the appearance of the drug's *peak plasma concentrations* varies primarily according to the route of administration and absorption. A drug's *half-life* is the time it takes for one half of a drug's peak plasma concentration to be metabolized and excreted from the body. A general guideline is that, if a drug is administered repeatedly in doses separated by intervals shorter than its half-life, the drug will reach 97 percent of its steady-state plasma concentrations in a time equal to five times its half-life. The *first pass effect* refers to the extensive initial metabolism of some drugs within the portal circulation or liver, thereby reducing the amount of unmetabolized drug that reaches the systemic circulation. *Clearance* is a measure of the amount of drug excreted in each unit of time. If some disease process or other drug interferes with the clearance of a psychoactive drug, the drug may reach toxic concentrations.

Pharmacodynamics

The major pharmacodynamic considerations include the receptor mechanism; the dose-response curve; the therapeutic index; and the development of tolerance, dependence, and withdrawal phenomena.

The *receptor* for a drug can be defined generally as the cellular component that binds to the drug and initiates the drug's pharmacodynamic effects. A drug can be an agonist for its receptor, thereby stimulating a physiological effect; conversely, a drug can be an antagonist for the receptor, most often by blocking the receptor so that an endogenous agonist cannot affect the receptor. The receptor site for most psychotherapeutic drugs is also a receptor site for an endogenous neurotransmitter. For example, the primary receptor site for chlorpromazine is the dopamine receptor. However, for other psychotherapeutic drugs that may not be the case. The receptor for lithium may be the enzyme inositol-l-phosphatase, and the receptor for verapamil (Isoptin, Calan) is a calcium channel.

The *dose-response curve* plots the drug concentration against the effects of the drug (Figure 20–1). The potency of a drug refers to the relative dose required to achieve a certain effect. Haloperidol, for example, is more potent than chlorpromazine because approximately 5 mg of haloperidol is required to achieve the same therapeutic effect as 100 mg of chlorpromazine. Both haloperidol and chlorpromazine, however, are equal in their clinical efficacy—that is, the maximum clinical response achievable by the administration of a drug.

The side effects of most drugs are often a direct result of their primary pharmacodynamic effects and are better conceptualized as adverse effects. The *therapeutic index* is a relative measure of a drug's toxicity or safety. It is defined as the ratio of the median toxic dose (TD_{50}) to the median effective dose (ED_{50}). The TD_{50} is the dose at which 50 percent of patients experience toxic effects, and the ED_{50} is the dose at which 50 percent of patients have a therapeutic effect. Haloperidol, for

Examples of Dose-Response Curves

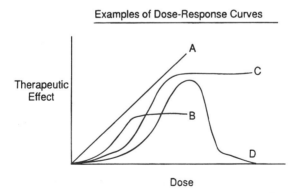

Figure 20–1. These dose-response curves plot the therapeutic effect as a function of increasing dose, often calculated as the log of the dose. Drug A has a linear dose response, drugs B and C have sigmoidal curves, and drug D has a curvilinear dose-response curve. Although smaller doses of drug B are more potent than are equal doses of drug C, drug C has a higher maximum efficacy than does drug B. Drug D has a therapeutic window, such that both low and high doses are less effective than are midrange doses.

example, has a very high therapeutic index, as evidenced by the wide range of doses in which it is prescribed. Conversely, lithium has a very low therapeutic index, thereby requiring careful monitoring of serum lithium concentrations when prescribing the drug. Both interindividual and intraindividual variation can be present in the response to a specific drug. An individual patient may be hyporeactive, normally reactive, or hyperreactive to a particular drug. For example, some patients with schizophrenia require 1 mg a day of haloperidol, others require a more typical 10 mg a day, and still others require 100 mg a day to achieve a therapeutic response. Idiosyncratic drug responses occur when a person experiences a particularly unusual effect from a drug. For example, some patients become quite agitated when given benzodiazepines, such as diazepam (Valium).

A person may become less responsive to a particular drug as it is administered over time, which is called *tolerance.* The development of tolerance is associated with the appearance of *physical dependence,* which may be defined as the necessity to continue administering the drug to prevent the appearance of withdrawal symptoms.

CLINICAL GUIDELINES

The practice of clinical psychopharmacology requires skill as both a diagnostician and a psychotherapist, knowledge of the available drugs, and the ability to plan a pharmacotherapeutic regimen. The selection and the initiation of drug treatment should be based on the patient's history, current clinical state, and the treatment plan. The psychiatrist should know the purpose or the goal of a drug trial, the length of time that the drug needs to be administered to assess its efficacy, the approach to be taken to reduce any adverse effects, alternative drug strategies should the current one fail, and whether long-term drug maintenance is indicated. In almost all cases the psychiatrist should explain the treatment plan to the patient and often to the family and other caregivers. The patient's reaction to and ideas about a proposed drug trial should be considered. However, if the psychiatrist believes that accommodating the patient's wishes would hinder treatment, that should be explained to the patient.

Choice of Drug

The first two steps in selecting drug treatment, the diagnosis and the identification of target symptoms, should be carried out when the patient has been in a drug-free state for one to two weeks. The drug-free state should include the absence of medications for sleep, such as hypnotics, as the quality of sleep can be both an important diagnostic guide and a target symptom. If a patient is hospitalized, however, insurance guidelines may make a drug-free period difficult or even impossible to obtain. Psychiatrists often evaluate symptomatic patients who are already receiving one or more psychoactive medications, and so it is usually necessary to wean the patient from the current medications and then to make an assessment. An exception to that practice occurs when a patient presents to the psychiatrist on a suboptimal regimen of an otherwise appropriate drug. In such cases the psychiatrist may decide to continue the drug at a higher dose to complete a full therapeutic trial.

From among the drugs appropriate to a particular diagnosis, the specific drug should be selected according to the patient's history of drug response (compliance, therapeutic response, and adverse effects), the patient's family history of drug response, and the psychiatrist's usual practice. If a drug has previously been effective in treating a patient or a family member, it should be used again unless there is some specific reason not to use the drug. A history of severe adverse effects from a specific drug is a strong indicator that the patient would not be compliant with that drug regimen. Unfortunately, patients and their families are often quite ignorant of what drugs have been used before, in what dosages, and for how long. That ignorance may reflect the tendency of psychiatrists not to explain drug trials to their patients; instead, psychiatrists should be encouraged to give their patients written records of drug trials for their personal medical records. A caveat to obtaining a history of drug response from patients is that, because of their mental disorders, they may inaccurately report the effects of a previous drug trial. If possible, therefore, the patients' medical records should be obtained as confirmation. Most psychotherapeutic drugs of a single class have been demonstrated to be equally efficacious; however, the drugs do differ in their adverse effects on individual patients. A drug should be selected that minimally exacerbates any of the patient's preexisting medical problems.

Combination Drugs.   Some combination drugs (Table 20-1) may increase the patient's compliance by simplifying the drug regimen. A problem with combination drugs, however, is that the clinician has less flexibility in adjusting the dosage of one component. That is, the use of combination drugs may cause two drugs to be administered when only one drug continues to be necessary for therapeutic efficacy.

Nonapproved Dosages and Uses.   Under the federal Food, Drug, and Cosmetic (FDC) Act, the Food and Drug Administration (FDA) has authority to control the initial availability of a drug by approving only those new drugs that demonstrate both safety and effectiveness and then to ensure that the drug's proposed labeling is truthful and contains all pertinent information for the safe and effective use of that drug.

Before the FDA can approve a new drug, the drug must be studied in humans. For the drug ultimately to be approved for commercial use, the sponsor must justify the safety and the effectiveness of the drug by submitting a New Drug Application (NDA) to the FDA. The NDA is approved or disapproved, depending on the clinical data accumulated. For approval, the FDA requires that adequate tests be conducted showing that the drug "is safe for use under the conditions prescribed, recommended, or suggested." There must also be "substantial evidence that the drug will have the effect it purports under the conditions of use prescribed, recommended, or suggested in the proposed labeling."

Use of FDA-approved drugs in private practice.   According to the Medical Liability Mutual Insurance Company (MLMIC), once a drug is approved for commercial use, the physician may, as part of the practice of medicine, lawfully prescribe

TABLE 20-1.
COMBINATION DRUGS USED IN PSYCHIATRY

Ingredients/ Preparation	Amount of Each Ingredient	Recommended Dosage	Indications	DEA† Control Level
Perphenozine and amitriptyline (Triavil, Etrafon)	Tablet—2:25, 4:25, 4:50, 2:10, 4:10	Initial therapy: tablet of 2:25 or 4:25 qid Maintenance therapy; tablet 2:25 or 4:25 bid or qid	Depression and associated anxiety	0
Meprobomate and benactyzine (Deprol)	Table—400:1	Initial therapy: one table qid Maintenance therapy: Initial dosage may be increased to six tablets a day, then gradually reduced to the lowest levels that provide relief	Depression and associated anxiety	IV
Chlordiazepoxide and clidinium bromide (Librax)	Capsule—5:25	One or two capsules tid or qid before meals and at bedtime	Peptic ulcer, gastritis, duodenitis, irritable bowel syndrome, spastic colitis, and mild ulcerative colitis	0
Chlordiazepoxide and amitriptyline (Limbitrol)	Tablet—5:12.5, 10:25	Tablet of 5:12.5 tid or qid Tablet of 10:25 tid or qid initially, then may increase to six tablets daily as required	Depression and associated anxiety	IV

†DEA, Drug Enforcement Administration.
bid: twice a day
tid: three times a day
qid: four times a day

a different dosage for a patient or otherwise vary the conditions of use from what is approved in the package labeling without notifying or obtaining FDA approval. Specifically, the FDC Act does not limit the manner in which a physician may use an approved drug. However, although physicians may treat patients with an approved drug for unapproved purposes—that is, indications not included on the drug's official labeling—without violating the FDC Act, the patient's right to redress for possible medical malpractice still remains. That is a significant concern because the failure to follow the FDA-approved label may create an inference that the physician was varying from the prevailing standard of care. Although the failure to follow the contents of the drug label does not impose liability per se and should not preclude a physician from using good clinical judgment in the interest of the patient, the physician should be aware that the drug label represents important information regarding safe and effective use (as determined by the scientific data submitted to the FDA).

In summary, psychiatrists may prescribe medication for any reason that they believe to be medically indicated for the welfare of a patient. That clarification is important in view of the increasing regulation of physicians by federal, state, and local government agencies and the intimidation many physicians experience in exercising their best medical judgment. When using a drug for an unapproved indication or in a dosage outside the usual range, the physician should document

TABLE 20-2
CHARACTERISTICS OF DRUGS AT EACH DEA LEVEL

DEA Control Level	Characteristics of Drug at Each Control Level	Examples of Drugs at Each Control Level
I	High abuse potential No accepted use in medical treatment in the United States at the present time and, therefore, not for prescription use Can be used for research	Lysergic acid diethylamide (LSD), heroin, marijuana, peyote, phencyclidine (PCP), mescaline, psilocybin, nicocodeine, nicomorphine, methyl-enedioxymethamphetamine (MDMA)
II	High abuse potential Severe physical dependence liability Severe psychological dependence liability No refills; no telephone prescriptions	Amphetamine, opium, cocaine, morphine, codeine, hydromorphine, phenmetrazine, amobarbital, secobarbital, pentobarbital, methylphenidate, dromabinol (tetrahydrocannibol), glutethimide
III	Abuse potential less than levels I and II Moderate or low physical dependence liability High psychological liability Prescriptions must be rewritten after six months or five refills	Methyprylon, nalorphine, sulfonmethane, benzphetamine, phendimetrazine, mazindol, chlorphentermine; compounds containing codeine, morphine, opium, hydrocodone, dihydrocodeine, naltrexone, diethylproplon
IV	Low abuse potential Limited physical dependence liability Limited psychological dependence liability Prescriptions must be rewritten after six months or five refills	Phenobarbital, benzodiazepines,* chloral hydrate, ethchlorvynol, ethinamate, meprobamate, paraldehyde
V	Lowest abuse potential of all controlled substances	Narcotic preparations containing limited amounts of nonnarcotic active medicinal ingredients

*In New York State, benzodiazepines are treated as schedule II substances, which require a triplicate prescription for a maximum of one month's supply.

the reasons for those treatment decisions in the patient's chart. If clinicians are in doubt about a drug treatment plan, they should consult with colleagues or suggest that the patient obtain a second opinion. The Drug Enforcement Agency (DEA) has classified drugs according to abuse potential (Table 20-2), and clinicians are advised to be cautious when prescribing any controlled substances.

Therapeutic Trials. A drug's therapeutic trial should last for a previously determined length of time. Because behavioral symptoms are more difficult to assess than other physiological symptoms, such as hypertension, it is particularly important for specific target symptoms to be identified at the initiation of a drug trial. The psychiatrist and the patient can then assess the target symptoms during the drug trial to help determine whether the drug has been effective. Some objective rating scales, such as the Brief Psychiatric Rating Scale (BPRS) and the Schedule for Affective Disorders and Schizophrenia (SADS), are available to help assess a patient's progress during a drug trial. If a drug has not been effective in reducing target symptoms within the specified length of time and if other reasons for the lack of response can be eliminated, the drug should be tapered and stopped. The brain is not a group of on-off neurochemical switches; rather, it is an interactive network of neurons in a complex homeostasis. Thus, the abrupt discontinuation of

TABLE 20–3
CONDITIONS THAT MAY REDUCE ADHERENCE TO RECOMMENDED TREATMENT

Excessively complex regimen (multiple agents, multiple small doses)
Early onset and persistence of side effects
Slow onset of beneficial effects
Low apparent relapse risk experienced if treatment is interrupted
Psychosis, confusion, dementia, pseudodementia, low intelligence, impaired hearing or vision, illiteracy
Simple lack of information, need for patient education
Financial hardship, conflicting obligations of time or money
Resentment, lack of confidence or trust
Specific psychopathology: paranoid delusions, hopelessness, masochism, anxiety and fear, ambivalence, control, splitting, passive aggression, passive dependence, denial, sociopathy, substance abuse or dependence
Involvement of multiple clinicians
Poor clinician-patient relationship
Inevitable human error

Table adapted from R J Baldessarini, J O Cole: Chemotherapy, In *The New Harvard Guide to Psychiatry*, A M Nicholi, editor, p 530. Belknap, Cambridge, MA, 1988. Used with permission.

virtually any psychoactive drug is likely to disrupt the brain's functioning further. Another common clinical mistake is the routine addition of medications without the discontinuation of a prior drug. Although this practice is indicated in specific circumstances, such as lithium potentiation of an unsuccessful trial of antidepressants, it often results in increased noncompliance and adverse effects. Also, the clinician will not know whether the second drug alone or the combination of drugs resulted in a therapeutic success or adverse effect.

Therapeutic Failures. The failure of a specific drug trial should prompt the clinician to consider a few possibilities. First, was the original diagnosis correct? That reconsideration should include the possibility of an undiagnosed mental disorder due to a general medical condition or substance-related disorder, including illicit drug abuse. Second, are the observed remaining symptoms actually the drug's adverse effects and not related to the original disease? Antipsychotic drugs, for example, can produce akinesia, which resembles psychotic withdrawal, or akathisia and neuroleptic malignant syndrome, which resemble increased psychotic agitation. Third, was the drug administered in sufficient dosage for an appropriate period? Patients can have vastly different drug absorption and metabolic rates for the same drug, and plasma drug concentrations should be obtained to assess that variable. Fourth, did a pharmacokinetic or pharmacodynamic interaction with another drug reduce the efficacy of the psychotherapeutic drug? Fifth, did the patient actually take the drug as directed? Drug noncompliance is a common clinical problem. Reasons for drug noncompliance are complicated drug regimens (more than one drug in more than one daily dose), adverse side effects (especially if unnoticed by the clinician), and poor patient education about the drug treatment plan (Table 20-3).

Drug Discontinuation. Sedative-hypnotic drugs are widely recognized as causing a withdrawal syndrome upon discontinuation. Other agents, including lithium and antidepressants, can produce discontinuation symptoms. Psychiatric drugs should be slowly withdrawn whenever possible.

Special Considerations

Children.   Special care must be given when administering psychotherapeutic drugs to children. Although the small volume of distribution in children suggests the use of lower dosages than in adults, children's higher rate of metabolism suggests that higher ratios of milligrams of drug to kilograms of body weight should be used. In practice it is best to begin with a small dose and to increase the dosage until clinical effects are observed (Table 20-4). The clinician, however, should not hesitate to use adult dosages in children if the dosages are effective and there are no side effects.

Geriatric Patients.   The two major concerns when treating geriatric patients with psychotherapeutic drugs are that elderly persons may be more susceptible to adverse side effects (particularly adverse cardiac effects) and may metabolize drugs more slowly, thus requiring lower dosages of medication (Tables 20-5 and 20-6). Another concern is that geriatric patients are often taking other medications, thereby requiring psychiatrists to consider possible drug interactions carefully. In practice, psychiatrists should begin treating geriatric patients with a small dose, usually about one half the usual dose. The dosage should be raised in small amounts more slowly than in middle-aged adults until either a clinical benefit is achieved or unacceptable adverse effects appear. Although many geriatric patients require a small dosage of medication, many others require the usual adult dosage.

Pregnant and Nursing Women.   The basic rule is to avoid administering any drug to a woman who is pregnant (particularly during the first trimester) or who is breast-feeding a child. That rule, however, occasionally needs to be broken when the mother's psychiatric disorder is severe. If psychotherapeutic medications need to be administered during a pregnancy, the possibility of therapeutic abortion should be discussed. The two most teratogenic drugs in the psychopharmacopeia are lithium and anticonvulsants. Lithium administration during pregnancy is associated with a high incidence of birth abnormalities, including Ebstein's anomaly, a serious abnormality in cardiac development. Other psychoactive drugs (antidepressants, antipsychotics, and anxiolytics), although less clearly associated with birth defects, should also be avoided during pregnancy if possible. The most common clinical situation occurs when a pregnant woman becomes psychotic. If a decision is made not to terminate the pregnancy, it is preferable to administer antipsychotics or ECT, rather than lithium.

The administration of psychotherapeutic drugs at or near delivery may cause the baby to be overly sedated at delivery, requiring a respirator, or to be physically dependent on the drug, requiring detoxification and treatment of a withdrawal syndrome. Virtually all psychotropic drugs are secreted in the milk of a nursing mother; therefore, mothers on these agents should be advised not to breast-feed their children.

Medically Ill Patients.   Considerations in administering psychotropic drugs to medically ill patients include a potentially increased sensitivity to side effects, either

TABLE 20-4
COMMON PSYCHOACTIVE DRUGS IN CHILDHOOD AND ADOLESCENCE

Drugs	Indications	Dosage	Adverse Reactions and Monitoring
Antipsychotics—also known as major tranquilizers, neuroleptics. Divided into (1) high-potency, low-dosage, e.g., haloperidol (Haldol), trifluoperazine (Stelazine), Thiothixene (Navane); (2) low-potency, high-dosage (more sedating), e.g., chlorpromazine (Thorazine), thioridazine (Mellaril); (3) clozapine (Clozaril); and (4) risperidone (Risperdal)	Psychoses; agitated, aggressive, self-injurious behaviors in mental retardation (MR), pervasive developmental disorders (PDD), and conduct disorder (CD) Studies support following indications: Haloperidol—schizophrenia, PDD, CD with severe aggression, Tourette's disorder Clozapine—refractory schizophrenia in adolescence Risperidone—anecdotal reports of success in PDD	All can be given in two to four divided doses or combined into one dose after gradual buildup Haloperidol—child 0.5–6 mg a day, adolescent 0.5–16 mg a day Thiothixene—5–12 mg a day Chlorpromazine and thioridazine—child 10–200 mg a day, adolescent 50–600 mg a day, over 16 years of age 100–700 mg a day Clozapine—dosage not determined in children; <600 mg a day in adolescents Risperidone—1–3 mg a day in several children with PDD	Sedation, weight gain, hypotension, lowered seizure threshold, constipation, extrapyramidal symptoms, jaundice, agranulocytosis, dystonic reaction, tardive dyskinesia; with clozapine, no extrapyramidal adverse effects Monitor: blood pressure, complete blood count (CBC), liver function tests (LFTs), electroencephalogram, if indicated; with thioridazine pigmentary retinopathy is rare but dictates ceiling of 800 mg in adults and proportionately lower in children; with clozapine, weekly white blood counts (WBCs) for development of agranulocytosis and electroencephalogram (EEG) monitoring due to lowering of seizure threshold.
Stimulants Dextroamphetamine (Dexedrine)—FDA-approved for children 3 years and older Methylphenidate (Ritalin) and pemoline (Cylert)—FDA-approved for children 6 years and older	In attention-deficit/hyperactivity disorder (ADHD) for hyperactivity, impulsivity, and inattentiveness	Dextroamphetamine and methylphenidate are generally given at 8 AM and noon (the usefulness of sustained-release preparations not proved) Dextroamphetamine—2.5–40 mg a day up to 0.5 mg per kg a day Methylphenidate—10–60 mg a day or up to 1.0 mg per kg a day Pemoline—37.5–112.5 mg given at 8 AM	Insomnia, anorexia, weight loss (and possibly growth delay), headache, tachycardia, precipitation or exacerbation of tic disorders With pemoline, monitor LFTS, as hepatoxicity is possible
Lithium—considered an antipsychotic drug, also has antiaggression properties	Studies support use in MR and CD for aggressive and self-injurious behaviors; can be used for some in PDD; also indicated for early-onset bipolar I disorder	600–2, 100 mg in two or three divided doses; keep serum concentrations to 0.4–1.2 mEq per L	Nausea, vomiting, enuresis, headache, tremor, weight gain, hypothyroidism Experience with adults suggests renal function monitoring

Drug	Indications	Dosage	Side Effects/Monitoring
Tricyclic drugs Imipramine (Tofranil) has been used in most child studies Nortriptyline (Pamelor) has been studied in children Clomipramine (Anafranil) is effective in child obsessive-compulsive disorder (OCD)	Major depressive disorder, separation anxiety disorder, bulimia nervosa, enuresis; sometimes used in ADHD, sleepwalking disorder, and sleep terror disorder Clomipramine is effective in child OCD and sometimes in PDD.	Imipramine—start with divided dosages totalling about 1.5 mg per kg a day; can build up to not more than 5 mg per kg a day and eventually combine in one dose; not FDA-approved for children except for enuresis; dosage is usually 50–100 mg before sleep Clomipramine—start at 50 mg a day; can raise to not more than 3 mg per kg a day or 200 mg a day	Dry mouth, constipation, tachycardia, drowsiness, postural hypotension, mania Electrocardiogram (ECG) monitoring is needed because or risk for cardiac conduction slowing: consider lowering dosage if PR interval >0.20 seconds of QRS interval >0.12 seconds; baseline EEG is advised, as it can lower seizure threshold (especially with clomipramine); blood levels of drug are sometimes useful
Serotonin-specific reuptake inhibitors—fluoxetine (Prozac) sertraline (Zoloff), and fluvoxamine (Luvox)	OCD; may be useful in major depressive disorder, anorexia, bulimia nervosa, repetitive behaviors in MR or PDD	Appears less than adult dosages	Nausea, headache, nervousness, insomnia, dry mouth, diarrhea, drowsiness
Carbamazepine (Tegretol)—an anticonvulsant	Aggression or dyscontrol in MR or CD, bipolar disorder	Start with 10 mg per kg a day; can build to 20–30 mg per kg a day; therapeutic serum concentration range appears to be 4–12 mg per L	Drowsiness, nausea, rash, vertigo, irritability Monitor: CBC and for possible blood dyscrasias and hepatoxicity; blood levels are necessary
Benzodiazepines—have been insufficiently studied in childhood and adolescence	Sometimes effective in parasomnias; sleepwalking disorder or sleep terror disorder; can be tried in generalized anxiety disorder Clonazepam (Klonopin) can be tried in all anxiety disorders, especially panic disorder Alprazolam (Xanax) can be tried in separation anxiety disorder	Parasomnias: diazepam (Valium) 2–10 mg before bedtime	Can cause drowsiness, ataxia, tremor, dyscontrol; can be abused
Fenfluramine (Pondimin)—an amphetamine congener	Well-studied in autistic disorder; generally ineffective, but some patients show improvement	Gradually increase to 1.0–1.5 mg per kg a day in divided doses	Weight loss, drowsiness, irritability, loose bowel movements
Propranolol (Inderal)—a β-adrenergic receptor antagonist	Aggression in MR, PDD, and cognitive disorder; awaits controlled studies	Effective dosage in children and adolescents is not yet established; range is probably 40–320 mg a day	Bradycardia, hypotension, nausea, hypoglycemia, depression; avoid in asthma

TABLE 20-4—continued

Drugs	Indications	Dosage	Adverse Reactions and Monitoring
Clonidine (Catapres)	Some success in ADHD; clonidine in Tourette's disorder	Clonidine—0.1-0.3 mg a day; 3-5.5 μg per kg a day Guanfacine (Tenex)—up to 3 mg a day	Orthostatic hypotension, sedation, dry mouth
Cyproheptadine (Periactin)	Anorexia nervosa	Dosages up to 8 mg four times a day	Antihistaminic side effects, including sedation and dryness of the mouth Sleepiness, aggressivity
Naltrexone (ReVia)	Self-injurious behaviors in MR and PDD; currently being studied in PDD	0.5-2.0 mg per kg a day	Monitor LFTs, as hepatotoxicity has been reported in adults at high dosages
Desmopressin (DDAVP)	Nocturnal enuresis	20-40 μg intranasally	Headache; hyponatremia seizures (rare)

Table by Richard Perry, MD

TABLE 20–5.
PHARMACOKINETICS AND AGING

Phase	Change	Effect
Absorption	Gastric pH increases Decreased surface villi Decreased gastric motility and delayed gastric emptying Intestinal perfusion decreases	Little overall change Absorption is slowed but just as complete
Distribution	Total body water and lean body mass decrease Increased total body fat, more marked in women than in men Albumin decreases, gamma globulin increases, alpha-acid glycoprotein unchanged	Volume of distribution (Vd) increases for lipid-soluble drugs, decreases for water-soluble drugs The free or unbound percentage of albumin-bound drugs increases
Metabolism	Renal: renal blood flow and glomerular filtration rates decrease Hepatic: decreased enzyme activity and perfusion	Decreased metabolism leads to prolonged half-lives, if Vd remains the same
Total body weight	Decreases	Think on a mg-per-kg basis
Receptor sensitivity	May increase	Increased effect

Table from L B Guttmacher: *Concise Guide to Somatic Therapies in Psychiatry*, p. 126. American Psychiatric Press, Washington, 1988. Used with permission.

increased or decreased metabolism and excretion of the drug, and interactions with other medications. As with children and geriatric patients, the most reasonable clinical practice is to begin with a small dose, increase it slowly, and watch for both clinical and adverse effects. The testing of plasma drug concentrations may be particularly helpful in those patients.

ADVERSE EFFECTS

Most psychotherapeutic drugs do not affect a single neurotransmitter system, nor are their effects localized to the brain. The effects of psychotherapeutic drugs on neurotransmitter systems result in the wide range of adverse effects. For example, some of the most common adverse effects of psychotherapeutic drugs are caused by the blockade of muscarinic acetylcholine receptors (Table 20-7). Many psychotherapeutic drugs antagonize dopaminergic, histaminergic, or adrenergic neurons, resulting in the adverse effects listed in Table 20-8. There are also several commonly observed adverse effects for which the neurotransmitters involved have not been specifically identified.

Patients generally have less trouble with adverse effects if they have previously been told to expect them. It is reasonable to explain the appearance of adverse effects as evidence that the drug is working. Nevertheless, clinicians should distinguish between probable or expected adverse effects and rare or unexpected adverse effects.

An extreme adverse effect of drug treatment is patients' attempts to commit suicide by overdosing on a psychotherapeutic drug. One psychodynamic theory of such behavior is that the patients are angry at their therapists for not having helped them. Whatever the motivation, psychiatrists should be aware of the risk and attempt

TABLE 20-6
GERIATRIC DOSAGES OF COMMON PSYCHOACTIVE DRUGS

Monoamine Oxidase Inhibitors (MAOIs)*		
Generic Name	**Trade Name**	**Geriatric Dosage Range (mg a day)**
Phenelzine	Nardil	15–45
Tranylcyprominet	Parnate	10–20

* Persons taking MAOIs should be on a tyramine-free diet.
† Not recommended in persons over 60 because of pressor effects.

Psychostimulants		
Generic name	**Trade Name**	**Geriatric Dosage Range (mg a day)**
Dextroamphetamine	Dexedrine	2.5–10
Pemoline	Cylert	18.75–37
Methylphenidate	Ritalin	2.5–20

Antipsychotics: Dopamine Receptor Antagonists		
Generic Name	**Trade Name**	**Geriatric Dosage Range (mg a day)**
Phenothiazines		
Aliphatic		
Chlorpromazine	Thorazine	30–300
Triflupromazine	Vesprin	1–15
Piperazine		
Perphenazine	Trilafon	8–32
Trifluoperazine	Stelazine	1–15
Fluphenazine	Prolixin	1–10
Piperidine		
Thioridazine	Mellaril	25–300
Mesoridazine	Serentil	50–400
Thioxanthenes		
Chlorprothixene	Taractan	30–300
Thiothixene	Navane	2–20
Dibenzoxazepine		
Loxapine	Loxitane	50–250
Dihydroindole		
Molindone	Mobon	50–225
Butyrophenone		
Haloperidol	Haldol	2–20
Benzisoxazole		
Risperidone	Risperdal	2–4

Tricyclic, Tetracyclic, and Unicyclic Antidepressants		
Generic Name	**Trade Name**	**Geriatric Dosage Range (mg a day)**
Tricyclics**		
Imipramine	Tofranil	25–300
Desipramine	Norpramin	10–300
Trimipramine	Surmontil	25–300
Amitriptyline	Elavil	25–300
Nortriptyline	Pamelor	10–150
Protriptyline	Vivactil	10–40
Doxepin	Sinequan	10–300
Tetracyclic		
Maprotiline	Ludiomil	25–150
Unicyclic		
Bupropion	Wellbutrin	75–450

** Exact range may vary among laboratories

TABLE 20-6—*continued*

Serotonin-Specific Reuptake Inhibitors and Phenylpiperazines		
Generic Name	**Trade Name**	**Geriatric Dosage Range (mg a day)**
Fluoxetine	Prozac	5–80
Fluvoxamine	Luvox	25–150
Nefazodone	Serzone	100–400
Paroxetine	Paxil	5–20
Sertraline	Zoloft	50–200
Trazadone	Desyrel	100–500

Drugs Used to Treat Bipolar Disorder		
Generic Name	**Trade Name**	**Geriatric Dosage Range (mg a day)**
Lithium carbonate	Eskalith Lithotabs	75–900
Carbamazepine	Tegretol	200–1,200
Valproate	Depakene, Depakote	250–1,000
Clonazepam (a benzodiazepine)	Klonopin	0.5–1.5

Drugs Used to Treat Anxiety and Insomnia		
Generic Name	**Trade Name**	**Geriatric Dosage Range (mg a day)**
Benzodiazepines		
Alprazolam	Xanax	0.5–6
Chlordiazepoxide	Librium	15–100
Chlorazepate	Tranxene	7.5–60
Diazepam	Valium	2–60
Flurazepam	Dalmane	15–30
Halazepam	Paxipam	60–160
Lorazepam	Ativan	2–6
Oxazepam	Serax	30–120
Prazepam	Centrax	20–60
Temazepam	Restoril	15–30
Triazolam	Halcion	0.125–0.25
Nonbenzodiazepines		
Buspirone	BuSpar	5–60
Secobarbital	Seconal	50–300
Meprobamate	Miltown	400–800
Chloral hydrate	Noctec	500–1,000
Zoplidem	Ambien	2.5–5
β-Adrenergic blockers		
Propranolol	Inderal	40–160
Atenolol	Tenormin	25–100

TABLE 20-7
**POTENTIAL ADVERSE EFFECTS CAUSED BY BLOCKADE OF MUSCARINIC
ACETYLCHOLINE RECEPTORS**

Blurred vision
Constipation
Decreased salivation
Decreased sweating
Delayed or retrograde ejaculation
Delirium
Exacerbation of asthma (through decreased bronchial secretions)
Hyperthermia (through decreased sweating)
Memory problems
Narrow-angle glaucoma
Photophobia
Sinus tachycardia
Urinary retention

TABLE 20-8
**POTENTIAL ADVERSE EFFECTS OF PSYCHOTHERAPEUTIC DRUGS AND ASSOCIATED
NEUROTRANSMITTER SYSTEMS**

Antidopaminergic
  Endocrine dysfunction
    Hyperprolactinemia
    Menstrual dysfunction
    Sexual dysfunction
  Movement disorders
    Akathisia
    Dystonia
    Parkinsonism
    Tardive dyskinesia
Antiadrenergic (primarily α)
  Dizziness
  Postural hypotension
Reflex tachycardia
Antihistaminergic
  Hypotension
  Sedation
  Weight gain
Multiple neurotransmitter systems
  Agranulocytosis (and other blood dyscrasias)
  Allergic reactions
  Anorexia
  Cardiac conduction abnormalities
  Nausea and vomiting
  Seizures

to prescribe the safest possible drugs. It is good clinical practice to write nonrefillable prescriptions for small quantities of drugs when suicide is a consideration. In extreme cases, attempts should be made to verify that patients are taking the medication and not hoarding the pills for a later overdose attempt. Patients may attempt suicide just as they are beginning to get better. Clinicians, therefore, should continue to be careful about prescribing large quantities of medication until the patient is almost completely recovered. Another consideration for psychiatrists is the possibility of accidental overdose, particularly by children in the household. Patients should be advised to keep psychotherapeutic medications in a safe place.

Treatment of Common Adverse Effects

Psychotherapeutic drugs are associated with many different adverse effects. The management of the adverse effects is similar, no matter which psychotherapeutic drug the patient is taking.

Dry Mouth. Dry mouth is caused by the blockade of muscarinic acetylcholine receptors. Patients who constantly suck on sugary hard candies to relieve dry mouth increase their risk of dental caries. They can avoid the problem by chewing sugarless gum or sucking on sugarless hard candies. Some clinicians recommend the use of a 1 percent solution of pilocarpine, a cholinergic agonist, as a mouth wash three times daily. Other clinicians suggest bethanechol (Urecholine) tablets, a cholinergic agonist, 10 to 30 mg, once to twice daily. It is best to start with 10 mg once a day and to increase the dosage slowly. Adverse effects of cholinomimetic drugs, such as bethanechol, include tremor, diarrhea, abdominal cramps, and excessive eye watering.

Blurred Vision. The blockade of muscarinic acetylcholine receptors causes mydriasis (pupillary dilation) and cycloplegia (ciliary muscle paresis), resulting in presbyopia (blurred near vision). Cholinomimetic eyedrops can relieve the symptom. A 1 percent solution of pilocarpine can be prescribed as one drop four times daily. Bethanechol can be used as for dry mouth as an alternative.

Urinary Retention. The anticholinergic activity of many psychotropics can lead to urinary hesitation, dribbling, urinary retention, and increased urinary tract infections. Elderly patients with enlarged prostates are at increased risk for urinary retention. Ten to 30 mg of bethanechol three to four times daily is usually effective in the treatment of that adverse effect.

Constipation. The anticholinergic activity of psychotropic drugs can result in the particularly disturbing adverse effect of constipation. The first line of treatment involves the prescribing of bulk-forming laxatives, such as Metamucil and Fiberall. If that treatment fails, cathartics, such as milk of magnesia, can be tried. Prolonged use of cathartics can result in a loss of their effectiveness. Bethanechol, 10 to 30 mg three to four times daily, can also be used.

Orthostatic Hypotension. Orthostatic hypotension is caused by the blockade of α_1-adrenergic receptors. It is necessary to warn patients of that possible adverse effect, particularly if the patient is elderly. The risk of hip fracture from falls is significantly elevated in patients who are taking psychotropic drugs. With patients at high risk of experiencing orthostatic hypotension, the clinician should choose a drug with low α_1-adrenergic activity. Most simply, the patient can be instructed to get up slowly and to sit down immediately if dizziness is experienced. The patient can also try support hose to help reduce venous pooling. Specific adjuvant medications have been recommended for specific pharmacotherapeutic agents.

Sexual Dysfunction. Psychotropic drug use can be associated with sexual dysfunctions—decreased libido, impaired ejaculation and erection, and inhibition of female orgasm. Warning a patient about those adverse effects may increase the patient's concerns. Alternatively, patients are not likely to report adverse sexual effects to the physician. Also, some sexual dysfunctions may be related to the primary psychiatric disorder. Nevertheless, if sexual dysfunctions emerge after pharmacotherapy has begun, attempting to treat them may be worthwhile. Neostigmine (Prostigmin), 7.5 to 15 mg taken orally 30 minutes before sexual intercourse, may help alleviate impaired ejaculation. Impaired erectile function may be helped with bethanechol given regularly. Cyproheptadine (Periactin), 4 mg every morning, can be used for the treatment of impaired female orgasm; 4 to 8 mg can be taken orally one to two hours before anticipated sexual activity for the treatment of impaired male orgasm secondary to serotonergic agents.

Weight Gain. Weight gain accompanies the use of many psychotropic drugs and can be the result of retained fluid, increased caloric intake, or decreased exercise. Edema can be treated by elevating the affected body parts or by administering a thiazide diuretic. If the patient is taking lithium or cardiac medications, the clinician must monitor drug concentrations, blood chemistries, and vital signs. The patient should also be instructed to minimize the intake of fats and carbohydrates and to exercise regularly. If the patient has not been exercising, however, the clinician should recommend that the patient start an exercise program at a modest level of exertion.

Extrapyramidal Side Effects. Neurological side effects—such as dystonias, parkinsonian effects (including so-called rabbit syndrome) and tardive dyskinesia— are discussed in Chapter 23, "Medication-Induced Movement Disorders."

DRUG-DRUG INTERACTIONS

Drug-drug interactions may be either pharmacokinetic or pharmacodynamic and vary greatly in their potential to cause serious problems. An additional consideration is one of phantom drug-drug interactions. The patient may be taking only drug A and then later receive both A and B. The clinician may notice some effect and attribute it to the induction of metabolism. What may have happened is that the patient was more compliant at one point in the observation period than in another, or there may have been some other effect of which the clinician was unaware. Thus, the clinical literature contains reports of phantom drug-drug interactions, but such interactions probably did not really take place.

Other interactions may be true but unproved, although reasonably plausible. Still other interactions have some modest effect and are well-documented. There are also well-studied, well-proved, clinically important drug-drug interactions. However, clinicians must remember that (1) animal pharmacokinetic data are not always readily generalizable to humans; (2) in vitro data do not necessarily replicate results obtained under in vivo conditions; (3) single-case reports can contain misleading information; and (4) acute studies should not be uncritically regarded as relevant to investigations of chronic steady-state conditions.

The informed clinician needs to keep those considerations in mind and to focus on the clinically important interactions—not on the ones that may be mild, unproved, or entirely phantom—and yet still maintain an open and receptive attitude toward drug-drug interactions.

For a more detailed discussion of this topic, see J A Grebb: General Principles of Psychopharmacology, Sec. 32.1, pp 1895, in CTP/VI.

21
Drugs Used in the Office Treatment of Psychiatric Disorders

The many pharmacological agents used to treat psychiatric disorders are referred to by three general terms used interchangeably: psychotropic drugs, psychoactive drugs, and psychotherapeutic drugs. Traditionally, those agents were divided into four categories: (1) antipsychotic drugs or neuroleptics used to treat psychosis, (2) antidepressant drugs, (3) antimanic drugs used to treat bipolar disorder, and (4) antianxiety drugs or anxiolytics used to treat anxious states (which were also effective as hypnotics in high dosages). That division, however, is less valid now than it was in the past for the following reasons: (1) Many drugs of one class are used to treat disorders previously assigned to another class. For example, many antidepressant drugs are used to treat anxiety disorders; and some antianxiety drugs are used to treat psychoses, depressive disorders, and bipolar disorders. (2) Drugs from all four categories are used to treat psychiatric disorders not previously treatable by drugs—for example, eating disorders, panic disorder, and impulse-control disorders. (3) Drugs such as clonidine (Catapres), propranolol (Inderal), and verapamil (Isoptin, Calan) can effectively treat a variety of disorders and do not fit easily into the traditional classification of drugs. (4) Some descriptive psychopharmacological terms overlap in meaning. For example, anxiolytics decrease anxiety, sedatives produce a calming or relaxing effect, and hypnotics produce sleep. However, most anxiolytics function as sedatives and at high doses can be used as hypnotics, and all hypnotics at low doses can be used for daytime sedation.

Tables 21-1 and 21-2 list the major drugs used in the treatment of the various psychiatric disorders.

INTOXICATION AND OVERDOSE

An extreme adverse effect of drug treatment is an attempt by patients to commit suicide by overdosing on a psychotherapeutic drug. One psychodynamic theory of such behavior is that the patients are angry at their therapists for not having been able to help them. Whatever the motivation, psychiatrists should be aware of the risk and attempt to prescribe the safest possible drugs. It is good clinical practice to write nonrefillable prescriptions for small quantities of drugs when suicide is a consideration. In extreme cases, an attempt should be made to verify that patients are taking the medication and not hoarding the pills for a later overdose attempt. Patients may attempt suicide just as they are beginning to get better. Clinicians, therefore, should continue to be careful about prescribing large quantities of medication until the patient is almost completely recovered. Another consideration for psychiatrists is the possibility of an accidental overdose, particularly by children in the household. Patients should be advised to keep psychotherapeutic medications in a safe place. A guide to the signs and symptoms and the treatment of overdoses with psychotherapeutic drugs is contained in Table 21-3.

TABLE 21-1
DRUGS USED IN PSYCHIATRY

Generic Name	Trade Name	Pharmacological Category
Alprazolam	Xanax	Benzodiazepine†
Armantadine	Symmetrel, Symadine	Dopamine agonist*
Amitriptyline	Endep, Elavil	Tricyclic
Amobarbital	Amytal	Barbiturates
Amoxapine	Asendin	Tetracyclic
Atenolol	Tenormin	β-Adrenergic receptor antagonist
Benztropine	Cogentin	Anticholinergic
Biperiden	Akineton	Anticholinergic
Bromocriptine	Partodel	Dopamine agonist–antagonist
Buproplon	Wellbutrin	Unicyclic
Buspirone	BuSpar	Azapirone†
Butabarbital	Butisol	Barbiturate
Carbamazepine	Tegretol	Carbamazepine
Carisoprodol	Soma	Carbamate†
Chloral hydrate	Noctec	Chloral Hydrate
Chlordiazepoxide	Librium	Benzodiazepine
Chlorpromazine	Thorazine	Dopamine receptor antagonist
Clomipramine	Anafranil	Tricyclic
Clonazepam	Klonopin	Benzodiazepine
Clonidine	Catapres	α-Adrenergic receptor agonist
Clorazepate	Tranxene	Benzodiazepine
Clozapine	Clazaril	Dibenzodiazepine (serotoxin-dopamine antagonist)*
Cyproheptadine	Periactin	Anthistamine
Dantrolene	Dantrium	Aldehyde dehydrin
Desipramine	Norpramin	Tricyclic
Dextroamphetamine	Dexedrine	Sympathomimetic
Dexfenfluramine	No trade name	Sympathometic amine
Diazepam	Valium	Benzodiazepine
Diltiazem	Cardizem	Calcium channel inhibitor
Diphenhydramine	Benadryl	Antihistamine
Disulfiram	Antabuse	Aldehyde dehydrogenase inhibitor
Doxepin	Sinequan	Tricyclic
Droperidol	Inapsine	Dopamine receptor antagonist
Estazolam	ProSom	Benzadiazepine
Ethchlorvynol	Placidyl	Tertiary carbinol†
Fenfluramine	Pondimin	Sympathometic amine
Flumazenil	Romazicon	Benzodiazepine receptor antagonist
Fluoxetine	Prozac	Serotonin-specific reuptake inhibitor
Fluphenazine	Prolixin	Dopamine receptor antagonist
Flurazepam	Dalmane	Benzodiazepine
Fluvaxamine	Luvox	Serotonin-specific reuptake inhibitor
Glutethimide	No trade name	Liperichinedione†
Halazepam	Paxipam	Benzodiazepine
Haloperidol	Haidol	Dopamine receptor antagonist
Hydroxyzine	Atarax, Vistaril	Antihistamine
Imipramine	Tofranil	Tricyclic
Levodopa	Larodopa	Dopamine agonist
Lithium	Eskalith, Lithobid	Lithium
Lorazepam	Ativan	Benzodiazepine
Loxapine	Loxitane	Dopamine receptor antagonist
Maprofiline	Ludiomil	Tetracyclic
Mephobarbital	Mebaril	Barbiturate
Meprobamate	Miltown, Equanil	Carbamate
Mesoridazine	Serentil	Dopamine receptor antagonist
Methadone	Dolophine	Opioid
Methylphenidate	Ritalin	Sympathomimetic
Metoprolol	Lopressor	β-Adrenergic receptor antagonist
Midazolam	Versed	Benzodiazepine
Molindone	Moban	Dopamine receptor antagonist

TABLE 21-1—*continued*

Generic Name	Trade Name	Pharmacological Category
Nadolol	Corgard	β-Adrenergic receptor antagonist
Naloxone	Narcan	Opioid antagonist
Naltrexone	ReVia	Opioid antagonist
Nefazodene	Serzone	Phenylpiperazine
Nifedipine	Procardia	Calcium channel inhibitor
Nimodipine	Nimotop	Calcium channel inhibitor
Nortriptyline	Pamelor	Tricyclic
Oxazepam	Serax	Benzodiazepine
Paraldehyde	Paral	Cyclic ether†
Paroxetine	Paxil	Serotonin-specific reuptake inhibitor
Pemoline	Cylert	Sympathomimetic
Pentobarbital	Nembutal	Barbiturate
Perphenazine	Tritafon	Dopamine receptor antagonist
Phenelzine	Nardil	Monoamine oxidase inhibitor
Phenobarbital	No trade name	Barbiturate
Pimozide	Orap	Dopamine receptor antagonist
Pindolol	Visken	β-Adrenergic receptor antagonist
Prazepam	Cenfrax	Benzodiazepine
Prochlorperazine	Compazine	Dopamine receptor antagonist
Procyclidine	Kemadrin	Anticholinergic
Propranolol	Inderal	β-Adrenergic receptor antagonist
Protriptyline	Vivactil	Tricyclic
Quazepam	Doral	Benzodiazepine
Reserpine	No trade name	Dopamine receptor antagonist
Risperidone	Risperdal	Serotonin-dopamine antagonist*
Secobarbital	Seconal	Barbiturate
Selegiline	Eldepryl	Monoamine oxidase inhibitor
Sertraline	Zoloft	Serotonin-specific reuptake inhibitor
Sodium divalproex	Depakote	Valproate (valproic acid)
Sodium valproate	Depakene	Valproate (valproic acid)
Tacrine	Cognex	Acetylcholine inhibitor
Temazepam	Restoril	Benzodiazepine
Thioridazine	Melfaril	Dopamine receptor antagonist
Thiothixene	Navane	Dopamine receptor antagonist
L-Thyroxine	Levoxyl, Levothroid, Synthroid	Thyroid hormone
Tranylcypromine	Parnate	Monoamine oxidase inhibitor
Trazadone	Desyrel	Phenylpiperazine
Triazolam	Halcion	Benzodiazepine
Trifluoperazine	Stelazine	Dopamine receptor antagonist
Triflupromazine	Vesprin	Dopamine receptor antagonist
Trihexyphenidyl	Artane	Anticholinergic
L-Triiodothyronine	Cytomel	Thyroid hormone
Trimipramine	Surmontil	Tricyclic
L-Tryptophan	No trade name	Serotonin agonist
Valproate	Depakene	Valproate (valproic acid)
Venlafaxine	Effexor	Phenylethylame
Verapamil	Calan, isoptin	Calcium channel inhibitor
Yohimbine	Yocon	α_2-Adrenergic antagonist
Zolpidem	Ambien	Benzodiazepine receptor agonist

* Antipsychotic
† Sedative, hypnotic, or anxiolytic

Nontoxic substances are listed in Table 21-4.

For a more detailed discussion of this topic, see J A Grebb: General Principles of Psychopharmacology, Sec. 32.1, p 1895, in CTP/VI.

TABLE 21–2
MAJOR MENTAL DISORDERS AND THE DRUGS AND CLASSES OF DRUGS USED IN THEIR TREATMENT

Aggression and agitation (see Intermittent explosive disorder)
Akathisia (see Medication-induced movement disorders)
Alcohol-related disorders
  β-Adrenergic receptor antagonists
  Benzodiazepines
  Carbamazepine
  Disulfiram
  Lithium
  Naltrexone
Anorexia nervosa (see Eating disorders)
Anxiety (see also specific anxiety disorders)
  Antihistamines
  Barbiturates and similarly acting drugs
  Benzodiazepines
  Buspirone
Bipolar disorders
  Benzodiazepines (especially clonazepam)
  Calcium channel inhibitors
  Carbamazepine
  Clozapine
  Dopamine receptor antagonists
  Lithium
  Thyroid hormones (L-thyroxine)
  L-Tryptophan
  Valproate
Bulimia nervosa (see Eating disorders)
Catatonic disorder due to a general medical condition
  Barbiturates
  Benzodiazepines
  Clozapine
  Dopamine receptor antagonists
Cyclothymic disorder (see Bipolar disorders)
Delusional disorder (see Schizophrenia)
Dementia of the Alzheimer's type (cognitive symptoms)
  Tacrine
Depressive disorders
  Benzodiazepines (especially alprazolam)
  Bromocriptine
  Bupropion
  Carbamazepine
  Lithium
  Monoamine oxidase inhibitors
  Serotonin-specific reuptake inhibitors
  Sympathomimetics
  Thyroid hormones
  Trazodone and nefazodone
  Tricyclics and tetracyclics
  L-Tryptophan
  Venlafaxine
Dysthymic disorder (see Depressive disorders)
Dystonia (see Medication-induced movement disorders)
Eating disorders
  Fenfluramine
  Lithium
  Monoamine oxidase inhibitors
  Serotonin-specific reuptake inhibitors
  Tricyclics and tetracyclics
Generalized anxiety disorder
  β-Adrenergic receptor antagonists
  Barbiturates and similarly acting drugs
  Benzodiazepines
  Buspirone
  Tricyclics and tetracyclics
Insomnia (see Sleep disorders)

TABLE 21-2—*continued*

Intermittent explosive disorder
  β-Adrenergic receptor antagonists
  Barbiturates (primarily for acute agitation)
  Buspirone
  Carbamazepine
  Dopamine receptor antagonists
  Lithium
  Valproate
Medication-induced movement disorders (see also Neuroleptic malignant syndrome)
  β-Adrenergic receptor antagonists
  Amantadine
  Anticholinergics
  Antihistamines
  Benzodiazepines
  L-Dopa
Neuroleptic malignant syndrome
  Bromocriptine
  Dantrolene
Obsessive-compulsive disorder
  Serotonin-specific reuptake inhibitors
  Tricyclics and tetracyclics (especially clomipramine)
Opioid use disorders
  Clonidine
  Methadone
  Naltrexone and Naloxone
Panic disorder (with and without agoraphobia)
  β-Adrenergic receptor antagonists
  Benzodiazepines (especially alprazolam and clonazepam)
  Monoamine oxidase inhibitors
  Serotonin-specific reuptake inhibitors
  Tricyclics and tetracyclics
Parkinsonism (see Medication-induced movement disorders)
Phobias (see also Panic disorder)
  β-Adrenergic receptor antagonists
  Benzodiazepines
  Monoamine oxidase inhibitors
Posttraumatic stress disorder
  Carbamazepine
  Monoamine oxidase inhibitors
  Serotonin-specific reuptake inhibitors
  Tricyclics and tetracyclics
  Valproate
Psychosis (see Schizophrenia)
Rabbit syndrome (see Medication-induced movement disorders)
Schizoaffective disorder (see Depressive disorders, Bipolar disorders, and Schizophrenia)
Schizophrenia
  Benzodiazepines
  Carbamazepine
  Clozapine
  Dopamine receptor antagonists
  Lithium
Sexual dysfunctions
  Antihistamines (cyproheptadine)
  Yohimbine
Sleep disorders
  Antihistamines
  Barbiturates and similarly acting drugs
  Benzodiazepines
  Chloral hydrate
  Sympathomimetics (for narcolepsy)
  Trazodone
  L-Tryptophan
  Zolpidem
Tic disorder
  Clonidine
  Dopamine receptor antagonists
Violence (see Intermittent explosive disorder)

TABLE 21–3
INTOXICATION AND OVERDOSE WITH PSYCHOTHERAPEUTIC DRUGS

Drug	Toxic or Lethal Dose*	Signs and Symptoms	Treatment
β-Adrenergic receptor antagonists	Propranolol 1 g	Hypotension, bradycardia, seizures, loss of consciousness bronchospasm, cardiac failure	Supportive care; emesis or gastric lavage after ingestion. If needed (comatose, seizures, absent gag), lavage with endotracheal tube with inflated cuff in place; intravenous (IV) atropine for symptomatic bradycardia. IV isoproterenol for persistent cases, a pacemaker if refractory; norepinephrine or dopamine for severe hypotension; IV diazepam for seizures; glucagon may be useful for hypotension and myocardial depression, theophylline or β₂-agonist for bronchospasm, a diuretic or cardiac glycoside for heart failure
Amantadine	2.5 g	Disorientation, visual hallucinations, confusion, aggressive behavior, minimally reactive and slightly dilated pupils, urinary retention, acid-base disturbances, coma	Induce emesis or use gastric lavage in recent overdose; supportive measures, including airway maintenance, cardiovascular monitoring, control of respiration and oxygen administration; monitoring urine pH, urinary output, serum electrolytes; acidifying agents can increase the rate of excretion, force fluids (IV if needed); observe for hypotension, seizures, psychosis, urinary retention, arrhythmias, hyperactivity, which should be treated appropriately; physostigmine may be useful in treating central nervous system (CNS) toxicity; chlorpromazine may be useful for toxic psychosis; adrenergic agents may predispose the patient to ventricular arrhythmias
Amphetamine	100 mg	Elation, irritability, hyperactivity, rapid speech, anorexia, hyperreflexia, insomnia, dry mouth, chest pain, arrhythmia, heart block, poor concentration, restlessness, psychotic symptoms	Emesis or lavage can be effective long after ingestion because of recycling through gastric mucosa; reduce external stimuli; treat cerebral edema and hyperthermia; peritoneal dialysis; sedate with chlorpromazine 0.5% 1 mg/kg intramuscular (IM) or by mouth every 30 minutes as needed; use 1/2 the dose for mixed amphetamine-barbiturate overdose
Anticholinergics	700 mg/7 g (doses vary, depending an agent involved)	Hot, dry, flushed skin; unreactive dilated pupils; blurred vision; dry mucous membranes; foul breath; difficulty in swallowing; urinary retention; decreased bowel sounds; tachycardia; nausea; vomiting; rash; anticholinergic delirium with delusions, hallucinations, disorientation	Supportive and symptomatic therapy; continuous electrocardiograph (ECG) monitoring; empty stomach immediately by inducing emesis if patient is conscious, has gag reflex and no seizures; otherwise, gastric lavage and activated charcoal can be used with endotracheal tube with inflated cuff in place; saline cathartics may be used; exchange transfusions can be considered in extreme cases; fluid therapy should be used for shock; cold packs, mechanical cooling devices, or sponging with tepid water can be used for hyperthermia; diazepam can be used for agitation; can reverse adverse effects with 1–2 mg of physostigmine; IV propranolol may be useful for supraventricular tachyarrhythmias; avoid dopamine receptor antagonists

Drug	Toxic dose	Symptoms	Treatment
Antihistamines	2.8 g (diphenhydramine); 1,750–17,500 mg (hydroxyzine)	Disorientation, drowsiness, excitation or depression, hallucinations, anxiety, delirium, hyperthermia, tachycardia, arrhythmias, seizures	Empty stomach with ipecac emesis or gastric lavage; support cardiorespiratory function; physostigmine may be useful for anticholinergic effects; diazepam for seizures; sponge baths with tepid water (not alcohol) or cold packs for hyperthermia
Barbiturates	10 times the daily therapeutic dose (e.g., 1–2 g of secobarbital)	Delirium, confusion, excitement, headache, CNS and respiratory depression from somnolence to coma, areflexia, circulatory collapse	Supportive treatment, including maintaining airway and respiration and treating shock as needed; within 30 minutes of ingestion, use activated charcoal; gastric lavage and aspiration can be used within 4 hours of ingestion; nasogastric administration of charcoal in multiple doses can shorten coma; maintain vital signs, fluid balances; alkalinizing the urine increases the excretion of mephobarbital, aprobarbital, phenobarbital; forced diuresis may be of use if renal function is normal; hemodialysis or peritoneal dialysis may be useful in severe cases
Benzodiazepines	Toxic dose: diazepam: 2 g; chlordiazepoxide: 6 g	Slurred speech, incoordination, somnolence, confusion coma, hyperreflexia, hypotension	General supportive care; induce emesis for recent ingestions in fully conscious patients; gastric lavage with endotracheal tube with inflated cuff if comatose; after above, use a saline cathartic and activated charcoal; maintain airway, monitor vital signs, give IV fluids; norepinephrine or metaraminol can be used for hypotension; flumazenil can be used with extreme caution.
Bromocriptine	Survival of 225 mg dose reported	Severe hypotension, nausea, vomiting, psychosis	Empty stomach by lavage and aspiration; IV fluids for hypotension
Bupropion	Ingestions of 850–4,200 mg have been survived; deaths have been reported in massive overdoses	Seizures, loss of consciousness, hallucinations, tachycardia	Ipecac emesis if conscious; gastric lavage with endotracheal tube in place with indicated out if there are seizures or a decreased level of consciousness; during first 12 hours after ingestion, use activated charcoal every 6 hours, provide fluids; electroencephalogram (EEG) and ECG monitoring for 48 hours; seizures can be treated with IV benzodiazepines
Buspirone	Toxic dose of 375 mg (used in studies); lethal dose unknown	Dizziness, drowsiness, nausea, vomiting, miosis, gastric distention	Symptomatic and supportive care; empty stomach with emesis or lavage in large ingestions; if needed, perform lavage with endotracheal tube in place with cuff inflated; monitor vital signs
Calcium channel inhibitors	9.6 g of verapamil has resulted in death; patients have survived ingestion of 8 to 10 g of diltiazem and 9 g of nifedipine (case reports)	Confusion, headache, nausea, vomiting, seizures, flushing, constipation, bradycardia, hypotension, atrioventricular block, hyperglycemia, metabolic acidosis	Emesis followed by gastric lavage with activated charcoal; calcium gluconate or calcium chloride 10–20 mg/kg in 10% solution with normal saline IV given over 30 minutes and repeated as needed; atropine or isoproterenol for atrioventricular block; a pacemaker may be needed

TABLE 21-3—continued

Drug	Toxic or Lethal Dose*	Signs and Symptoms	Treatment
Carbamazepine	Lowest known lethal dose in adults: 60 g; highest doses survived: children 10 g, adults 30 g	Drowsiness, stupor, dizziness, restlessness, ataxia, agitation, nausea, vomiting, involuntary movements, abnormal reflexes, adiadochokinesis, nystagmus, mydriasis, flushing, cyanosis, urinary retention, hypotension or hypertension, coma, cardiac arrhythmias	Induce emesis or gastric lavage; supportive measures: ECG monitoring
Carisoprodol	Patients have recovered from 3.4 g and 9.45 g ingestions	Stupor, shock, coma, respiratory depression, headache, diplopia, dizziness, drowsiness, nystagmus	Supportive treatment; induce emesis or use gastric lavage with endotracheal tube in place with cuff inflated if clinically indicated; activated charcoal after emptying stomach; maintain airway, respiration, and blood pressure; pressor agents can be used with caution if necessary; elimination may be enhanced by forced diuresis with hemodialysis, performed dialysis, or osmotic diuresis; avoid overhydration; monitor neurological status, electrolytes, and vital signs; continue monitoring for relapse secondary to delayed absorption and incomplete gastric emptying
Chloral hydrate	4–10 g	Coma, confusion, drowsiness, respiratory depression, hypotension, hypothermia, vomiting, miosis, gastric necrosis and perforation, esophageal stricture, hepatic injury, renal injury	General supportive measures; gastric lavage with endotracheal tube with inflated cuff in place; maintain airway, oxygenation, cardiorespiratory function, and body temperature; hemodialysis or peritoneal dialysis may be of use; saline enema if drug was administered rectally
Clonidine	No known deaths from overdoses of clonidine alone; 100 mg is the largest known overdose survived; two known deaths from mixed overdoses that included clonidine	Hypotension hyporeflexia or areflexia, vomiting, weakness, irritability, sedation coma, lethargy, hypothermia, constricted pupils, dry mouth, hypoventification, seizures, arrhythmia, cardiac conduction defects	Induce emesis or lavage followed by activated charcoal and a saline cathartic; lavage is preferred in patients with decreased levels of consciousness and should be used with endotracheal tube with inflated cuff in place if patient is comatose, has seizures, or lacks gag reflex; supportive and symptomatic measures; establish airway, IV fluids, and Trendelenburg's position for hypotension; if persistent, use dopamine; atropine IV for symptomatic bradycardia; tolazoline 10 mg IV every 30 minutes may reverse cardiovascular effects of clonidine; IV furosemide, α-blockers, or diazoxide for hypertension; IV benzodiazepines can be used for seizures.
Clozapine	Lethal dose: >2.5 g, although patients have survived ingestions of >4 g	Delirium, drowsiness, coma, respiratory depression, tachycardia, arrhythmics, hypotension, hypersalivation, seizures	Symptomatic and supportive care; establish and maintain airway, verification and oxygenation; activated charcoal with sorbitol (may be as effective as or more effective than lavage or emesis); monitor and adjust acid-base and electrolyte balance; physostigmine may be a useful adjunct for anticholinergic toxicity but is not for routine use; epinephrine, quinidine, procainamide are to be avoided; patient should be observed for several days for delayed effects

Drug	Lethal Dose / Fatality	Signs and Symptoms	Treatment
Dantrolene	No data available	Speech and visual disturbances, gastrointestinal (GI) upset or bleeding, liver damage, nausea, vomiting, CNS depression	Supportive measures: Immediate gastric lavage; ECG monitoring; large quantities of IV fluids; maintain airway; have artificial respiratory measures available; observe patient
Disulfiram	Six or more fatalities have occurred with ingestions of 0.5–1 g of disulfiram with blood alcohol levels of 1 mg/mL; a 30 g ingestion would produce serious toxicity	Headache, rash, peripheral or optic neuropathy, mucous membrane injury, psychotic behavior	Supportive treatment, gastric lavage or aspiration
Levodopa	Dose should not exceed 8 g a day in therapeutic use	Palpitations, arrhythmias, spasm or closing of eyes, psychosis	Symptomatic treatment: maintain airway, lavage; ECG monitoring; IV fluids; treat arrhythmias as necessary
Dopamine receptor antagonists	Fatal doses reported: chlorpromazine: 26 g (in an adult), 350 mg in a child; thiothixene: 2.5–4g; phenothiazines: 1,050 mg–10.5 g	Sedation hypertension, severe extrapyramidal symptoms, confusion, excitement, CNS depression, coma arrhythmias, miosis tremor, spasm, rigidity, seizures, dry mouth, ileus, difficulty in swallowing, muscular hypotonia, difficulty in breathing, hypothermia, vasomotor or respiratory collapse, sudden apnea	Symptomatic and supportive care: If clinically indicated, lavage may be performed with endotracheal tube with inflated cuff in place; emesis should not be induced; saline cathartic may be helpful; hypotension should be treated as necessary (avoid epinephrine); anticholinergics may be useful for extrapyramidal symptoms; exchange transfusions may be useful; oversedation and hypothermia should be treated as appropriate
Ethchlorvynol	6 g has been lethal; overdoses of 50 g and in one case 100 g have been survived	Hypotension, hypothermia, severe respiratory depression, apnea, deep coma (can last days to weeks), areflexia, mydriasis, bradycardia	Supportive treatment; gastric lavage with endotracheal tube with inflated cuff in place; maintain airway; give oxygen; maintain cardiorespiratory function and body temperature; monitor blood gases; provide pulmonary care; hemoperfusion with Amberlite XAD-4 resin hastens drug elimination; hemodialysis or peritoneal dialysis may be beneficial
Fenfluramine	2 g (460 mg in a child) was lowest reported fatal dose; 1.8 g in an adult is the highest reported nonfatal dose	Drowsiness, agitation, flushing, tremor, confusion, shivering, hyperventilation, dilated nonreactive pupils, tachycardia, hyperpyrexia, coma, seizures, cardiac arrest	Symptomatic and supportive care; gastric lavage; activated charcoal; endotracheal tube placement in consultation with an anesthesiologist is needed if trismus is present and lavage is to be performed; maintain cardiorespiratory function; cardiac monitoring; defibrillation, cardioversion, ventilatory support if needed; phenobarbital or diazepam for seizures or muscle hyperactivity; propranolol for severe tachycardia; lidocaine for ventricular extrasystoles; chlorpromazine may be useful for hyperthermia; forced acid diuresis with ammonium chloride may increase excretion rate

TABLE 21-3—*continued*

Drug	Toxic or Lethal Dose*	Signs and Symptoms	Treatment
Fluoxetine	Lethal dose unknown (one death reported)	Restlessness. Insomnia, agitation, tremor, hypomania, tachycardia, seizures, nausea, vomiting, hypertension, drowsiness, coma, nystagmus	Supportive and symptomatic care; keep airway open; maintain oxygenation and ventilation; monitor ECG and vital signs; gastric lavage (if clinically indicated) have endotracheal tube with cuff inflated during lavage) or emesis in recent ingestion, or use activated charcoal; IV diazepam for ongoing seizures; consider phenobarbital or phenytoin if refractory to diazepam
Glutethimide	5 g; severe intoxication; 10–20 g; often lethal	Hypotension, prolonged coma (up to days), shock, respiratory depression, hypothermia, fever, inadequate ventilation, apnea, cyanosis, fixed and dilated pupils, ileus, bladder atony, dry mouth, hyperreflexia, areflexia, intermittent spasticity or flaccidity	Supportive treatment; gastric lavage using 1 to 1 mixture of castor oil and water (may be more effective than aqueous lavage); perform with endotracheal tube in place with inflated cuff; leave 50 ml castor oil in stomach as a cathartic; activated charcoal may be of use; maintain airway and cardiorespiratory function; hemodialysis may be useful in severe cases (particularly with activated charcoal or soybean dialysate); hemoperfusion with Amberlite XAD–2 resin may be more effective than hemodialysis; charcoal hemoperfusion may be useful; continue drug removal procedures for at least 2 hours after the patient regains consciousness; maintain urinary output but avoid overhydration
Lithium	Lethal dose produces serum levels of >3.5 mEq/L 12 hours after ingestion	Diarrhea, vomiting, confusion, drowsiness, tremor, apathy, giddiness, nausea, ataxia, muscle rigidity, vertical nystagmus, impaired consciousness, cogwheel rigidity, coma, seizures, cardiovascular collapse	Induce emesis or lavage (lavage with endotracheal tube in place with cuff inflated if indicated); infuse 0.9% sodium chloride IV if toxicity is due to sodium depletion; hemodialysis for 8–12 hours if fluid and electrolyte imbalance does not respond to supportive measures; if levels is >2 mEq/L and patient is deteriorating or if level has not decreased 20% in 6 hours repeated courses of dialysis are often needed; goal is level of <1 mEq/L. 8 hours after dialysis is completed
Meprobamate	12 g is usually lethal; 40 g overdoses have been survived	Stupor, drowsiness, lethargy, ataxia, coma, respiratory depression, hypotension	Supportive treatment; induce emesis or use gastric lavage with endotracheal tube in place with cuff inflated if clinically indicated; use activated charcoal after emptying stomach; maintain airway, respiration, and blood pressure; pressor agents can be used with caution if necessary; elimination may be enhanced by forced diuresis with hemodialysis, peritoneal dialysis, or osmotic diuresis
Methadone	Lethal dose: 40–60 mg in nontolerant persons	CNS depression (stupor to coma), pinpoint pupils, shallow respiration, bradycardia, hypotension, hypothermia, cold and clammy skin, apnea, cardiac arrest, mydriasis in severe hypoxia or terminal narcosis	Establish and maintain airway and respiration; gastric lavage; supportive care with IV fluids; naloxone may be used to treat respiratory depression; initial adult dose is 0.4–2 mg IV every 2–3 minutes if needed; if there is no response after a total of 10 mg has been given, other diagnoses should be considered; repeated doses of naloxone may be needed, as narcotic induced respiratory depression may return as the effects of naloxone diminish; dosage regimens for continuous naloxone infusions are not well established and should be titrated to the patient's response; patients should be observed for sustained improvement after treatment

Drug	Toxic dose/concentration	Symptoms	Treatment
Methylphenidate hydrochloride	2 g	Delirium, confusion, psychosis, agitation, hallucinations, palpitations, arrhythmias, hypertension, vomiting, hyperpyrexia, mydriasis, sweating tremors, muscle twitching, seizures, coma	Emesis or lavage in mild cases; if patient is conscious, careful use of a short-acting barbiturate may be required before lavage in severe cases; supportive measures, including maintenance of respiratory and circulatory function; isolation to reduce external stimuli; protection against self-harm; external cooling procedures for hyperpyrexia
Methyprylon	Toxic blood concentration: 30 µg/mL	Confusion, somnolence, hypotension, tachycardia, edema, coma, shock, respiratory depression	Induce emesis or gastric lavage with endotracheal tube in place with cuff infected if clinically indicated; support cardiorespiratory function; barbiturates can be used with caution to control seizures and agitation
Monoamine oxidase inhibitors (MAOIs)	Single doses of 1.75-7 g have been fatal	Dizziness, drowsiness, irritability, ataxia, restlessness, insomnia, headache, tachycardia, hypotension, arrhythmia, confusion, fever, diaphoresis, hyperreflexia or hyperreflexia, respiratory depression, chest pain, shock, hypertension (rare)	Symptomatic and supportive care; induce emesis or use gastric lavage with endotracheal tube in place with inflated cuff if clinically indicated; maintain normal vital signs; correct fluid and electrolyte abnormalities with conservative measures; volume expansion for hypotension (pressor amines may be potentiated by MAOIs and may be of limited value); evaluate liver function immediately and 4-6 weeks later; barbiturates may relieve myoclonic reactions, but MAOIs may prolong their effect; phenothiazines can be used for agitation; hypertensive crisis mainly occurs in conjunction with tyramine; discontinue MAOIs and treat with phentolamine (5-10 mg by slow IV injection)
Pemoline	2 g	Excitement, agitation, restlessness, hallucinations, tachycardia, rhabdomyolysis, choreoathetosis	Gastric lavage in mild cases; symptomatic treatment; maintain respiratory on circulatory function; monitor cardiac function; reduce stimulation; haloperidol or chlorpromazine for psychosis and agitation; IV benzodiazepines can control choreoathetosis; hemodialysis may be of value
Sertraline	Three known overdoses at 750-2,100 mg; no deaths reported	Possible symptoms include confusion, ataxia, incoordination, hypotension, hypertension, seizures, arrhythmias, serotonin syndrome, coma, mydriasis	General symptomatic and supportive measures; establish and maintain airway; ensure adequate oxygenation and ventilation; use activated charcoal with sorbitol; monitor vital signs and cardiac function
Thyroid hormones	0.3 g per kg desiccated thyroid has caused severe toxicity (with recovery)	Nervousness, sweating, palpitations, abdominal cramps, diarrhea, tachycardia, hypertension, headache, arrhythmias, tremors, cardiac failure	Symptomatic and supportive treatment; induce emesis or use gastric lavage with endotracheal tube in place with cuff infated if clinically indicated; control fluid loss, fever, hypoglycemia; give oxygen and maintain ventilation; β-adrenergic receptor antagonists can be used to counteract increased sympathetic activity

TABLE 21-3—*continued*

Drug	Toxic or Lethal Dose*	Signs and Symptoms	Treatment
Trazodone	Patients have survived overdoses of 7.5 g and 9.2 g	Lethargy, vomiting, drowsiness, headache, orthostasis, dizziness, dyspnea, tinnitus, myalgias, tachycardia, incontinence, shivering, coma	Symptomatic and supportive treatment; induce emesis or use gastric lavage; forced diuresis may enhance elimination; treat hypotension and sedation as appropriate
Tricyclics and tetracyclics	700–1,400 mg: moderate to severe toxicity; 2.1–2.8 g: often fatal; one patient survived infestation of 10 g amitriptyline; lowest known fatal dose of amitriptyline: 500 mg; average lethal dose of imipramine; 30 mg per kg (fatalities occurred with 500 mg)	Initial CNS stimulation, confusion, agitation, hallucinations, hyperpyrexia, hypertension, nystagmus, hyperreflexia, parkinsonian symptoms, mydriasis, ileus, constipation, seizures, CNS depression (follows stimulation), hyperthermia, areflexia, respiratory depression, cyanosis, hypotension, coma, cardiac conduction abnormalities, tachycardia, quinidinelike effects (QRS prolongation, the degree of which may be the best indication of the severity of the overdose)	Symptomatic and supportive care; monitor ECG and vital signs; support vital functions; establish and maintain airway; treat and correct fluid, electrolyte, acidbase, and temperature abnormalities; minimize stimulation; gastric lavage with activated charcoal or ipecac emesis if gag reflex is present and patient is awake; treat hypotension supportively; IV diazepam (with caution) for seizures; lidocaine, phenytoin, propranolol for life-threatening arrhythmia, sodium bicarbonate IV to achieve pH of 7.4–7.6 to help treat arrhythmias and hypotension; use of multiple antiarrhythmics or pacemaker may be needed in some cases; physostigmine has been used for anticholinergic symptoms, but its use is controversial because of serious adverse effects, and it should be used only for life-threatening treatment-refractory anticholinergic toxicity
Valproic acid	One adult survived an ingestion of 36 g valproic acid as part of a polydrug overdose	Somnolence, coma	Supportive measures; lavage may be of limited value because of drug's rapid absorption; the value of emesis or lavage varies with time since ingestion if delayed-release preparations are ingested; maintain adequate urinary output; naloxone may reverse CNS depressant effects of overdose but may also reverse anticonvulsant effects and should be used with caution

*The toxic dose is the amount of the drug capable of producing signs and symptoms of an overdose. The same dose may also have lethal effects depending on such factors as the rate of administration, the rate of absorption, and the age and general health of the patient. A toxic dose for one patient may be lethal for another. The ranges given in this table are approximate, based on available scientific literature.
The clinician should always consult Physician's Desk Reference (PDR) or contact the manufacturer of the drug for the latest information on toxicity and lethality.
†A patient may have ingested more than one substance, and the signs and symptoms may represent polysubstance abuse or overdose. Treatment must be adjusted accordingly, and a history (from other persons, if necessary) and an inspection of all drugs should be obtained.

TABLE 21–4
SUBSTANCES GENERALLY NONTOXIC WHEN INGESTED*

Ball-point inks (amount in 1 pen)	Magnesium silicate (antacid)
Barium sulfate	Matches
Bathtub toys (floating)	Methylcellulose
Blackboard chalk (calcium carbonate)	Modeling clay
Candles (insect-repellent type may be toxic)	Paraffin, chlorinated
Carbowax (polyethylene glycol)	Pencil lead (graphite)
Carboxymethylcellulose (dehydrating material	Pepper, black (except inhaled in mass)
packed with drugs, film, etc.)	Petrolatum
Castor oil	Polyethylene glycols
Cetyl alcohol	Polyethylene glycol stearate
Crayons (children's: marked A.P., C.P.,	Polysorbate (Tweens®)
or C.S. 130-46)	Putty
Detergents, anionic and nonionic	Red oil (turkey-red oil, sulfated castor oil)
Dichloral (herbicide)	Silica (silicon dioxide)
Dry cell battery	Spermaceti
Glycerol	Stearic acid
Glyceryl monostearate	Sweetening agents
Graphite	Talc (except when inhaled)
Gums (acacia, agar, ghatti, etc)	Tallow
Hormones	Thermometer fluid or mercury
Kaolin	Titanium oxide
Lanolin	Triacetin (glyceryl triacetate)
Lauric acid	Vitamins, children's multiple (with or without
Linoleic acid	iron)
Linseed oil (not boiled)	Vitamins, multiple without iron
Lipstick	

*Substances listed here may, however, be present in combination with phenol, petroleum distillate vehicles, or other toxic chemicals. Since manufactured products may be changed in their composition, this table is intended only as a guide, and prudence requires that a poison center be consulted for up-to-date information.
Table from *Merck Manual*, ed 16, p 2682. Merck Sharp & Dohme Research Laboratories, Rahway, NJ 1992. Used with permission.

22
Combined Psychotherapy and Pharmacotherapy

One of the fastest growing practices in psychiatry is the use of pharmacological agents in combination with individual or group psychotherapy. This approach should not be attempted if the therapist meets with the patient only on an occasional or irregular basis to monitor the effects of medication or to make notations on a rating scale to assess progress or side effects. Instead, both therapies are integrated and synergistic. In many cases it has been demonstrated that the results of combined therapy are superior to either type of therapy used alone. The term "pharmacotherapy-oriented psychotherapy" is used by some practitioners to refer to the combined approach. The methods of psychotherapy used with pharmacotherapy vary immensely.

HISTORY

Before the introduction of antipsychotic medication in the 1950s, psychotherapy for schizophrenia was limited in its usefulness. Schizophrenic patients were unpredictable and sometimes aggressive, leaving many psychiatrists hesitant to start psychotherapy for fear of physical assault. In addition, schizophrenic patients were often withdrawn, uncommunicative, and unable to talk about their thoughts and feelings, factors that interfered with the conduct of psychotherapy. The use of medication helped reduce aggression and enhanced communication, making psychotherapy a potentially more effective treatment for those patients. To some extent, managing aggression and enhancing communication remain among the most significant reasons to use medication in combination with psychotherapy, whatever the diagnosis.

QUALIFICATIONS OF THERAPISTS

Besides having extensive training in one or more psychoanalytic or psychotherapeutic techniques, the psychiatrist who practices pharmacotherapy-oriented psychotherapy must have a comprehensive knowledge of psychopharmacology. That knowledge must include a thorough understanding of the indications for each drug, the contraindications, the pharmacokinetics, the pharmacodynamics, the drug-drug interactions (with all pharmacological agents, not only the psychoactive agents), and the adverse effects. The psychiatrist must also be able to diagnose and treat the adverse effects. Nonpsychiatric physicians often use psychoactive agents inaccurately because they lack the requisite psychopharmacological knowledge, training, and experience. Psychiatrists must have a high level of confidence and assurance in the combined-therapy approach. They must view emotional disorders as biopsychosocial events and must not separate mind from body. A unitary model in which illness is conceptualized as an interaction between biological and psychological processes allows the therapist to use combined therapy most effectively.

COUNTERTRANSFERENCE

As in all types of psychotherapy, psychiatrists must be aware of countertransference, their conscious and unconscious feelings toward their patients. A noncompliant patient may anger some psychiatrists. If unaware of that anger, the therapist may become, to the detriment of the therapy, punitive, authoritarian, or even rejecting. It is unwise, for example, to threaten a patient with termination because the patient will not take a prescribed drug. In those instances the resistance of the patient should be examined.

Psychiatrists must also be aware of their own psychological attitudes toward drugs (Table 22-1). Medications cannot replace the therapeutic alliance. They are not a shortcut to a cure and are no substitute for the intense concentration and involvement by the psychiatrist who is conducting psychotherapy. Therapists who are pessimistic about the value of psychotherapy or who misjudge the patient's motivation may prescribe medications out of their own nihilistic belief. Others may withhold medication if they overvalue psychotherapy or devalue pharmacological agents. Withholding medication is most likely to occur with borderline personality disorder patients, suicidal patients, and patients with a history of substance abuse. Each case must be evaluated individually, and the risk-benefit ratio must be carefully assessed so that the patient is not undeservedly punished, deprived, or mistreated.

INDICATIONS FOR COMBINED THERAPY

The primary indication for combined therapy is as a treatment for the specific disorder. As mentioned above, psychotropics reduce the hostility and the aggression that may be directed toward the therapist and, thus, improve the patient's capacity to communicate and to participate in the psychotherapeutic process. Another indication for combined therapy is to relieve distress when the signs and the symptoms of the patient's disorder are so prominent that they require more rapid relief than psychotherapy alone may be able to offer. In addition, each technique may facilitate the other; psychotherapy may enable the patient to accept a much-needed pharmacological agent, and the psychoactive drug may enable the patient to overcome resistance to entering or continuing psychotherapy.

TABLE 22–1
COUNTERTRANSFERENCE ISSUES IN COMPLIANCE

1. Overprescribing related to anger and helplessness
2. Inducing guilt in the patient
3. Colluding with noncompliance to demonstrate how ill the patient will get
4. Bullying the patient
5. Failures of empathy
6. Dread of the patient's anger

Table from G O Gobbard: Dynamic pharmacotherapy of depression. In *Psychiatric Times Medicine and Behavior*, p 52, 1991. Used with permission.

TYPES OF PSYCHOTHERAPY

Psychoanalysis

The therapist's ability to tolerate frustration and to delay gratification is a part of all psychotherapies, but especially so in psychoanalysis, which requires that regressive patterns emerge as a transference neurosis. This is the phenomenon in which the patient has a strong emotional attachment to the therapist because of the patient's feelings toward persons in his or her past. Many psychoanalysts are reluctant to use medication for fear that it will interfere with the development of the transference neurosis. However, if the analyst examines the meaning of the medication for the patient, it can provide material for further analysis. For example, in the technique of free association, one patient may view the analyst's prescribing medication as equivalent to receiving nurturance from an all-giving mother. Conversely, another patient may view the giving of medication as an act of control by an authoritarian father.

Analysts opposed to using medication believe that it violates, in theory, the rule of abstinence, in which patients can recognize their infantile needs only when they are not gratified. However, in actual practice, if interpretations of the patient's unconscious drives are timely and relevant and if the mental representation of the prescribed medication is explored, insights can be gained, often expeditiously. For example, transference may be expressed through the patient's attitude to the drug. In such cases, feelings are usually displaced from the therapist onto the medication and are subject to examination and interpretation. In some surveys 60 percent of psychoanalysts reported prescribing medication for some of their patients. Transference issues affecting compliance are listed in Table 22-2.

Psychoanalytic Psychotherapy

Psychoanalytic psychotherapy relies on psychoanalytic principles but focuses on current conflicts in the patient's life to a greater degree than does classic psychoanalysis. It is commonly divided into insight-oriented or expressive psychotherapy and supportive or relationship-oriented psychotherapy. Pharmacotherapy is used more often within this therapeutic framework than in psychoanalysis. Because this type of therapy is usually associated with guidance, advice giving, therapeutic leadership, and other relationship factors, both patients and therapists are generally less conflicted about using medication than they are in classic psychoanalysis. When the

TABLE 22–2
TRANSFERENCE ISSUES IN COMPLIANCE

---

1. The doctor is experienced as authoritarian or controlling.
2. The doctor threatens the patient's counterdependent stance.
3. The patient experiences the doctor as a mothering figure who will take care of all needs. Inducing passivity in the patient.
4. The patient rejects help as a way of defeating the doctor.
5. The doctor is experienced as giving up on psychotherapeutic approaches.
6. The patient develops transference to the medication itself.

Table from G O Gabbard: Dynamic pharmacotherapy of depression. In *Psychiatric Times: Medicine and Behavior,* p 51, 1991. Used with permission.

psychiatrist deals with issues related to the use of medications, many patients gain new insights into their behavior. For example, some patients are so frightened of becoming dependent on the therapist that they categorically refuse all medications.

Behavior Therapy

Behavior therapies include systematic desensitization, relaxation training, and social skills training. Various drugs have been used successfully to hasten the process in which the patient learns to decrease anxiety and to develop new patterns of behavior. Drugs such as methohexital (Brevital) and diazepam (Valium) relax most patients to the point that exposure to the stimulus that normally elicits the anxiety response instead desensitizes the patients to anxiety. Medications can also be used to increase assertiveness and overcome shyness, especially if such avoidant behavior is associated with depression or anxiety.

Cognitive Therapy

This short-term structured therapy has been used most often to treat patients with depression, including those with suicidal ideation. Therapy can be augmented with antidepressants and psychostimulants to overcome apathy, anhedonia, abulia, and feelings of helplessness.

Interpersonal Therapy

This type of psychotherapy is used primarily to treat depression. The therapy consists of weekly meetings held over a three-to-four-month period. The therapist attempts to clarify feeling states and to improve interpersonal relations. Medication is often used to deal with the sense of hopelessness and the feelings of anxiety that frequently accompany the the patient's depression.

Group Therapy

The concomitant use of medication can reduce withdrawal, isolation, avoidance, shyness, hostility, and other signs and symptoms of psychiatric disorders that interfere with social interactions. These interactions are crucial if cohesiveness, interpersonal learning, instillation of hope, identification, and other therapeutic factors in group psychotherapy are to be effective.

Triangular Therapy

In triangular therapy, also known as cotherapy, one therapist (who may be a psychologist or a social worker) conducts psychotherapy while the other therapist (always a psychiatrist) prescribes medications. The method requires that the two therapists regularly exchange information. Some patients split the transference between the two; one therapist may be seen as giving and nurturing and the other as withholding and aloof. Similarly, countertransference issues, such as one therapist's identifying with the patient's idealized or devalued image of the other therapist, can interfere with therapy. For triangular therapy program to succeed, cotherapists must be compatible, resolve countertransferance issues, and be respectful of each other's orientation.

THERAPEUTIC CONSIDERATIONS

Motivation for Psychotherapy

The reduction of symptoms, especially anxiety, does not decrease the patient's motivation for psychoanalysis or other insight-oriented psychotherapy. In practice, drug-induced symptom reduction improves communication and motivation. All therapies have a cognitive base, and anxiety generally interferes with the patient's ability to gain cognitive understanding of the illness. Drugs that decrease anxiety facilitate cognitive understanding. They also increase other functions of the ego, such as attention, concentration, memory, and learning. If resistance to combined therapy is persistent, the therapist should consider the factors listed in Table 22-3.

Self-Esteem

It may be a blow to the patient's self-esteem when the therapist introduces the need for a drug. Some patients may conclude that they are sicker than they thought, and others may feel themselves as failures unsuitable for psychotherapy. If those reactions are explored, they usually lead to previously unexpressed fears and feelings of inadequacy and self-deprecation. In most instances drugs help raise patients' self-esteem by improving functioning and allowing patients to better cope with the stresses of life.

Symptom Substitution

According to Sigmund Freud, symptom formation is the result of a conflict between the id, the superego, and the ego that produces anxiety, which is then channeled into a symptom. Although medication reduces the symptom, the conflict remains and can be analyzed; the drug does not cause symptom substitution. Thus, in a phobic patient whose phobia is diminished by medication, another symptom

TABLE 22-3
RESISTANCE ISSUES IN COMPLIANCE

1. Illness may be preferable to health.
2. Punishment is felt to be deserved.
3. Illness is denied because of stigmatization.
4. Unconscious identification with a depressed relative is being warded off.
5. Psychological factors override pharmacological effects.

Table from G O Gabbard: Dynamic pharmacotherapy of depression. In *Psychiatric Times: Medicine and Behavior,* p 62. 1991. Used with permission.

does not develop in its place; the insight-oriented therapy continues to make the unconscious conflict accessible to conscious reality.

Defense Mechanisms

Some processes relieve conflict and anxiety arising from one's impulses and drives. The ego uses defense mechanisms to guard against or to reduce the strength of an impulse, which is usually sexual or aggressive in nature. Mentally ill patients tend to use immature defense mechanisms to deal with those impulses. If a drug can lower instinctual anxiety, the patient may be able to use a mature defense mechanism in place of a primitive or immature defense. For example, a delusional patient using the immature defense of projection (attributing to another person unacceptable thoughts or feelings) may be able to use the mature defense of suppression (conscious controlling and inhibiting of unacceptable impulses or ideas), thus eliminating those unwanted ideas from consciousness and gaining more normal functioning.

Linkage Phenomenon

At some point patients may view the improvement being made in therapy as the result of a conscious or unconscious linkage between the psychopharmacological agent and the therapist. In fact, after being weaned from medication, patients often carry a pill with them for reassurance. In that sense the pill acts as a transitional object between the patient and the therapist.

Some patients with anxiety disorders, for example, may carry a single benzodiazepine tablet, which they take when they think they are about to have an anxiety attack. The patient may then report that the attack was aborted immediately—before the medication could even have been absorbed into the bloodstream. In other cases the pill is never taken because the patient knows that the pill is available and thus gains reassurance. The linkage phenomenon is usually not seen unless the patient is in a positive transference to the therapist. The therapist may use the phenomenon to his or her advantage by suggesting that the patient carry medication to use as needed. Eventually, the behavior has to be analyzed, and one often finds that the patient has attributed magical properties to the therapist that are then transferred to the medication. Some clinicians believe the effect to be the result of conditioning. After repeated trials the sight of the medicine can decrease anxiety.

CHOICE OF DRUG

The psychiatrist identifies and elicits from patients signs and symptoms of psychiatric disorders. *Signs* are objective findings observed by the clinician—for example, tachycardia and flat affect. *Symptoms* are the patient's subjective complaints—for example, palpitations and depressed mood. In many conditions, such as anxiety disorder, signs and symptoms overlap. The sign or the symptom can be targeted as a specific criterion that both the psychiatrist and the patient can use to determine whether the psychotropic agent is having the desired effect.

Placebo Effect

In pharmacology the *placebo effect* is that phenomenon in which a person exhibits a clinically significant response to a pill containing a physiologically inert substance. The response is purely psychological and is not due to any psychopharmacological property of the drug. In some cases the placebo effect can be measured objectively. For example, not only does the patient state that he or she feels less anxious, but there is less autonomic nervous system arousal, evidenced by lower blood pressure and a decrease in heart rate. Placebo effects are common in patients with dissociative disorders, hypochondriasis, somatoform disorders, anxiety disorders, and sexual disorders.

COMPLIANCE AND PATIENT EDUCATION

Compliance is the degree to which a patient carries out the recommendations of the treating physician. A positive doctor-patient relationship is the best assurance of compliance, and the patient's refusal to take medication may provide insight into a negative transferential situation. In some cases the patient acts out hostilities by noncompliance, rather than becoming aware of and ventilating such negative feelings toward the doctor. Medication noncompliance may give the psychiatrist the first clue that a negative transference is present in an otherwise compliant patient who had appeared to be nothing but agreeable and cooperative.

Patients should know the target signs and symptoms that the drug is supposed to reduce, the length of time that they will be taking the drug, both the expected and the unexpected adverse effects, and the treatment plan to be followed if the current drug is unsuccessful. Although some psychiatric disorders interfere with patients' ability to comprehend that information, the psychiatrist should relay as much of the information as possible. The clear presentation of the material is often less frightening than are patients' fantasies about drug treatment. The psychiatrist should tell patients when they will begin to receive benefits from the drug. That information is perhaps most critical when the patient has a mood disorder and may not observe any therapeutic effects for three to four weeks (Table 22-4).

Some patients' ambivalent attitudes toward drugs often reflect the confusion in the field of psychiatry about drug treatment. Patients often believe that taking a psychotherapeutic drug means that they are not in control of their lives or that they

TABLE 22-4
SPECIFIC INSTRUCTIONS FOR PATIENTS

- Name of the medication (brand name and generic name)
- Whether it is meant to treat the disease or the symptoms and, therefore, how important it is to take it
- How to tell if it is working and what to do if it appears not to be working
- When and how to take it—before or after meals
- What to do if a dose is missed
- How long to take it
- Side effects that are important for the patient and what to do about them
- Possible effects on driving, on work, and so on, and what precautions to take
- Interactions with alcohol and other drugs

Table adapted from N G Ward. In *Integrating Pharmacotherapy and Psychotherapy*, B D Bellman, G L Klerman, editors, p 87. American Psychiatric Press. Washington, 1991. Used with permission.

may become addicted to the drug and have to take it forever. Psychiatrists should explain the difference between drugs of abuse that affect the normal brain and psychiatric drugs used to treat emotional disorders. Psychiatrists should also point out to patients that antipsychotics, antidepressants, and antimanic drugs are not addictive in the way that, for example, heroin is addictive. The psychiatrist's clear and honest explanation of how long the patient should take the drug will help the patient adjust to the idea of chronic maintenance medication if that is, indeed, the treatment plan. In some cases the psychiatrist may appropriately give the patient increasing responsibility for adjusting the medications as the treatment progresses. Doing so often helps the patient feel less controlled by the drug and in a collaborative role with the therapist.

COMBINED THERAPY IN SPECIFIC DISORDERS

Depressive Disorders

Some patients and clinicians fear that medication will cover over the depression and that psychotherapy will be impeded. Medication should be viewed as a facilitator in overcoming the anergia that may inhibit communication between doctor and patient. The psychiatrist should also explain to the patient that depression interferes with interpersonal activity in a variety of ways. For instance, depression produces withdrawal and irritability, which alienates significant others who may otherwise gratify the strong dependency needs that make up much of depressive psychodynamics.

The psychiatrist should be alert for signs and symptoms of a recurrent major depressive episode. Medication may have to be reinstituted. Before doing so, however, one should carefully review any stress, especially rejections, that may have precipitated recurrent major depressive disorder. A major episode may also occur because the patient is in a stage of negative transference, and the psychiatrist must try to elicit negative feelings. In many cases the ventilation of angry feelings toward the therapist without an angry response can serve as a corrective emotional experience, and a major depressive episode necessitating medication can thereby be forestalled. Depressed patients are generally maintained on their medication for six months or longer after clinical improvement. The cessation of pharmacotherapy before that time is likely to result in a relapse.

Suicidal Behavior

The possibility of suicide must be considered in treating patients with schizophrenia, bipolar I disorder, depressive disorders, and anxiety disorders (especially those who have panic attacks). If the psychiatrist decides that the patient is in imminent risk for suicidal behavior, hospitalization is always indicated. If the patient can be managed outside a hospital, medication should be given to a responsible family member who can monitor the dosage and the frequency of the prescribed medication. As a further precaution, the psychiatrist may treat the patient with a drug known to have little or no lethal potential when taken in an overdose attempt. Medication is almost always indicated in suicidally depressed patients.

Bipolar I Disorder

Patients taking lithium (Eskalith) or other treatments for bipolar I disorder are usually medicated for an indefinite time to prevent episodes of either mania or depression. Most psychotherapists insist that patients with bipolar I disorder be medicated before starting any insight-oriented therapy. Without such premedication, most bipolar I disorder patients cannot make the necessary therapeutic alliance. When those patients are depressed, their abulia seriously disrupts their flow of thoughts, and the sessions are nonproductive. When they are manic, their flow of associations can be rapid and their speech pressured; the therapist may be flooded with material and unable to make appropriate interpretations or unable to assimilate the material into the patient's disrupted cognitive framework.

Anxiety Disorders

Anxiety disorders encompass obsessive-compulsive disorder, posttraumatic stress disorder, generalized anxiety disorder, phobic disorders, and panic disorder with or without agoraphobia. Many drugs are effective in managing distressing signs and symptoms. As medication controls the symptoms, patients are reassured and develop confidence that the disorder will not incapacitate them. That effect is particularly strong in panic disorder, which is often associated with anticipatory anxiety about the attack. Depression may also complicate the symptom picture in patients with anxiety disorders and has to be addressed both pharmacologically and psychotherapeutically.

Schizophrenia and Other Psychotic Disorders

Included in this group of disorders are schizophrenia, delusional disorder, schizo-affective disorder, schizophreniform disorder, and brief psychotic disorder. Drug treatment for those disorders is always indicated, and hospitalization is often necessary for diagnostic purposes, to stabilize medication, to prevent danger to self or others, and to establish a psychosocial treatment program that may include individual psychotherapy. In attempting individual psychotherapy, the therapist must establish a treatment relationship and a therapeutic alliance with the patient. The schizophrenic patient defends against closeness and trust and often becomes suspicious, anxious, hostile, or regressed in therapy. Before the arrival of psychotropics, many psychiatrists were fearful for their own safety when working with such patients. Indeed, many assaults occurred.

Individual psychotherapy for schizophrenia is labor-intensive, expensive, and still not often attempted. The recognition that combined psychotherapy-pharmacotherapy has a greater chance of success than does either type of therapy alone may reverse that situation. The psychiatrist who conducts such combined therapy must be especially empathic and able to tolerate the bizarre manifestations of the illness. The schizophrenic patient is exquisitely sensitive to rejection, and individual psychotherapy should never be started unless the therapist is willing to make a total commitment to the process.

Substance Abuse

Patients who abuse alcohol or drugs present the most difficult challenge in combined therapy. They are often impulsive and, though they promise not to abuse a substance, may do so repeatedly. In addition, they frequently withhold information from the psychiatrist about episodes of abuse. For that reason some psychiatrists do not prescribe any medication to such patients, especially not substances with a high abuse potential, such as benzodiazepines, barbiturates, and amphetamines. Drugs with no abuse potential—such as thioridazine (Mellaril), amitriptyline (Elavil), and fluoxetine (Prozac)—have an important role in treating the anxiety or depression or both that almost always accompanies substance-related disorders. The psychiatrist conducting psychotherapy with such patients should have no reservations about sending the patient to a laboratory for random urine toxicological tests. As in all forms of insight-oriented psychotherapy, the psychological significance of such tests should be examined.

An overview of the medication issues in the combined therapy approach is given in Table 22-5.

ETHICAL AND LEGAL ISSUES

Informed Consent

Informed consent is a legal term indicating that the patient has agreed to a particular treatment program—for example, a drug trial—after having been advised of the potential benefits of treatment, the risks of treatment, and alternative treatments. Some states require patients to sign a document stating that they have given informed consent, and some clinicians have adopted that practice in states that do not require such a form. In either case the physician should make a notation in the patient's chart that the issue has been discussed. Clearly, the capacity of a psychiatric patient to understand the information is often difficult to assess. The problem represents an ethical dilemma that can best be met by clinicians' attempting to meet the letter and the spirit of the law to the best of their abilities. When in doubt about a patient's ability to make such a decision, the physician should consult the patient's family, friends, or legal counsel.

Hospital Care

In hospitals, especially hospitals in the public sector, medication is often the major form of treatment offered. The shortage of psychiatrists and the excessive number of patients in the city and state mental hospital system prevent the use of psychotherapy for patients who are, for the most part, either psychotic or demented. Those patients unwilling to take medication can be forced to do so under certain circumstances. For example, if they are imminently dangerous to themselves or others, medication can be given against their will and forcibly, if necessary.

TABLE 22-5
THE STAGES OF INDIVIDUAL PSYCHOTHERAPY: A MEDICATION EMPHASIS

Stage	Engagement	Pattern Search	Change	Termination
Goals	Trust Credibility Self-observer alliance	To define problem patterns that, if changed, would lead to a desirable outcome	1. Relinquish old pattern (s) 2. Initiate new pattern(s) 3. Practice new pattern (s)	To separate efficiently
Techniques	Convey empathic understanding Effective suggestions Effective medications	Questionnaires Homework-idiosyncratic meanings ascribed to medication	Interpretation Reforming Behavioral suggestion Medications-induced change	Mutually agreed Patient initiates Therapist initiates Medication-influenced
Content	Medication responsive Diagnosis	Does response to medication reflect a problem pattern?	Medication effects or insight around medication use accelerates change	Medications may prolong termination
Resistance	Are excessive side effects resistance to treatment?	Does pattern of nonadherence to medication regimen reflect a problem pattern?	Do new side effects suggest resistance to change?	Symptom reoccurrence not necessarily indication for medication change
Transference	Physician seen as malevolent or all-powerful	Is key interpersonal pattern reflected in meaning of medication?	Unresolved distortions may be signaled by a new medication issue inhibiting change	Desire for new or more medication reflects desire to keep therapist
Countertransference	Physician failure to prescribe appropriately	Medication prescription reflects distorted response to patient	Sudden change in regimen reflects an attempt to undermine change	New medication reflects desire to keep contact

Table by B D Bellman. In *Integrating Pharmacotherapy and Psychotherapy*, B D Bellman, G I Klerman, editors, p 22. American Psychiatric Press, Washington, 1991. Used with permission.

Treatment Records

In addition to making any process notes regarding psychotherapy, the psychiatrist should keep detailed records of prescription dates, dosages, directions, warnings about side effects, and physical and psychological responses to the drug.

Most malpractice cases against psychiatrists result from the adverse effects of psychotropic drugs, but some suits have been brought because doctors withheld medication. In one case a severely depressed patient was treated with insight-oriented psychotherapy and long-term hospitalization. The patient's attorney argued that, if psychotropic medication had been prescribed, the patient's depression would have lifted more rapidly than it did and his stay in the hospital would have been shortened. The parties settled the case out of court.

DURATION OF MEDICATION USE

The length of time a patient is expected to take medication depends on several factors: (1) the purpose of the medication (for example, symptom removal), (2) the disorder being treated (for example, depression or schizophrenia), (3) the type of associated psychotherapeutic program (for example, psychoanalysis), and (4) the characteristics of the drug (for example, whether it is associated with adverse effects, such as withdrawal symptoms). In some cases medication can and should be taken indefinitely, and in others it is used only as a short-term adjuvant.

Antidepressant Drugs

A wide range of antidepressant compounds are used to treat depression, and clinical improvement can occur in more than 50 percent of depressed patients so treated. An untreated depressive episode lasts 6 to 12 months on average. Because of that, the withdrawal of antidepressant medication before three months almost always results in the return of symptoms. Most psychiatrists keep giving medication to a depressed patient for six months after clinical improvement occurs. Long-term antidepressant drug treatment is often indicated as a prophylactic measure in patients with a history of recurrent serious depression. However, a relapse or a recurrence of depressive symptoms may occur. For that reason, combined drug therapy and psychotherapy is the treatment of choice.

Antimanic Drugs

Although most patients with manic episodes also experience depressive intervals, lithium and the anticonvulsants are the mainstays of treatment for mania. An untreated manic episode lasts about three months, and discontinuing drugs before that time is unwise. As the illness progresses, the time between manic episodes decreases, and most patients with bipolar disorder keep taking lithium indefinitely. As with all pharmacological agents, the risk of adverse effects must be considered—for example, lithium is contraindicated in pregnancy. Patients in psychotherapy whom a psychiatrist observes frequently (once or twice a week) may be treated with lithium intermittently because the physician can assess an impending manic episode based on an ongoing assessment of the patient.

Antipsychotic Drugs

Antipsychotic medication is the mainstay of treatment for schizophrenia and related disorders. Antipsychotic drugs are relatively safe and are prescribed indefinitely for most patients. Maintenance dosages of antipsychotics are usually lower than dosages for acute episodes. Schizophrenic patients receiving combined drug and psychosocial therapy do better than those treated with medication alone and are less likely to relapse.

Antianxiety Drugs

The most frequently used class of drugs in the treatment of anxiety disorders are the benzodiazepines. Most patients with generalized anxiety disorder are treated for about two to three months for their acute symptoms, at which point the drug is gradually withdrawn. Some patients require long-term administration of benzodiazepines. There is no evidence of tolerance or a need to increase the dosage of the drug when such patients are receiving concomitant individual psychotherapy. Long-term treatment is especially useful in patients with hyperactive autonomic nervous systems or with autonomic nervous system arousal syndromes. The risk of abuse in such patients is minimal when the drugs are used in an integrated therapy program.

Sympathomimetics

The sympathomimetics include dextroamphetamine (Dexedrine), methylphenidate (Ritalin), and pemoline (Cylert). They are used mainly in attention-deficit/ hyperactivity disorder (ADHD) in children and in adults when residual symptoms of ADHD are present. The drugs are also useful in certain patients with chronic depressive states, though psychostimulants are not labeled for that use by the Food and Drug Administration (FDA). Because sympathomimetics are subject to abuse if not used judiciously, they should always be prescribed in conjunction with a course of psychotherapy. Many patients with anhedonia, low energy levels, and abulia can be maintained with small dosages of amphetamines (5 to 15 mg a day) for long periods of combined treatment without risk of abuse or tolerance.

For a more detailed discussion of this topic, see T B Karasu: Psychoanalysis and Psychoanalytic Psychotherapy, Sec. 31.1, p 1767 in CTP/VI.

23
Medication-Induced Movement Disorders and Their Management

The antipsychotic drugs and other drugs with dopamine-antagonist properties (for example, amoxapine [Asendin], an antidepressant drug) are associated with several uncomfortable and potentially serious neurological adverse effects. They include (1) neuroleptic-induced parkinsonism, (2) neuroleptic-induced acute dystonia, (3) neuroleptic-induced acute akathisia, (4) neuroleptic-induced tardive dyskinesia, (5) neuroleptic malignant syndrome, (6) medication-induced postural tremor, and (7) hypothermic syndromes. Those disorders are discussed in this chapter. Other movement disorder symptoms can result from the use of antipsychotic drugs but, because they also may be symptoms of psychiatric disorders, are discussed in Chapter 19: akinesia (Section 19.1), dyskinesia (Section 19.5), and tremor (Section 19.21).

NEUROLEPTIC-INDUCED PARKINSONISM

Parkinsonian adverse effects occur in about 15 percent of patients who are treated with antipsychotics, usually in 5 to 90 days after the initiation of treatment. Symptoms include muscle stiffness (lead-pipe rigidity), cogwheel rigidity, shuffling gait, stooped posture, and drooling. The pill-rolling tremor of idiopathic parkinsonism is rare, but a regular, coarse tremor similar to essential tremor may be present. A focal, perioral tremor, sometimes called *rabbit syndrome* is another parkinsonian effect seen with antipsychotics, although perioral tremor differs from other extrapyramidal side effects in that it typically occurs only after prolonged treatment. Rabbit syndrome may be misdiagnosed as a negative symptom of schizophrenia (flattened affect).

Women are affected by neuroleptic-induced parkinsonism about twice as often as men, and the disorder can occur at all ages, although it is most common after age 40. All antipsychotics can cause the symptoms, especially high-potency drugs with low anticholinergic activity (for example, trifluoperazine [Stelazine]). Chlorpromazine (Thorazine) and thioridazine (Mellaril) are not likely to be involved. The blockade of dopaminergic transmission in the nigrostriatal tract is the cause of neuroleptic-induced parkinsonism. The differential diagnosis of the parkinsonian symptoms should include idiopathic parkinsonism, other medical causes of parkinsonism, and depression, which can also be associated with parkinsonian symptoms.

Treatment

The disorder can be treated with anticholinergic agents, amantadine (Symadine, Symmetrel), or diphenhydramine (Benadryl) (Table 23-1). Anticholinergics should be withdrawn after four to six weeks to assess whether the patient has developed

TABLE 23–1
DRUG TREATMENT OF EXTRAPYRAMIDAL DISORDERS

Generic Name	Trade Name	Usual Daily Dosage	Indications
Anticholinergic			
Benztropine	Cogentin	PO 0.5–2mg tid; IM or IV 1–2 mg	Acute dystonic reaction, parkinsonism, akinesia, akathisia
Biperiden	Akineton	PO 2–6 mg tid; IM or IV 2 mg	
Procyclidine	Kemadrin	PO 2.5–5 mg bid–qid	
Trihexyphenidyl	Artane	PO 2–5 mg tid	
Ethopropazine	Parsidol	PO 50–100 mg bid–qid	Rabbit syndrome
Orphenadrine	Norflex	PO 50–100 mg bid–qid; IV 60 mg	
Antihistamine			
Diphenhydramine	Benadryl	PO 25 mg qid; IM or IV 25 mg	Acute dystonic reaction, parkinsonism, akinesia, rabbit syndrome
Dopamine agonist			
Amantadine	Symmetrel	PO 100–200 mg bid	Parkinsonism, akinesia, rabbit syndrome
β-Adrenergic antagonist			
Propranolol	Inderal	PO 20–40 mg tid	Akathisia, tremor
α-Adrenergic antagonist			
Clonidine	Catapres	PO 0.1 mg tid	Akathisia
Benzodiazepines			
Clonazepam	Klonopin	PO 1 mg bid	Akathisia, acute dystonic reactions
Lorazepam	Ativan	PO 1 mg tid	
Buspirone	BuSpar	PO 20–40 mg qid	Tardive dyskinesia
Vitamin E	—	PO 1,200–1,600 IU od	Tardive dyskinesia

PO, orally; *IM*, intramuscular; *IV*, intravenous; *od*, per day; *bid*, twice a day; *tid*, three times a day; *qid*, four times a day.

a tolerance for the parkinsonian effects; about 50 percent of patients with neuroleptic-induced parkinsonism need continued treatment. Even after the antipsychotics are withdrawn, parkinsonian symptoms may last up to two weeks and even up to three months in elderly patients. With such patients the clinician may continue the anticholinergic drug after stopping the antipsychotic until the parkinsonian symptoms have completely resolved.

NEUROLEPTIC-INDUCED ACUTE DYSTONIA

About 10 percent of all patients experience dystonia as an adverse effect of antipsychotics, 50 percent of those in the first two days of treatment. It is a less common side effect than parkinsonism and akathisia. Acute dystonia is the slow, involuntary contraction of one or more muscle groups. Dystonia can involve the neck (spasmodic torticollis or retrocollis), the jaw (forced opening resulting in a dislocation of the jaw or trismus), the tongue (protrusions, twisting), and the entire body (opisthotonos). Involvement of the eyes can result in an oculogyric crisis, characterized by the eyes' upward lateral movement. Blepharospasm, grimacing, dysphagia, and respiratory stridor may also occur. Laryngeal dystonia can be life-threatening. Writhing movements of the limbs or the trunk may be a form of dystonia. Children are particularly likely to evidence opisthotonos, scoliosis, lordosis, and writhing movement. It is a frightening and often painful experience for the patient, and a common reason for future noncompliance with antipsychotic medications. Patients who refer to having had an allergic reaction to past treatment with an antipsychotic are often referring to an episode of dystonia.

Dystonia is most common in young men (less than 40 years old) but can occur at any age in either sex. Although it is most common with intramuscular (IM) dosages of high-potency antipsychotics, dystonia can occur with any conventional dopamine receptor antagonist antipsychotic. It is least common with thioridazine and is uncommon with risperidone (Risperdal). The mechanism of action is thought to be the dopaminergic hyperactivity in the basal ganglia that occurs when the central nervous system (CNS) levels of the antipsychotic drug begin to fall between doses. Dystonia can fluctuate spontaneously, responding to reassurance and resulting in the clinician's false impression that the movement is hysterical or completely under conscious control. The disorder must be differentiated from seizures, tetany, tetanus, tardive dyskinesia that does not involve spastic muscle contraction, encephalitis, metabolic illness, and hysterical or psychotic posturing. Some patients simulate dystonia to obtain antiparkinsonian agents, which can produce euphoria.

Other causes of dystonia include (1) dystonia musculorum deformans (torsion dystonia), a rare disorder in children marked by bizarre postures; (2) focal dystonia of a single muscle group, typically presenting in adulthood; (3) spastic torticollis, caused by dystonia of the sternocleidomastoid muscle; and (4) occupational spasms that result from the repeated use of a particular muscle group (for example, writer's cramp).

Treatment

Treat antipsychotic-induced dystonia rapidly with benztropine (Cogentin) 1 to 2 mg IM or intravenously (IV); with other anticholinergic medications; or with antihistamines, such as diphenhydramine 25 to 50 mg by mouth, IM, or IV. For the most rapid relief, an IM or an IV injection usually relieves the symptoms within several minutes. The dose can be repeated in 15 minutes. Suspect another diagnosis if three doses are ineffective. For dystonia that does not respond to anticholinergic drugs, give methylphenidate (Ritalin), caffeine sodium benzoate, a benzodiazepine, or a barbiturate.

Laryngeal dystonias are medical emergencies that should be treated with benztropine 2 mg IV at once, with a repeat dose in 5 to 10 minutes if the patient does not respond. If the patient still does not respond, try lorazepam (Ativan) 1 to 2 mg by slow IV. The patient rarely requires intubation.

Prophylaxis with anticholinergics or related drugs (Table 23-1) usually prevents the development of dystonia, although the risks of prophylactic treatment weigh against that benefit. Prophylactic treatment may be indicated for several days when starting to give high-potency antipsychotics to patients at high risk for dystonia (for example, brain-damaged patients, young men, children).

Although tolerance for the adverse effect usually develops, changing the antipsychotic is sometimes prudent if the patient is particularly concerned that the reaction may recur.

NEUROLEPTIC-INDUCED ACUTE AKATHISIA

Akathisia is a subjective feeling of muscular discomfort that can cause the patient to be agitated, pace relentlessly, alternately sit and stand in rapid succession, and feel generally dysphoric. The symptoms are primarily motor and cannot be controlled by the patient's will. Akathisia is an extrapyramidal symptom most commonly caused by high-potency antipsychotics. An estimated 50 percent of the people with akathisia also show evidence of other extrapyramidal side effects, such as parkinsonism, dystonias, cogwheeling, rigidity, and flattened affect. The condition is difficult to treat and may not respond to any treatment. Akathisia is commonly mistaken for worsening agitation, especially since it is aggravated by stress and anxiety, and it may be mistakenly and incorrectly treated with increased dosages of antipsychotic medication. Akathisia is a common reason for noncompliance with antipsychotic medication. An estimated 20 to 50 percent of patients taking antipsychotic medications experience akathisia.

Treatment

If both akathisia and agitation are present, consider sedating the patient with a benzodiazepine—for example, lorazepam 2 mg IM—and then reevaluating the patient in one to two hours. A typical dosage of lorazepam is 1 mg three times a day.

If akathisia, alone is present, reduce the antipsychotic dosage if the target symptoms of antipsychotic treatment allow it. β-Blockers, such as propranolol (Inderal) 10 to 40 mg three times a day, may be helpful.

Clonidine (Catapres) has also been reported to be effective. It may be given parenterally in severe cases or orally 0.1 mg three times a day.

Anticholinergic medication—for example, benztropine 2 mg by mouth, IM, or IV—can be tried. Anticholinergic drugs are much less effective in treating akathisia than they are in treating other extrapyramidal syndromes.

Amantadine, a dopamine agonist, 100 to 300 mg, may also be tried. If those interventions are not effective, akathisia may warrant changing the medication to a low-potency antipsychotic.

NEUROLEPTIC-INDUCED TARDIVE DYSKINESIA

Tardive dyskinesia is a delayed effect of antipsychotics; it rarely occurs until after six months of treatment. The disorder consists of abnormal, involuntary, irregular choreoathetoid movements of the muscles of the head, the limbs, and the trunk. The severity of the movements ranges from minimal—often missed by patients and their families—to grossly incapacitating. Perioral movements are generally the earliest and most common signs and include darting, twisting, and protruding movements of the tongue; chewing and lateral jaw movements; lip puckering; and facial grimacing. Finger movements and hand clenching are also common. Even relatively minor movements of the upper extremities may interfere with coordination and result in disability. Torticollis, retrocollis, trunk twisting, and pelvic thrusting are seen in severe cases. Respiratory dyskinesia has also been reported. Dyskinesia is exacerbated by stress and disappears during sleep.

About 10 to 20 percent of patients treated with antipsychotics for more than a year develop tardive dyskinesia. About 15 to 20 percent of long-term hospital patients have tardive dyskinesia. Women are more likely to be affected than are men, and patients more than 50 years of age, patients with brain damage, children, and patients with mood disorders are also at high risk.

The risk increases with the length of antipsychotic treatment. However, the course of tardive dyskinesia is variable. It may remain stable on the same antipsychotic dosage or progress; if antipsychotics are discontinued, the movements may diminish or disappear completely, particularly in mild cases detected in the early stages.

Prevention is best achieved by using antipsychotic medications only when clearly indicated and in the lowest effective dosages. The new antipsychotics (for example, risperidone) are associated with less tardive dyskinesia than the old antipsychotics. Patients who are receiving antipsychotics should be examined regularly for the appearance of abnormal movements, preferably by using a standardized rating scale such as the Abnormal Involuntary Movement Scale (Table 23-2).

TABLE 23–2
ABNORMAL INVOLUNTARY MOVEMENT SCALE (AIMS) EXAMINATION PROCEDURE

Patient identification	Date
Rated by	

Either before or after completing the examination procedure, observe the patient unobtrusively at rest (eg, in waiting room).

The chair to be used in this examination should be a hard, firm one without arms.

After observing the patient, rate him or her on a scale of 0 (none), 1 (minimal), 2 (mild), 3 (moderate), and 4 (severe) according to the severity of the symptoms.

Ask the patient whether there is anything in his or her mouth (ie, gum, candy, etc.) and, if so, to remove it.

Ask the patient about the *current* condition of his or her teeth. Ask patient if he or she wears dentures. Do teeth or dentures bother patient now.

Ask patient whether he or she notices any movement in mouth, face, hands, or feet. If yes, ask patient to describe and indicate to what extent they *currently* bother patient or interfere with his or her activities.

0 1 2 3 4 Have patient sit in chair with hands on knees, legs slightly apart, and feet flat on floor. (Look at entire body for movements while in this position.)

0 1 2 3 4 Ask patient to sit with hands hanging unsupported. If male, between legs, if female and wearing a dress, hanging over knees. (Observe hands and other body areas.)

0 1 2 3 4 Ask patient to open mouth. (Observe tongue at rest within mouth.) Do this twice.

0 1 2 3 4 Ask patient to protrude tongue. (Observe abnormalities of tongue movement.) Do this twice.

0 1 2 3 4 Ask the patient to tap thumb, with each finger, as rapidly as possible for 10 to 15 seconds; separately with right hand, then with left hand. (Observe facial and leg movements.)

0 1 2 3 4 Flex and extend patient's left and right arms. (One at a time.)

0 1 2 3 4 Ask patient to stand up. (Observe in profile. Observe all body areas again, hips included.)

0 1 2 3 4 *Ask patient to extend both arms outstretched in front with palms down. (Observe trunk, legs, and mouth.)

0 1 2 3 4 Have patient walk a few paces, turn and walk back to chair. (Observe hands and gait.) Do this twice.

* Activated movements

Consider a number of other diagnoses: perioral (rabbit) syndrome; bruxism; Parkinson's disease; Huntington's disease; and Tourette's disorder. Abnormal movements sometimes emerge when the antipsychotic dosage is reduced. The relation of withdrawal emergent dyskinesias to tardive dyskinesia is unclear, but the withdrawal dyskinesias are generally regarded as early tardive dyskinesia masked by high dosages but uncovered by dosage reduction. Tardive movements can be suppressed, at least temporarily, by increasing the antipsychotic dosage. Antiparkinsonian agents may worsen tardive dyskinesia.

Treatment

Once tardive dyskinesia is recognized, the clinician should consider reducing the dosage of the antipsychotic or even stopping the medication altogether. Alternatively, the clinician may switch the patient to clozapine (Clozaril) or to one of the new dopamine receptor antagonists, such as risperidone. Vitamin E and high dosages of buspirone (BuSpar) (up to 160 mg a day) may be effective.

Between 5 and 40 percent of all cases of tardive dyskinesia eventually remit, and between 50 and 90 percent of all mild cases remit. However, tardive dyskinesia is less likely to remit in elderly patients than in young patients.

Tardive dyskinesia has no single effective treatment. Lowering the dosage of the antipsychotic and switching to a new antipsychotic, including clozapine, are the primary treatment strategies. In patients who cannot continue taking any antipsychotic medication, lithium (Eskalith), carbamazepine, or benzodiazepines may be effective in reducing both the movement disorder symptoms and the psychotic symptoms.

NEUROLEPTIC MALIGNANT SYNDROME

Neuroleptic malignant syndrome is an uncommon but life-threatening complication that usually occurs within the first ten days of starting an antipsychotic or increasing the dosage, although it may occur at any time during treatment. The motor and behavioral symptoms include muscular rigidity and dystonia, akinesia, mutism, obtundation, and agitation. The autonomic symptoms include hyperpyrexia (up to 107°F), sweating, and increased pulse and blood pressure. Laboratory findings include increased white blood cell count, creatinine phosphokinase, liver enzymes, plasma myoglobin, and myoglobinuria, occasionally associated with renal failure. The symptoms usually evolve over 24 to 72 hours, and the untreated syndrome lasts 10 to 14 days. The diagnosis is often missed in the early stages, and the withdrawal or agitation may mistakenly be considered to reflect increased psychosis. Men are affected more frequently than are women, and young patients (20 to 40 years) are affected more commonly than are elderly patients. The mortality rate can reach 20 to 30 percent or even higher when depot antipsychotic medications are involved. Incidence estimates range from 1 to 10 in 10,000 episodes of antipsychotic treatment. The disorder can also occur when the patient is withdrawn from dopaminergic agonists—for example, carbidopa (Sinemet), levodopa (Larodopa), amantadine, and bromocriptine (Parlodel). Concomitant treatment with lithium and an antipsychotic has been associated with several cases of neuroleptic malignant syndrome. The pathophysiology is unknown.

Treatment

If the patient's mild rigidity does not respond to conventional anticholinergic agents—for example, benztropine 2 mg by mouth or IM—and if the fever does not have an obvious origin, a provisional diagnosis of neuroleptic malignant syndrome is warranted. Discontinue the patient's prescribed antipsychotic immediately and monitor vital signs. Order the needed laboratory tests. Creatinine phosphokinase (CPK) is usually markedly elevated and is directly related to the severity of the neuroleptic malignant syndrome. Leukocytosis is also common. Also order routine blood tests, including a complete blood count (CBC) with differential white blood count, a chemistry profile, a test for blood urea nitrogen (BUN) and creatinine, and liver function tests. Emergency cooling with an ice bath or evaporative cooling helps reduce the patient's fever. Antipyretics are not usually useful. Vigorous hydration may prevent shock and decrease the likelihood of renal impairment. Neuroleptic malignant syndrome usually lasts about 15 days.

Anticholinergics and benzodiazepines are generally not effective in neuroleptic malignant syndrome. Dantrolene (Dantrium) 1 mg per kilogram four times a day or 1 to 5 mg per kilogram IV directly prevents the contraction of the skeletal muscles and may prevent rigidity and myoglobinuria. Bromocriptine—2.5 to 5 mg by mouth three times a day through a nasogastric tube and repeated if not effective, up to 60 mg a day—is a dopaminergic agonist that may help reduce the severity of the syndrome. Amantadine may also be of use. Other supportive treatments and close monitoring are indicated. The patient often needs treatment in an intensive care unit.

After recovery, the difficult decision remains of whether to reinstitute an antipsychotic agent. Conventional clinical wisdom suggests trying an antipsychotic of a different class and potency, but the benefits must be weighed against the risk of not using the original antipsychotic, which may have been effective.

MEDICATION-INDUCED POSTURAL TREMOR

Tremor is a rhythmical alteration in movement that is usually faster than one beat a second. Typically, tremors decrease during periods of relaxation and sleep and increase with stress or anxiety. Whereas all the above diagnoses specifically include an association with an antipsychotic, a range of psychiatric medications can produce tremor—most notably lithium.

Treatment

The treatment of tremor involves four general steps: (1) The lowest possible dosage of the psychiatric drug should be taken. (2) Patients should minimize their caffeine consumption. (3) The psychiatric drug should be taken at bedtime to

TABLE 23-3
DRUG-INDUCED CENTRAL HYPERTHERMIC SYNDROMES[a]

Condition (and Mechanism)	Common Drug Causes	Frequent Symptoms	Possible Treatment[b]	Clinical Course
Hyperthermia (↓ heat dissipation) (↑ heat production)	Atropine, lidocaine, meperidine NSAID toxicity, pheochromocytoma, thyrotoxicosis	Hyperthermia, diaphoresis, malaise	Acetaminophen per rectum (325 mg every 4 hours), diazepam oral or per rectum (5 mg every 8 hours) for febrile seizures	Benign, febrile seizures in children
Malignant hyperthermia (↑ heat production)	NMJ blockers (succinylcholine), halothane (1:50,000)	Hyperthermia, **muscle rigidity, arrhythmias,** ischemia,[c] hypotension, **rhabdomyolysis;** disseminated intravascular coagulation	Dantrolene sodium (1–2 mg/kg/ min IV infusion)[d]	Familial, 10% mortality if untreated
Tricyclic overdose (↑ heat production)	Tricyclic antidepressants, cocaine	Hyperthermia, confusion, visual hallucinations, agitation, **hyperreflexia, muscle relaxation, anticholinergic effects** (dry skin, pupil dilation), arrhythmias	**Sodium bicarbonate** (1 mEq/kg IV bolus) if arrhythmias are present, physostigmine (1–3 mg IV) with cardiac monitoring	Fatalities have occurred if untreated
Autonomic hyperreflexia (< heat production)	CNS stimulants (amphetamines)	Hyperthermia excitement, hyperreflexia	Trimethaphan (0.3–7 mg/ minute IV infusion)	Reversible
Lethal catatonia (↓ heat dissipation)	Lead poisoning	Hyperthermia, intense anxiety, **destructive behavior, psychosis**	Lorazepam (1–2 mg IV every 4 hours), antipsychotics may be contraindicated	High mortality if untreated
Neuroleptic malignant syndrome (mixed hypothalamic, ↓ head dissipation, ↑ heat production)	Antipsychotics (neuroleptics), methyldopa, reserpine	Hyperthermia, **muscle rigidity, diaphoresis** (60%), **leukocytosis, delirium, rhabdomyolysis, elevated CPK,** autonomic deregulation, **extrapyramidal symptoms**	**Bromocriptine (2–10 mg every 8 hours PO or NG tube),** lisuride (0.02–0.1 mg/hour IV infusion), Sinemet (carbidopa: levodopa (25/ 100) PO every 8 hours), dantrolene sodium (0.3–1 mg/ kg IV every 6 hours)	Rapid onset, 20% mortality if untreated

[a]Boldface indicates features that may be used to distinguish one syndrome from another. NSAID, nonsteroidal antiinflammatory drugs; MAOI, monoamine oxidase inhibitors; NMJ, neuromuscular junction; CNS, central nervous system; DO, dopamine; CPK, creatine phosphokinase; IV, intravenously; PO, orally; NG, nasogastric.
[b]Gastric lavage and supportive measures, including cooling, are required in most cases.
[c]Oxygen consumption increases by 7% for every 1°F up in body temperature.
[d]Has been associated with idiosyncratic hepatocellular injury, as well as severe hypotension in one case.
Table from T C Theoharides, R S Harris, D Weckstein; Neuroleptic malignant-like syndrome due to cyclobenzaprine? (letter). J Clin Psychopharmacol 15: 80, 1995. Used

minimize the amount of daytime tremor. (4) β-adrenergic receptor antagonists (for example, propranolol) can be given in the treatment of drug-induced tremors.

HYPERTHERMIC SYNDROMES

Hyperthermia is a heat illness associated with an elevated body temperature. All antipsychotics can induce hyperthermia, particularly low-potency antipsychotics, which have prominent anticholinergic effects (Table 23-3). Typically, the patient has also been exposed to heat or has engaged in physical activity. Children, the elderly, and the medically ill are the most susceptible.

Symptoms of hyperthermia begin with sweating, thirst, fatigue, giddiness, ataxia, and hysteria. As the condition progresses, the body's temperature rises, eventually leading to delirium. The patient may be hypoactive or hyperactive. If the patient becomes dehydrated, sweating may stop, and symptoms of profound CNS disturbance may develop, including restlessness, rigidity, seizures, coma, and death.

Antipsychotic drugs can decrease the body's central thermoregulation. In addition, sweating is impaired, further reducing the patient's ability to dissipate heat. Hyperthermia is most likely to develop shortly after the patient starts taking an antipsychotic or after the dosage is changed.

Hyperthermia may also accompany substance abuse withdrawal (for example, withdrawal from alcohol or opioids).

Treatment

Is it a drug-induced fever? Does the patient have a skin rash? An uncommon side effect of antipsychotics, drug fever is commonly caused by antibiotics, antihistamines, barbiturates and other anticonvulsants, and antiarrhythmics. Discontinue any drugs that could be causing even mild side effects.

Does the fever have a medical cause? Perform a full fever workup. Also perform a full battery of laboratory screening tests, including CPK, erythrocyte sedimentation rate (ESR), CBC, chemistry panel, electrolytes, glumatic acid, (Glu), BUN, creatinine, hepatic enzymes, and blood and urine cultures.

Place the patient in an air-conditioned environment. In severe cases, consider either an ice bath or evaporative cooling by spraying the patient with lukewarm water and then blowing with a fan. Evaporative cooling may be more effective, since it produces less peripheral vasoconstriction than do ice packs or ice baths.

If the fever is mild, follow the temperature closely, consider discontinuation of the antipsychotic, and encourage the patient to drink liberal amounts of fluids.

Treat neuroleptic malignant syndrome immediately. Supportive measures, such as cooling, monitoring in an intensive care unit, and the maintenance of vital functions, are necessary. Antipyretics (for example, acetaminophen and aspirin) may be helpful, but they are of little use in treating heat exhaustion and heatstroke. Moreover, those drugs do not reduce the patient's elevated temperature when the hyperthermia involves an antipsychotic medication.

For a more detailed discussion of this topic, see J A Grebb: Medication-Induced Movement Disorders, Sec 32.2, p 1909, in CTP/VI.

24

The Primary Care Physician and Brief Psychotherapy

The relationship between primary care physicians and their patients can be a potent force in ameliorating emotional and interpersonal problems. The primary aim of psychotherapy is to alter pathological behavior, with treatment goals ranging from relieving specific symptoms, such as bed-wetting, to making fundamental changes in character structure and behavior patterns that affect important aspects of life, such as work, love, sex and interpersonal relationships. Primary care physicians who learn of a patient's psychological problems may choose to intervene by using one of the psychotherapeutic treatment methods described in this section.

These therapies are suitable only for those primary care physicians who are committed to learning the techniques and devoting the necessary time to implement them. The physician using short-term or brief therapies can expect to conduct weekly psychotherapy sessions with the patient for 5 to 20 weeks. By comparison, insight-oriented psychotherapies, including psychoanalysis, require 1 to 4 sessions per week during a period of years. This type of treatment should be provided by a psychiatrist, who has the time, training, and skills to conduct the therapy.

INTERPERSONAL PSYCHOTHERAPY FOR DEPRESSION

Interpersonal psychotherapy (IPT) for depression is a brief weekly treatment (12 to 16 sessions) for ambulatory, nonbipolar, nonpsychotic depressed persons. It is based on the premise that understanding and renegotiating the interpersonal context of a depressive episode will facilitate recovery and prevent relapse. The effectiveness of IPT, alone and in combination with pharmacological treatments, has been verified by numerous controlled clinical trials, including the National Institute of Mental Health (NIMH) Collaborative Study on the treatment of depression.

IPT Theory of Depression

The conceptual and technical roots of IPT are eclectic, representing a combination of clinical approaches. The scientific bases for understanding and treating depression in an interpersonal context have been derived from various research studies. Some of these studies conclude:

1. Despair and depression may result from disturbances in the formation, maintenance, or renewal of affectional attachment bonds, in both past and present contexts.
2. An intimate confiding relationship can protect against the development of depression in the face of life stressors and may reduce the severity of psychological symptoms that occur.

3. Marital problems are the most common event reported by depressed patients prior to the onset of their depression.
4. Loss of relationships in the 6 months preceding the depressive episode occurred more often among depressed persons than among nondepressed persons.
5. Depression has been associated with global deficits in social functioning as a worker, spouse, parent, family member, and friend, and these impairments diminish substantially upon recovery from depressive symptoms.

Four basic interpersonal problems are commonly associated with acute depression: (1) abnormal grief reaction, or grief in excess of normal bereavement; (2) role disputes, in which patients and their significant other have conflicting expectations about their relationship; (3) role transitions, which involve attempts to cope with life changes of developmental or traumatic origin; and (4) interpersonal deficits, which include isolation and self-defeating patterns of interpersonal interaction.

In IPT, depression is viewed from three perspectives:

1. Symptom formation, including depressive affect and vegetative signs;
2. Social and interpersonal relations, based on current interactions and emphasizing the four common problems—grief, role disputes, role transitions, and interpersonal deficits; and
3. Personality, in the form of enduring traits, such as inhibitions of expressing anger and other emotions and tendencies toward perfectionism and self-criticism.

Techniques

IPT relies on traditional techniques such as clarification of internal emotional states, improvement of communication skills, support of interpersonal reality testing, and reassurance. The techniques and guidelines are described in detail by Myrna M. Weissman and John C. Markowitz (Interpersonal psychotherapy: Current status. Arch Gen Psychiatry *51*: 599, 1994). Primary care physicians who wish to conduct IPT should familiarize themselves with the article. IPT therapists conduct a systematic analysis of the patient's relationships with significant others, emphasizing current problems, conflicts, frustrations, and wishes. The therapeutic relationship is an active collaborative exploration. Primitive or regressed transference is neither encouraged nor interpreted. Though remaining nonjudgmental, the therapist is viewed as an advocate rather than a neutral screen on which the patient projects transferential themes and conflicts. Early childhood contributions to current problems may be recognized by historical reconstructions, but are de-emphasized in favor of here-and-now formulations. Partly because IPT is a brief therapy that emphasizes rational problem solving rather than exploration of unconscious dynamics, the therapist makes no claims about its effectiveness in changing enduring aspects of personality structure.

Goals

The first goal of IPT is to reduce immediate depressive symptoms and improve self-esteem, which can be accomplished rather quickly by using the following methods:

1. Thoroughly review the symptoms of depression with the patient, using, for example, the interview version of the Hamilton Depression Rating Scale as a guide (Table 24-1).
2. Make a diagnosis and name the symptoms as depression. Give the patient permission to assume a temporary sick role.
3. Educate the patient about depression: its epidemiology, course, prognosis, and treatment. That educational collaboration establishes the nature of the expected therapeutic relationship.
4. Evaluate the need for medication. If medication is recommended, explain that it will help relieve the depressive affect and vegetative symptoms, while the concurrent psychotherapy will address the interpersonal problems that initiate and maintain depression and that may produce a relapse.
5. Identify specific interpersonal problems to be worked on in the psychotherapy sessions.

After assessing and relieving the immediate depressive symptoms, the therapist can identify the patients interpersonal problems by using the following techniques:

1. Develop strategies for exploration, clarification, and systematic data gathering.
2. Encourage experience, acceptance, and insightful use of affect.
3. Analyze communication failures and teach effective communications skills.
4. Explore the therapeutic relationship as a tool for learning about patterns of interaction with others and as a means to correct negative therapeutic reactions.
5. Apply specific behavior-change techniques—including education, setting limits and making contracts, role playing, and practice in generating alternatives and systematic decision making—and direct help and advice when it is necessary.

IPT assumes that every patient is unique and that each will require a different combination of techniques. As a rule, the least intrusive techniques are preferred so long as adequate progress is being made.

Efficacy

Controlled clinical trials of IPT, both alone and in combination with drug therapy, have been conducted at a number of sites with hundreds of patients—all of whom met the diagnostic criteria for major depressive disorder—of both sexes, different races, and various educational levels.

Results of the trials support the following conclusions:

1. After 4 to 8 weeks, patients who receive IPT improve significantly more than those who have no treatment, and IPT is as effective as antidepressant medication with respect to overall symptom improvement. However, drug therapy primarily affects vegetative signs and symptoms (for example, lethargy, anhedonia), whereas IPT mainly affects mood, work performance, activity interest, guilt, and suicidal ideation.
2. Because of the different effects of antidepressant drug therapy and IPT, combined treatment is more effective than either treatment alone. Furthermore, patients

TABLE 24-1
HAMILTON RATING SCALE FOR DEPRESSION

For each item select the "cue" which best characterizes the patient.

1: DEPRESSED MOOD (Sadness, hopeless, helpless, worthless)
  0 Absent
  1 These feeling states indicated only on questioning
  2 These feeling states spontaneously reported verbally
  3 Communicates feeling states nonverbally—i.e., through facial expression, posture, voice, and tendency to weep
  4 Patient reports VIRTUALLY ONLY these feeling states in his spontaneous verbal and nonverbal communication

2: FEELINGS OF GUILT
  0 Absent
  1 Self-reproach, feels he has let people down
  2 Ideas of guilt or rumination over past errors or sinful deeds
  3 Present illness is a punishment. Delusions of guilt
  4 Hears accusatory or denunciatory voices and/or experiences threatening visual hallucinations

3: SUICIDE
  0 Absent
  1 Feels life is not worth living
  2 Wishes he were dead or any thoughts of possible death to self
  3 Suicide ideas or gesture
  4 Attempts at suicide (any serious attempt rates 4)

4: INSOMNIA EARLY
  0 No difficulty falling asleep
  1 Complains of occasional difficulty falling asleep—i.e., more than 1/4 hour
  2 Complains of nightly difficulty falling asleep

5: INSOMNIA MIDDLE
  0 No difficulty
  1 Patient complains of being restless and disturbed during the night
  2 Waking during the night—any getting out of bed rates 2 (except for purpose of voiding)

6: INSOMNIA LATE
  0 No difficulty
  1 Waking in early hours of the morning but goes back to sleep
  2 Unable to fall asleep again if gets out of bed

7: WORK AND ACTIVITIES
  0 No difficulty
  1 Thoughts and feelings of incapacity, fatigue or weakness related to activities, work, or hobbies
  2 Loss of interest in activity, hobbies, or work—either directly reported by patient, or indirect in listlessness, indecision and vacillation (feels he has to push self to work or activities)
  3 Decrease in actual time spent in activities or decrease in productivity. In hospital, rate 3 if patient does not spend at least three hours a day in activities (hospital job or hobbies) exclusive of ward chores
  4 Stopped working because of present illness. In hospital, rate 4 if patient engages in no activities except ward chores, or if patient fails to perform ward chores unassisted

8: RETARDATION (Slowness of thought and speech; impaired ability to concentrate; decreased motor activity)
  0 Normal speech and thought
  1 Slight retardation at interview
  2 Obvious retardation at interview
  3 Interview difficult
  4 Complete stupor

9: AGITATION
  0 None
  1 "Playing with" hands, hair, etc.
  2 Hand-wringing, nail biting, hair pulling, biting of lips

10: ANXIETY PSYCHIC
  0 No difficulty
  1 Subjective tension and irritability
  2 Worrying about minor matters
  3 Apprehensive attitude apparent in face or speech
  4 Fears expressed without questioning

TABLE 24-1—*continued*

11: ANXIETY SOMATIC
   0 Absent   Physiological concomitants of anxiety, such as:
   1 Mild   Gastrointestinal—dry mouth, wind, indigestion, diarrhea,
   2 Moderate   cramps, belching
   3 Severe   Cardiovascular—palpitations, headaches
   4 Incapacitating   Respiratory—hyperventilation, sighing
                           Urinary frequency
                           Sweating
12: SOMATIC SYMPTOMS GASTROINTESTINAL
   0 None
   1 Loss of appetite but eating without staff encouragement. Heavy feelings in abdomen
   2 Difficulty eating without staff urging. Requests or requires laxatives or medication for bowels
     or medication for G.I. symptoms
13: SOMATIC SYMPTOMS GENERAL
   0 None
   1 Heaviness in limbs, back or head. Backaches, headache, muscle aches. Loss of energy
     and fatigability
   2 Any clear cut symptom rates 2
14: GENITAL SYMPTOMS
   0 Absent   Symptoms such as:
   1 Mild   Loss of libido
   2 Severe   Menstrual disturbances
15: HYPOCHONDRIASIS
   0 Not present
   1 Self-absorption (bodily)
   2 Preoccupation with health
   3 Frequent complaints, requests for help, etc.
   4 Hypochondriacal delusions
16: LOSS OF WEIGHT
   A: WHEN RATING BY HISTORY
   0 No weight loss
   1 Probable weight loss associated with present illness
   2 Definite (according to patient) weight loss
   B: ON WEEKLY RATINGS BY WARD PSYCHIATRIST, WHEN ACTUAL WEIGHT CHANGES ARE MEASURED
   0 Less than 1 lb. weight loss in week
   1 Greater than 1 lb. weight loss in week
   2 Greater than 2 lb. weight loss in week
17: INSIGHT
   0 Acknowledges being depressed and ill
   1 Acknowledges illness but attributes cause to bad food, climate, overwork, virus, need for
     rest, etc.
   2 Denies being ill at all
18: DIURNAL VARIATION

A.M.	P.M.		
0	0	Absent	If symptoms are worse in the morning or evening,
1	1	Mild	note which it is and rate severity of variation
2	2	Severe	

19: DEPERSONALIZATION AND DEREALIZATION
   0 Absent
   1 Mild   Such as:
   2 Moderate   Feelings of unreality
   3 Severe   Nihilistic ideas
   4 Incapacitating
20: PARANOID SYMPTOMS
   0 None
   1
     Suspiciousness
   2
   3 Ideas of reference
   4 Delusions of reference and persecution
21: OBSESSIONAL AND COMPULSIVE SYMPTOMS
   0 Absent
   1 Mild
   2 Severe

TABLE 24-1—*continued*

22:	HELPLESSNESS
	0 Not present
	1 Subjective feelings which are elicited only by inquiry
	2 Patient volunteers his helpless feelings
	3 Requires urging, guidance, and reassurance to accomplish ward chores or personal hygiene
	4 Requires physical assistance for dress, grooming, eating, bedside tasks, or personal hygiene
23:	HOPELESSNESS
	0 Not present
	1 Intermittently doubts that "things will improve" but can be reassured
	2 Consistently feels "hopeless" but accepts reassurances
	3 Expresses feelings of discouragement, despair, pessimism about future, which cannot be dispelled
	4 Spontaneously and inappropriately perseverates "I'll never get well" or its equivalent
24:	WORTHLESSNESS (Ranges from mild loss of esteem, feelings of inferiority, self-depreciation to delusional notions of worthlessness)
	0 Not present
	1 Indicates feelings of worthlessness (loss of self-esteem) only on questioning
	2 Spontaneously indicates feelings of worthlessness (loss of self-esteem)
	3 Different from 2 by degree. Patient volunteers that he is "no good," "inferior," etc.
	4 Delusional notions of worthlessness—i.e., "I am a heap of garbage" or its equivalent

Table from M Hamilton: A rating scale for depression. J Neurol Neurosurg Psychiatry *23:* 56, 1960.

receiving combined treatment are less likely to refuse treatment initially and are less likely to drop out before completion of the 16-week protocol.

3. Follow-up studies indicate that the full effects of IPT on patients' social and interpersonal functioning may take from 6 to 8 months to develop even though they experience some relief within 2 months.

COGNITIVE THERAPY

Cognitive therapy is a short-term structured therapy that uses active collaboration between the patient and the therapist to achieve the therapeutic goals. It is oriented toward resolving current problems. Cognitive therapy is usually conducted on an individual basis, although group methods are sometimes used. Medication may be used in conjunction with cognitive therapy, if necessary.

Cognitive therapy has been applied mainly to depressive disorders (with or without suicidal ideation); however, it is also used to treat other conditions, such as panic disorder, obsessive-compulsive disorder, paranoid personality disorder, and somatoform disorders. The treatment of depression can serve as a paradigm of the cognitive approach.

Cognitive Theory of Depression

The cognitive theory of depression holds that cognitive dysfunctions are at the core of depression and that affective and physical changes and other symptoms of depression are the consequence of cognitive dysfunctions. For example, apathy and low energy result from the person's expectation of failure in all areas. Similarly, paralysis of will (that is, abulia) stems from a person's pessimism and feelings of hopelessness.

TABLE 24-2.
PRIMITIVE VERSUS MATURE THINKING

Primitive Thinking	Mature Thinking
Nondimensional and global: I am fearful	Multidimensional: I am moderately fearful, quite generous, and fairly intelligent.
Absolutistic and moralistic: I am a despicable coward.	Relativistic and nonjudgmental: I am more fearful than most people I know.
Invariant: I always have been and always will be a coward.	Variable: My fears vary from time to time and from situation to situation.
Character diagnosis: I have a defect in my character	Behavioral diagnosis: I avoid situations too much, and I have many fears.
Irreversibility: Since I am basically weak, there's nothing that can be done about it.	Reversibility: I can learn ways of facing situations and fighting my fears.

Table from A T Beck, A J Rush, B F Shaw, G Emery: *Cognitive Therapy of Depression,* p 31. Guilford, New York, 1979. Used with permission.

The cognitive triad of depression consists of (1) a negative self-percept that one is defective, inadequate, deprived, worthless, and undesirable; (2) a tendency to experience the world as a negative, demanding, and self-defeating place in which failure and punishment, are expected; and (3) an expectation that hardship, suffering, deprivation, and failure will continue.

The goal of therapy is to alleviate depression and to prevent its recurrence by helping the patient (1) to identify and test negative thoughts, (2) to develop alternative and more flexible schemas, and (3) to rehearse both new cognitive and behavioral responses. The goal is to change the way a person thinks which will alleviate the depressive disorder. Table 24-2 gives examples of typical depressive thinking (termed primitive thinking by Aaron Beck), contrasted with the adaptive (mature) thinking that cognitive therapy attempts to foster.

Techniques

Overall, therapy is relatively short, lasting up to about 25 weeks. If the patient does not improve in that time, the diagnosis should be reevaluated. Maintenance therapy can be carried out over a period of years.

As with other psychotherapies, the therapists' attributes are important to successful outcome. Therapists must be able to exude warmth, understand the life experience of each patient, and be truly honest with themselves and their patients. Therapists must be able to relate skillfully and interact effectively with their patients.

At the beginning of each session, the cognitive therapist sets the agenda, assigns homework to be performed between sessions, and teaches new skills.

The cognitive approach includes four processes: (1) eliciting automatic thoughts, (2) testing automatic thoughts, (3) identifying maladaptive underlying assumptions, and (4) testing the validity of these assumptions.

Eliciting Automatic Thoughts. Automatic thoughts are cognitions that intervene between external events and the person's emotional reaction to the event. An example of an automatic thought is the belief that "everyone is going to laugh at me when they see how badly I bowl"—a thought that occurs to someone who has been asked to go bowling and responds negatively. Another example is the thought

TABLE 24-3
COGNITIVE PROFILE OF PSYCHIATRIC DISORDERS

Disorder	Specific Cognitive Content
Depressive disorder	Negative view of self, experience, and future
Hypomanic episode	Inflated view of self, experience, and future
Anxiety disorders	Fear of physical or psychological danger
Panic disorder	Catastrophic misinterpretation of bodily and mental experiences
Phobias	Danger in specific, avoidable situations
Paranoid personality disorder	Negative bias, interference, and so forth by others
Conversion disorder	Concept of motor or sensory abnormality
Obsessive-compulsive disorder	Repeated warning or doubting about safety and repetitive acts to ward off threat
Suicidal behavior	Hopelessness and deficit in problem solving
Anorexia nervosa	Fear of being fat or unshapely
Hypochondriasis	Attribution of serious medical disorder

Table adapted from Aaron Beck, MD., and A. John Rush, MD.

that "she doesn't like me," if someone passes the person in the hall without saying hello.

Automatic thoughts are also called cognitive distortions. Every psychopathological disorder has its own specific cognitive profile of distorted thought, which, if known, provides a framework for specific cognitive interventions (Table 24-3).

Testing Automatic Thoughts. Acting as a teacher, the therapist helps patients test the validity of automatic thoughts. The goal is to encourage patients to examine automatic thoughts carefully and reject inaccurate or exaggerated thoughts.

Identifying Maladaptive Assumptions. As the patient and the therapist continue to identify automatic thoughts, patterns usually become apparent. The patterns represent rules or maladaptive general assumptions that guide the patient's life. Examples of such rules are "In order to be happy, I must be perfect" and "If anyone doesn't like me, I'm not lovable." Such rules inevitably lead to disappointments and then to depression.

Testing the Validity of Maladaptive Assumptions. Testing the accuracy of maladaptive assumptions is conducted in a manner similar to testing the validity of automatic thoughts. One particularly effective test is for the therapist to ask the patient to defend the validity of an assumption. For example, if a patient states that he should always work up to his potential, the therapist might ask, "Why is that so important to you?"

Efficacy

Studies have clearly shown that cognitive therapy is as effective and, in some cases, superior to drug treatment alone. It is one of the most useful psychotherapeutic interventions currently available for depressive disorders.

BEHAVIOR THERAPY

Behavior therapy focuses on overt behavior, emphasizing the removal of overt symptoms, without examining the patients' inner conflicts. The therapeutic goal is straightforward and concrete: the extinction of maladaptive habits or attitudes and the substitution of new, appropriate, nonanxiety-provoking behavior. The methods inherent in behavior therapies are based on the fundamental belief that persistent maladaptive behaviors and anxieties have been conditioned (or learned); therefore, successful treatment consists of various forms of deconditioning (or unlearning)— that is, whatever bad behavior has been learned can be unlearned.

Behavior therapy is based on the principles of learning theory—in particular, operant and classical conditioning. Behavior therapy is most often used to change specific, delineated habits of reacting with anxiety (for example, phobias, compulsions, psychophysiological reactions, and sexual dysfunctions) to objectively nondangerous stimuli. Specific types of behavior therapy follow.

Systematic Desensitization

A core method used in behavior therapy is systematic desensitization, in which the patient attains a state of complete relaxation and is then exposed to the stimulus that elicits anxiety. The negative reaction is then inhibited by the relaxed state, a process called *reciprocal inhibition.*

Rather than use the actual situation or object that elicits fear, the patient and therapist prepare a graded list or hierarchy of anxiety-provoking scenes. Then, the learned relaxation state and the anxiety-provoking scenes are systematically paired. Thus, systematic desensitization consists of three steps: relaxation training, hierarchy construction, and desensitization of the stimulus.

Relaxation Training. Relaxation produces physiological effects that are opposite to those of anxiety—slower heart rate, increased peripheral blood flow, and neuromuscular stability. A variety of relaxation methods have been developed, although some, such as yoga and Zen, have been known for centuries.

Most methods of achieving relaxation are based on progressive relaxation. The patient relaxes major muscle groups in a fixed order, beginning with the small muscle groups of the feet and working up toward the head, or vice versa. Some clinicians use hypnosis to facilitate relaxation during the session or use tape-recorded procedures to enable patients to practice relaxation on their own.

Another relaxation method is mental imagery, in which patients are instructed to imagine themselves in a place associated with pleasant, relaxing memories. Those images allow the patients to enter a relaxed state or experience.

Hierarchy Construction. When constructing the hierarchy, the clinician determines which conditions elicit anxiety; then the patient creates a hierarchy of 10 to 12 scenes in order of increasing anxiety. For example, the acrophobic hierarchy may begin with the patient's imagining standing near a window on the second floor

TABLE 24-4
HIERARCHY CONSTRUCTION FOR DOG PHOBIA

1. Looking at a picture of a dog in a children's picture book.
2. Cuddling the children's toy dog.
3. Seeing a poodle on a leash (a) 10 yards away.
                                 (b) 5 yards away.
                                 (c) passing by.
4. Touching a puppy behind a wire mesh in the market.
5. Looking at the neighbor's spaniel, Kim, held in the arms of its mistress.
6. Touching Kim when the dog is quiet and held in the arms of its mistress.
7. Touching Kim when the dog is quiet.
8. Stroking Kim.
9. Kim putting up her paws.
10. Looking at an Alsatian dog.
11. Watching Kim jumping on the road when the patient is indoors and the windows are closed.
12. Watching Kim walk around the room.
13. Feeding Kim a biscuit.
14. Kim held by its mistress and then jumping onto the ground.
15. Kim running.
16. Kim jumping from a chair onto the floor.
17. Kim jumping onto the floor and then putting up her paw.
18. Kim wagging her tail.
19. Kim wagging her tail and then putting her paw up.
20. Kim running down the corridor.
21. Kim running away from the patient.
22. Kim running toward the patient.
23. Kim roaming around the house without a lead.
24. Knocking on the door of the neighbor, and Kim running toward her, barking.
25. Dogs fighting.

and end with being on the roof of a 20-story building, leaning on a guard rail and looking straight down. Table 24-4 provides an example of an hierarchy construction.

Desensitization of the Stimulus. Desensitization is achieved systematically by having patients proceed through the list, from the least anxiety-provoking scene to the most anxiety-provoking one, while in a deeply relaxed state. The rate at which patients progress through the list is determined by their responses to the stimuli. When patients can vividly imagine the most anxiety-provoking scene of their hierarchy with equanimity, they should be able to experience little anxiety in the corresponding real-life situation.

Adjunctive Use of Drugs. Various drugs have been used to hasten desensitization, but they should be used with caution and only by psychiatrists trained and experienced in potential adverse effects. The most commonly used drug is the rapid-acting barbiturate, sodium methohexital (Brevital), which is given intravenously in subanesthetic doses. Usually, up to 60 mg of the drug is given in divided doses during a session. Intravenous diazepam (Valium) may also be used cautiously. If the procedural details are carefully followed, almost all patients find the procedure pleasant, with few unpleasant side effects. The advantages of pharmacological desensitization are that preliminary training in relaxation can be shortened, almost all patients are able to become adequately relaxed, and the treatment proceeds more rapidly than when drugs are not used.

Indications. Systematic desensitization works best when there is a clearly identifiable anxiety-provoking stimulus. Phobias, obsessions, compulsions, and certain sexual disorders have been successfully treated with the technique.

Graded Exposure

Graded exposure is similar to systematic desensitization except that relaxation training is not involved and treatment is usually carried out in a real-life context. For example, a person with an elevator phobia will be accompanied by the therapist in the feared situation.

Flooding

Flooding is based on the premise that escaping from an anxiety-provoking experience reinforces the anxiety through conditioning. Therefore, by not allowing the person to escape, the clinician can extinguish the anxiety and prevent the conditioned avoidance behavior.

This technique encourages patients to confront their feared situation directly, without a gradual build-up as in systematic desensitization or graded exposure. No relaxation exercises are used, as in systematic desensitization. Patients experience fear, which gradually subsides after a time. The success of the procedure depends on patients' ability to remain in the fear-generating situation until they are calm and feel a sense of mastery. Prematurely withdrawing from the situation or prematurely terminating the fantasized scene is equivalent to an escape, in which both the conditioned anxiety and the avoidance behavior are reinforced, the opposite of what is intended. A variant of flooding is called *implosion,* in which the feared object or situation is confronted only in the imagination, rather than in real life.

Many patients refuse flooding because of the psychological discomfort involved. It is also contraindicated in patients for whom intense anxiety would be hazardous (for example, patients with heart disease or fragile psychological adaptation). The technique works best with specific phobias.

Participant Modeling

Participant modeling is a method in which patients learn by imitation. Patients learn a new behavior primarily by observation, without having to perform the behavior until they feel ready. This method is based on the premise that irrational fears are acquired by learning, thus they may be unlearned by observing a fearless model confront the feared object. The technique has been useful with phobic children, who are placed with other children of their own age and sex who approach the feared object or situation. With adults, the therapist may describe the feared activity in a calm manner with which the patient can identify, or the therapist may perform the feared activity with the patient. Sometimes a hierarchy of activities is established, with the least anxiety-provoking activity performed first. The participant-modeling technique has been used successfully to treat agoraphobia by having the therapist accompany the patient into the feared situation.

A variant of participant modeling is called *behavior rehearsal,* in which real-life problems are acted out under the therapist's observation or direction. The technique is useful for complex behavioral patterns, such as shyness, and may be used to help patients perform well in such situations as job interviews.

Assertiveness and Social Skills Training

To be assertive requires that persons have confidence in their judgment and sufficient self-esteem to express their opinions. Assertiveness and social skills training teaches people how to respond appropriately in social situations, to express their opinions in acceptable ways, and to achieve their goals. A variety of techniques—including role modeling, desensitization, and positive reinforcement (reward of desired behavior)—are used to increase assertiveness. Social skills training includes assertiveness, but also attends to a variety of real-life tasks, such as food shopping, looking for work, interacting with other people, and overcoming shyness.

Efficacy

Behavior therapy has been successful in treating a variety of disorders (Table 24-5) and can be easily learned (Table 24-6). It requires less time to produce results than other therapies and is less expensive to administer. A limitation of the method is that it is useful for circumscribed behavioral symptoms, rather than for global areas of dysfunction (for example, neurotic conflicts, personality disorders).

As with other forms of treatment, an evaluation of the patient's problems, motivation, and psychological strengths should be made before instituting any behavior therapy approach. Table 24-7 summarizes behavior therapy.

BRIEF DYNAMIC THERAPY AND CRISIS INTERVENTION

Brief dynamic psychotherapy has assumed greater importance than long-term dynamic therapy for several reasons: Long-term treatment extending over several years has become too expensive for many patients; third-party payers have pressed the psychiatric profession to develop brief psychotherapies; and this type of therapy has been proved effective for a wide range of psychiatric disorders.

Most of the basic characteristics of brief dynamic psychotherapy were identified by Franz Alexander and Thomas French in 1946. They described a therapeutic experience that puts the patient at ease, manipulates the transference, and uses trial interpretations in a flexible manner.

Principles of Short-Term Dynamic Psychotherapy

Brief dynamic therapy emphasizes developing a corrective emotional experience capable of repairing traumatic events of the past and convincing the patient that new ways of thinking, feeling, and behaving are possible.

TABLE 24–5
SOME COMMON CLINICAL APPLICATIONS OF BEHAVIOR THERAPY

Disorder	Comments
Agoraphobia	Graded exposure and flooding can reduce the fear of being in crowded places. About 60 percent of patients so treated are improved. In some cases the spouse can serve as the model while accompanying the patient into the fear situation; however, the patient cannot get a secondary gain by keeping the spouse nearby and displaying symptoms.
Alcohol dependence	Aversion therapy in which the alcohol-dependent patient is made to vomit (by adding an emetic to the alcohol) every time a drink is ingested is effective in treating alcohol dependence. Disulfiram (Antabuse) can be given to alcohol-dependent patients when they are alcohol-free. Such patients are warned of the severe physiological consequences of drinking (e.g., nausea, vomiting, hypotension, collapse) with disulfiram in the system.
Anorexia nervosa	Observe eating behavior; contingency management; record weight.
Bulimia nervosa	Record bulimic episodes; log moods
Hyperventilation	Hyperventilation test; controlled breathing; direct observation.
Other phobias	Systematic desensitization has been effective in treating phobias, such as fears of heights, animals, and flying. Social skills training has also been used for shyness and fear of other people.
Paraphilias	Electric shocks or other noxious stimuli can be applied at the time of a paraphilic impulse, and eventually the impulse subsides. Shocks can be administered by either the therapist or the patient. The results are satisfactory but must be reinforced at regular intervals.
Schizophrenia	The token economy procedure, in which tokens are awarded for desirable behavior and can be used to buy ward privileges, has been useful in treating inpatient schizophrenic patients. Social skills training teaches schizophrenic patients how to interact with others in a socially acceptable way so that negative feedback is eliminated. In addition, the aggressive behavior of some schizophrenic patients can be diminished through those methods.
Sexual dysfunctions	Dual-sex therapy, developed by William Masters and Virginia Johnson, is a behavior therapy technique used for various sexual dysfunctions, especially male erectile disorder, orgasm disorders, and premature ejaculation. It uses relaxation, desensitization, and graded exposure as the primary techniques.
Shy bladder	Inability to void in a public bathroom; relaxation exercises.
Type A behavior	Physiological assessment; muscle relaxation, biofeedback (on EMG)

TABLE 24–6
SOCIAL SKILLS COMPETENCE CHECKLIST OF THERAPIST-TRAINER BEHAVIORS

1. Actively helps the patient in setting and eliciting specific interpersonal goals.
2. Promotes favorable expectations, a therapeutic orientation, and motivation before role playing begins.
3. Assists the patient in building possible scenes in terms of: "What emotion or communication?" "Who is the interpersonal target?" "Where and when?"
4. Structures the role playing by setting the scene and assigning roles to the patient and surrogates.
5. Engages the patient in behavioral rehearsal—getting the patient to role-play with others.
6. Uses self or other group members in modeling appropriate alternatives for the patient.
7. Prompts and cues the patient during the role playing.
8. Uses an active style of training through coaching, shadowing, being physically out of a seat, and closely monitoring and supporting the patient.
9. Gives the patient positive feedback for specific verbal and nonverbal behavioral skills.
10. Identifies the patient's specific verbal and nonverbal behavioral deficits or excesses and suggests constructive alternatives.
11. Ignores or suppresses inappropriate and interfering behavior.
12. Shapes behavioral improvements in small, attainable increments.
13. Solicits from the patient or suggests an alternative behavior for a problem situation that can be used and practiced during the behavioral rehearsal or role playing.
14. Evaluates deficits in social perception and problem solving and remedies them.
15. Gives specific attainable and functional homework assignments.

Table by Robert Paul Liberman, MD., and Jeffrey Bedell, PhD.

TABLE 24-7
BEHAVIOR THERAPY

Goal	Modify learned maladaptive behavior patterns that lead to pathological symptoms
Selection criteria	Specific, well-delineated, circumscribed, easily identified maladaptive behaviors (e.g., phobias, overeating, sexual dysfunctions)
	Psychophysiological disorders in which manifestations of symptoms are affected by stress (e.g., asthma, pain, hypertension)
Duration	Generally time-limited, specific to specific behavior
Techniques	Based on learning theory principles (e.g., operant and classical conditioning)
	Relaxation training
	Reinforcements
	Aversive therapy
	Systematic desensitization
	Flooding
	Participant modeling
	Token economies

Table by Rebecca Jones, MD.

Selection Criteria

The most valuable predictor for a successful outcome is the patients' motivation for treatment. In addition, patients must be able to understand psychological concepts, to respond to interpretation, and to concentrate on and resolve the conflict around the central issue or focus that underlies their basic problem. Patients must also be able to develop a therapeutic alliance and work with the therapist toward achieving emotional health.

Techniques.   The techniques of brief dynamic psychotherapy include the therapeutic alliance or dynamic interaction between the therapist and the patient, the use of transference, the active interpretation of a therapeutic focus or central issue, the repetitive links between parental and transference issues, and the early termination of the therapy.

The treatment can be divided into four major phases: patient-therapist encounter, early therapy, height of the treatment, and evidence of change and termination. The therapist applies the techniques previously mentioned during these four phases.

Patient-therapist encounter.   The therapist establishes a working alliance by quickly establishing rapport and generating positive feelings. Judicious use of open-ended and forced-choice questions enables the therapist to outline and concentrate on a therapeutic focus. The therapist specifies the minimum expectations of outcome to be achieved by the therapy.

Early therapy.   As transference occurs, feelings for the therapist are clarified as soon as they appear, leading to the establishment of a true therapeutic alliance.

Height of the treatment.   This final phase emphasizes actively focusing on the conflicts that have been chosen by asking provoking questions and confrontating the patient; avoiding, at all costs, a transference neurosis; repeatedly demonstrating patients' neurotic ways or maladaptive patterns of behavior; concentrating on the anxiety-laden material, even before the defense mechanisms have been clarified; repeatedly identifying parent-transference links by using properly timed interpretations based on material given by the patient; establishing a corrective emotional experience; encouraging and supporting the patients, who become anxious while struggling to understand their conflicts; establishing new learning and problem-solving patterns; and repeatedly presenting and recapitulating the patient's psychodynamics until the defense mechanisms used in dealing with conflicts are understood.

Evidence of change and termination of psychotherapy. This phase emphasizes the tangible demonstration of change in the patient's behavior outside the therapy sessions. If the therapist finds evidence that more adaptive behavior patterns are being used, discussion about terminating the treatment may begin.

Efficacy

The outcome of brief dynamic treatment has been investigated more extensively than that of any other form of psychotherapy. The results support five major generalizations: (1) The capacity for genuine recovery in certain patients is far greater than was previously thought. (2) Certain patients receiving brief psychotherapy may benefit greatly from working out their nuclear conflicts through transference. (3) Such patients can be recognized in advance through a process of dynamic interaction, because they are responsive, motivated, and able to face disturbing feelings of living independently of therapy. (4) The more radical the technique is, in terms of transference, depth of interpretation, and link to childhood, the more radical the therapeutic effects will be. (5) For some disturbed patients, a carefully chosen partial focus can be therapeutically effective. Table 24-8 lists 15 lessons that can be learned in brief dynamic therapy.

CRISIS INTERVENTION

Crisis intervention is a treatment method offered to persons who are incapacitated or severely disturbed by a crisis.

Theory

A crisis is a response to hazardous events and is experienced as a painful state. Consequently, it tends to mobilize powerful reactions to help the person alleviate the discomfort and return to the state of emotional equilibrium that existed before its onset. If these reactions take place, the crisis can be overcome and the person can learn how to use adaptive reactions to avoid future crises. Furthermore, it is possible that by resolving the crisis, patients may achieve a better emotional state than they had before the crisis. If, on the other hand, the patient uses maladaptive reactions, the painful state will intensify, the crisis will deepen, and a regressive deterioration, producing psychiatric symptoms, will take place. These symptoms, in turn, may crystallize into a neurotic pattern of behavior that restricts the patient's ability to function freely. At times, however, the situation cannot be stabilized; new maladaptive reactions are introduced; and the consequences can be of catastrophic proportions, leading at times to suicide. Those psychological crises are painful experiences that may be viewed as turning points for a better or worse emotional condition.

TABLE 24–8
FIFTEEN LESSONS LEARNED IN BRIEF DYNAMIC PSYCHOTHERAPY

1. The world is not such a bad place after all. People are more reliable and trustworthy than one had previously experienced. In some respects people are "bad" (that is, not satisfying to the patient), but in other ways they are much more valuable than one had believed.
2. One has to be less demanding of people; others resent and react negatively to exploitation. One must modify (infantile) demands and expectations to be "happier." This idea means giving up some things one always wanted (for example, praise, adulation); that is, one has to reduce one's narcissism and accept limitations in oneself and others.
3. If one achieves something or gets pleasure from some activity or experience, one's own satisfaction must be sufficient. One cannot expect others to praise and applaud and cannot bask in the glory of reflected feelings because if so one will be continually disappointed. This disappointment tends to breed hostility and resentment, which in turn set in motion vicious cycles.
4. A primary lesson one learns is to delay gratification. This learning is painful because often one cannot get what one wants when one wants it. One must modify wishes and desires, learn to accept "half a loaf," and in general get along with less (for instance, narcissistic supplies of all kinds). One also has to learn to endure tension, frustration, and privation.
5. Separation is painful but it need not last forever. One can hope (sometimes against great odds) that gratification will eventually be forthcoming. The gratification of interpersonal closeness need not be physical; it can be symbolic.
6. If one wants to reach a goal one has to institute realistic action. Sitting back and wishing is not likely to produce results. A large part of the satisfaction in any achievement is commensurate with the effort invested. By the same token, some things are realistically unattainable; therefore, the wish has to be abandoned or modified.
7. Tension, suffering, anxiety, or depression are not quite as bad as one had thought. One has greater strength than one had believed. Phobic fears have to be endured, and inevitably one gains greater strength and self-confidence in the process. Ultimately, it does not help to avoid painful, difficult, and anxiety-provoking situations; avoidance may provide temporary relief but essentially it is a pseudo (neurotic) solution which intensifies rather than solves the problem. One has to learn to stand one's ground.
8. Certain interpersonal maneuvers do not work and are self-defeating. At the same time, they are not as dangerous as one had considered one's be, either when used by oneself or others. An example is anger and hostile feelings in oneself which, the person learns will not destroy the other person or, via retaliation, oneself.
9. Cooperation as a technique for getting along with others generally brings the greatest returns. One cannot "buy" others, but one can cooperate with those who are willing. Others are not obligated to cooperate, and efforts to subjugate them are not likely to "pay off." It is wise to avoid persons whose exploitative tendencies have been identified. One is neither beholden to others, nor are others likely to enjoy being obligated (except for neurotic reasons of their own).
10. Honesty about one's feelings and motives, no matter how unpleasant or immoral they may seem, is a good policy. However, one does not need to broadcast one's less desirable tendencies—although they are universal—or wallow in guilt or self-pity because one is not perfect. Those feelings have to be accepted as part of people's primitive strivings, which are present throughout life. At the same time, recognition of their existence is no justification for acting on them. In the end, a person is judged by actions, not by fantasies. By recognizing one's motivations, one can often take more appropriate action. On the other hand, one is responsible for one's actions; they cannot be blamed on others, and the therapist cannot absolve the patient from guilt. One has to forgive oneself.
11. Every person has rights, and one needs to learn how to stand up for them. By doing so, one can learn to respect others and oneself, learning to gratify one's wishes more effectively.
12. One needs to respect, accept, and subordinate oneself to higher authority. It is futile to try to topple persons in higher positions, aggress, compete with, rebel against them, or defeat them in other ways. Their power is never complete, and ordinarily one has the choice of leaving the domain of oppressors to search for a more congenial climate.
13. Accepting authority, however, does not entail abandoning one's freedom, a false belief frequently held by patients. On the contrary, accepting authority frees the patient from struggles with others.
14. It is crucial to accept full responsibility for one's psychological processes and for one's actions. The past is irreversible, but a person usually has considerable latitude in shaping the present. Blaming others for one's predicament is self-defeating and ineffectual.
15. Implicit in several preceding items is the process of achieving a clearer understanding of one's identity and role functions, whose central importance in personality development has long been recognized. One learns not only to see oneself more clearly as an adult, but also acquires greater flexibility. Depending upon the circumstances, one can function as an authority or as a subordinate, a person who in some conditions is dependent and in others independent, who can assert and submit, who can compete when it is appropriate or abstain when it is inappropriate.

Adapted from various writings of Hans Strupp, Ph.D.

A crisis is self-limited and can last anywhere from a few hours to about 6 weeks. The crisis, as such, is characterized by an initial phase, in which anxiety and tension rise. That phase is followed by another phase in which problem-solving mechanisms are set in motion. The mechanisms may be successful, depending on whether they are adaptive or maladaptive.

Energy conservation is another feature of a person in a crisis state. All available resources are used for only one purpose: resolution of the crisis and the dimunition of pain. A successful resolution has important mental health implications. The person who can use resources efficiently, either alone or with the help of another person, not only learns how to handle the crisis and devise ways to resolve it, but has also discovers how to anticipate future trouble and prevent its recurrence. In this way, crisis resolution is also a preventive intervention.

During a period of turmoil patients are receptive to minimal help and obtain meaningful results. All sorts of services, therefore, have been devised for such purposes. Some are open-ended; others limit the length of treatment.

Crisis theory helps one understand healthy normal people, as well as to develop therapeutic tools aimed at preventing future psychological difficulties.

Selection Criteria

The criteria used to select patients are (1) a history of a specific hazardous situation of recent origin that produced the anxiety, a precipitating event that intensified this anxiety; (2) clear-cut evidence that the patient is in a state of psychological crisis, as previously defined; (3) high motivation to overcome the crisis; (4) a potential for making a psychological adjustment equal or superior to the one that existed before the crisis; and (5) a certain degree of psychological sophistication—an ability to recognize psychological reasons for the present predicament.

Techniques

Because crisis intervention is used for persons in the midst of a crisis, rapid treatment is crucial. The therapy is based on helping patients understand the psychodynamics involved and how they contributed to the crisis. Patients and therapists work together to resolve the crisis as quickly as possible.

The techniques used in crisis intervention include reassurance, suggestion, environmental manipulation, and psychotropic medications, and the treatment may include brief hospitalization, if necessary. All therapeutic maneuvers are aimed at decreasing the patient's anxiety. The length of crisis intervention varies from 1 or 2 sessions to several interviews over a period of 1 or 2 months. The required steps for successful outcome of crisis intervention include rapidly establishing rapport with the patient to foster a therapeutic alliance; reviewing the steps that have led to the crisis; understanding the maladaptive reactions the patient is using to deal with the crisis; preventing development of new symptoms; using the positive transference as a learning tool; teaching the patient how to avoid hazardous situations that are likely to produce future crises; and ending the intervention as soon as the crisis has been resolved and the patient clearly understands the steps that led to its development and resolution.

Efficacy

The most striking result of crisis therapy is that the patient becomes better equipped to avoid hazardous situations, or, if necessary, to handle these situations adequately. On the basis of some patients' observations, this therapeutic experience has enabled them to attain a better level of emotional functioning than they had before the crisis.

For a more detailed discussion of this topic, see M M Weissman, J C Markowitz: Interpersonal Psychotherapy: Current Status. Arch Gen Psychiatry 51: 599, 1994.

Index

Note: Page numbers followed by a *t* indicates tables.

of control, definition, 23–24
definition, 23
erotomanic, 197*t*
grandiose (of grandeur), 197*t*, 198–199
  definition, 23
of infidelity, definition, 24
jealous, 197*t*
mixed, 197*t*
mood-congruent, definition, 23
mood-incongruent, definition, 23
nihilistic, definition, 23
paranoid, definition, 23
persecutory (of persecution), 197*t*, 205
  definition, 23
of poverty, definition, 23
of reference, definition, 23
of self-accusation, definition, 23
somatic, 197*t*
  definition, 23
systematized, definition, 23
Delusional disorder, 196–198
  clinical features, 196–197
  combined therapy for, 407
  definition, 196
  diagnosis, 196–197
  diagnostic criteria for, 197*t*
  drug treatment, 198
  evaluation, 197
  interviewing and psychotherapeutic
    guidelines with, 197
  management, 197
  persecutory type, 206
Delusional jealousy, definition, 24
Dementia, 86–90
  in AIDS, 103
  alcohol-related. *See* Alcohol dementia
  of the Alzheimer's type, drug
    treatment, 388*t*
  vs. anger, 332
  causes, 87, 88*t*
  clinical features, 86–89
  definition, 28–29, 86
  vs. delirium, 87, 87*t*
  vs. depression, 87, 88*t*
  diagnosis, 86–89
  diagnostic criteria for, 87*t*
  drug treatment, 90
  dysprosody with, 338
  evaluation, 89–90
  interviewing and psychotherapeutic
    guidelines with, 89
  management, 89–90
  vs. normal aging, 87
Dementia syndrome of depression,
  definition, 29
Demerol. *See* Meperidine
Denial, definition, 39*t*
Depakene. *See* Valproate

Depakote. *See* Divalproex
Depersonalization, 260–262
  clinical features, 260–261
  definition, 27, 260
  diagnosis, 260–261
  diagnostic criteria, 261*t*
  in disaster survivors, 334–335
  drug treatment, 262
  evaluation, 261
  interviewing and psychotherapeutic
    guidelines with, 261
  management, 261
  in schizophrenia, 212
Depot medication, akinesia secondary to,
  331
Deprenyl, for Parkinson's disease, 128
Depression, 219–225
  in adolescence, 55
  vs. anger, 332
  anorexia nervosa and, 299–300
  with anxiety, 241
  in borderline personality disorder,
    328–329
  breathlessness in, 44–45
  causes
    medical, 222*t*
    neurological, 222*t*
    pharmacological, 222*t*
  in children, 62
  clinical features, 219–220
  with cocaine withdrawal, 165–166
  cognitive profile of, 430*t*
  cognitive theory of, 428–429
  cognitive therapy for, 428–430
  cognitive triad, 429
  combined therapy in, 406
  definition, 19, 219
  vs. dementia, 87, 88*t*
  diagnosis, 219–220
  in disaster survivors, 334–335
  drug treatment, 223–225, 388*t*. *See
    also* Antidepressant(s)
  dysprosody with, 338
  in epilepsy, 114
  evaluation, 221
  vs. grief, 226, 226*t*
  with hemodialysis, 122
  hospitalization for, 221
  with hyperthyroidism, 130–131
  in hypochondriacal patient, 268
  with hypothyroidism, 130–131
  with inanition, 129–130
  insomnia related to, 306*t*
  interpersonal context of, 423–424
  interpersonal psychotherapy for,
    423–428

Diet pills. *See* Phenylpropanolamine
Differential diagnosis, 36
Digoxin (Lanoxin)
  confusion caused by, 82*t*
  male sexual dysfunction and, 287*t*
Dihydroindoles, geriatric dosage range, 380*t*
Dilaudid. *See* Hydromorphone
Dildo, 296
Diltiazem (Cardizem), pharmacological category, 386*t*
Dimethyltryptamine, 169, 170*t*
Diphenhydramine (Benadryl), 337
  anxiolytic effects, 242
  for extrapyramidal disorders, 413, 414*t*, 415
  for parkinsonism, 128*t*
  pharmacological category, 386*t*
  for separation anxiety, 65
  for tremor, 362
Diplopia, 44
Dipsomania, definition, 20
Disaster survivors
  clinical features, 334
  definition, 334
  diagnosis, 334
  drug treatment, 335
  evaluation and management, 335
  interviewing and psychotherapeutic guidelines with, 335
Disorders usually first diagnosed in infancy, childhood, or adolescence, 55–69
Disorientation, 91–92
  clinical features, 91
  definition, 17, 91
  diagnosis, 91
  drug-related, 91–92
  drug treatment with, 92
  evaluation, 91–92
  interviewing and psychotherapeutic guidelines with, 91
  management, 91–92
  medical causes, 92
  medical workup with, 92
Dispal. *See* Orphenadrine
Displacement, definition, 39*t*
Dissociation, definition, 39*t*
Dissociative identity disorder, definition, 27
Dissociative phenomena, definition, 27
Distractibility, definition, 18
Distribution, drug, 368
  age-related changes in, 379*t*
Disulfiram (Antabuse), 134
  cognitive impairment with, 91
  indications for, 388*t*
  intoxication or overdose, 393*t*

pharmacological category, 386*t*
Divalproex (Depakote), 365
  for mania, 230
  pharmacological category, 387*t*
Doctor–patient relationship, 3–4
  models of, 3, 4*t*
    active-passive, 4*t*
    general considerations, 4
    intimate model, 4*t*
    mutual participation, 4*t*
    teacher-student, 4*t*
Doll's-eye maneuver, 109
Dolophine. *See* Methadone
DOM. *See* Methyldimethoxyamphetamine
Don Juanism, 285
L-Dopa. *See also* Levodopa (Dopar, Larodopa)
  intoxication, 166–167
Dopamine agonist(s). *See also specific agent*
  for extrapyramidal disorders, 414*t*
  for parkinsonism, 127, 128*t*
  withdrawal, neuroleptic malignant syndrome with, 418
Dopamine antagonist(s)
  for brief psychotic disorder, 194
  indications for, 388*t*–389*t*
  intoxication or overdose, 393*t*
Dopar. *See* Levodopa
Doral. *See* Quazepam
Doriden. *See* Glutethimide
Dose-response curve, 369, 369*f*
Doxepin (Sinequan)
  for cocaine dependence, 166
  dosage and administration, 224*t*
  geriatric dosage range, 380*t*
  for pain control, 273*t*
  pharmacological category, 386*t*
Dreamlike state, definition, 17
Droperidol (Inopsine), pharmacological category, 386*t*
Drug(s). *See also* Substance
  abstinence syndrome, 361
  anticholinergic effects, 149
  choice of, 370–374
    in combined therapy, 404
  combination, 371, 372*t*
  confusion caused by, 82*t*
  countertransference and, 400
  delusions with, 199
  discontinuation, 374
  implicated in anorgasmia, 283, 284*t*
  implicated in male sexual dysfunction, 287*t*
  nocturia caused by, 349
  nonapproved dosages and uses, 371–373
  used in psychiatry, 385–397, 386*t*–387*t*
  withdrawal syndrome, 374

Encephalitis lethargica, 69*t*
Encephalopathy
  hepatic, confusion caused by, 81*t*
  Wernicke's, 76, 92–94
  confusion caused by, 81*t*
Enuresis. *See* Bed-wetting
Epidural hematoma, confusion caused by,
  81*t*
Epilepsy, 111–116. *See also* Seizure(s)
  causes, 114
  clinical features, 111–113
  comorbidity with psychiatric
    conditions, 111
  definition, 111
  depression in, 114
  diagnosis, 111–113
  drug treatment, 116. *See also*
    Anticonvulsant(s)
    drugs of choice for, 116*t*
  evaluation, 114
  hypersexuality in, 285
  ictal event in, 113
  impaired cognition in, 115
  interviewing and psychotherapeutic
    guidelines with, 113–114
  management, 114
  personality changes in, 114
  postictal events in, 113
  preictal events in, 113
  prevalence, 111
  psychosis in, 115
  temporal lobe, 113
  violence in, 115–116
Epileptoid personality, 313
Epivir. *See* Lamivudine
Equanil. *See* Meprobamate
Erectile difficulty, 45. *See also* Impotence
Ergot alkaloids, for migraine, 119
Erotomania, definition, 24
Erythrophobia, definition, 24
Eskalith. *See* Lithium
Essential tremor, 361
  dyskinesia with, 336–337
Estazolam (ProSom)
  for amphetamine (or amphetaminelike)
    intoxication or overdose, 148
  for anxiety
    with drug flashback, 168
    with nutmeg intoxication, 178
  for anxiety with arrhythmias, 106
  for aphasic patient, 75
  for brief psychotic disorder, 194
  for clonidine withdrawal, 162
  for cocaine withdrawal, 166
  for depersonalization disorder, 262
  for disaster survivors, 335
  dosage and administration, 243*t*
  for grandiosity, 199

  for grieving patient, 228
  for insomnia, 309
  pharmacological category, 386*t*
  pharmacology, 243*t*
  for phencyclidine intoxication, 185
  for phobia, 253–254
  for posttraumatic stress disorder, 259
  for psychogenic urinary retention, 275
  for thyrotoxicosis, 131
Ethchlorvynol (Placidyl)
  intoxication or overdose, 393*t*
  pharmacological category, 386*t*
Ethopropazine (Parsidol)
  for extrapyramidal disorders, 414*t*
  for parkinsonism, 128*t*
Etrafon. *See* Perphenazine and
    amitriptyline
Euphoria, definition, 19
Excretion, drug, 368
Exhibitionism, 296
Explanation, in interview, 8*t*
Extrapyramidal disorders, drug treatment,
  414*t*

Face, assessment, 47
Facilitation, in interview, 8*t*
Factitial dermatitis, 279–280
Factitious disorder(s), 279–280
  clinical features, 279
  definition, 279
  diagnosis, 279
  differential diagnosis, 279
  drug treatment, 280
  evaluation, 280
  interviewing and psychotherapeutic
    guidelines with, 280
  management, 280
Fainting. *See* Syncope
Family history, in psychiatric history, 33*t*
Fausse reconnaissance, definition, 28
Fear
  definition, 19
  in disaster survivors, 334–335
Febrile illness. *See* Fever
Female orgasmic disorder, 283–284
Fenfluramine (Pondimin)
  indications for, 388*t*
  intoxication or overdose, 393*t*
  for pediatric patients
    adverse effects, 377*t*
    dosage and administration, 377*t*
    indications for, 377*t*
    monitoring, 377*t*
  pharmacological category, 386*t*
Fever
  confusion caused by, 81*t*
  workup, 421

Somnambulism. *See* Sleepwalking
Somnolence
  definition, 17
  excessive daytime, 310
Speaking in tongues, definition, 22
Speech
  assessment, 48
  definition, 25
  disturbances in, 25
  excessively loud or soft, definition, 25
  impairment. *See* Dysarthria
  in mental status examination, 34*t*
  nonspontaneous, definition, 25
  poverty of, 74
    definition, 25
  poverty of content of, definition, 25
  pressure of, definition, 25
Spironolactone (Aldactone), male sexual
    dysfunction and, 287*t*
Splitting, definition, 40*t*
Spouse abuse, 320–322
  clinical features, 321
  definition, 320
  diagnosis, 321
  drug treatment and, 322
  epidemiology, 320
  evaluation, 321–322
  interviewing and psychotherapeutic
    guidelines for, 321
  management, 321–322
  risk factors for, 320
Starvation, 128–130
  clinical features, 129
  definition, 128
  diagnosis, 129
  drug treatment, 130
  evaluation, 129
  hospitalization for, 129
  interviewing and psychotherapeutic
    guidelines with, 129
  management, 129
  physical symptoms with, 128
  psychiatric symptoms with, 128
  in schizophrenia, 129
Status epilepticus, 115
  drug treatment, 116*t*
Stavudine (Zerit), 105*t*
Stelazine. *See* Trifluoperazine
Stereotypy, definition, 20
Sternbach, Richard, 366
Steroid(s)
  for cluster headache, 119
  cognitive impairment with, 91
  delusions with, 199
  for temporal arteritis, 119
Stimulant(s). *See also specific agent*
  for narcolepsy, 311
  for pediatric patients

  adverse effects, 376*t*
  dosage and administration, 376*t*
  indications for, 376*t*
  monitoring, 376*t*
  psychotic symptoms with, 194, 202–203
STP. *See* Methyldimethoxyamphetamine
Stress(es)
  extraordinary, 334
  overwhelming psychic, death from, 345
Stroke, confusion caused by, 81*t*
Stupor, 108*t*
  with catatonia, 77
  catatonic, 109*t*
  definition, 17
Stuttering, definition, 25
Subacute sclerosing panencephalitis, 337
Subarachnoid hemorrhage, 44
Subdural hematoma, 44
  confusion caused by, 81*t*
Sublimation, definition, 40*t*
Substance abuse
  vs. anger, 332
  combined therapy for, 408
Substance intoxication, 172–174
  clinical features, 172
  definition, 172
  diagnosis, 172
  diagnostic criteria, 173*t*
  drug treatment, 174
  evaluation, 173–174
  interviewing and psychotherapeutic
    guidelines for, 173
  management, 173–174
Substance-related disorders, 133–191. *See
    also specific substance*
Substance use disorder, dysprosody with,
    338
Sudden death. *See* Death, impending
Suggestibility, disturbances in, 18
Suicidal ideation, definition, 234
Suicide/suicidal patient, 14, 234–237, 344
  in adolescence, 55
  and alcohol dependence, 140
  associated psychiatric conditions, 234
  attempts, in borderline personality
    disorder, 328
  clinical features, 234–235
  cocaine withdrawal and, 165–166
  cognitive profile of, 430*t*
  combined therapy for, 406
  definition, 234
  diagnosis, 234–235
  drug treatment, 236–237
  evaluation, 236
  hospitalization, 236
  interviewing and psychotherapeutic
    guidelines for, 235–236
  management, 236

BOOKS BY HAROLD I. KAPLAN, M.D., AND BENJAMIN J. SADOCK, M.D.

Published by Williams & Wilkins

Comprehensive Textbook of Psychiatry

1st edition, 1967 (with A.M. Freedman)
2nd edition, 1975 (with A.M. Freedman)
3rd edition, 1980 (with A.M. Freedman)
4th edition, 1985
5th edition, 1989
6th edition, 1995

Synopsis of Psychiatry

1st edition, 1972 (with A.M. Freedman)
2nd edition, 1976 (with A.M. Freedman)
3rd edition, 1981
4th edition, 1985
5th edition, 1988
6th edition, 1991
7th edition, 1994 (with J. Grebb)

Study Guide and Self-Examination Review for Synopsis of Psychiatry

1st edition, 1983
2nd edition, 1985
3rd edition, 1989
4th edition, 1991
5th edition, 1994

Comprehensive Group Psychotherapy

1st edition, 1971
2nd edition, 1983
3rd edition, 1993

The Sexual Experience

1976 (with A.M. Freedman)

Clinical Psychiatry

1988

Concise Textbook of Clinical Psychiatry

1996

Pocket Handbook of Clinical Psychiatry

1st edition, 1990
2nd edition, 1996

Comprehensive Glossary of Psychiatry and Psychology

1991

Pocket Handbook of Psychiatric Drug Treatment
   1st edition, 1993
   2nd edition, 1996

Pocket Handbook of Emergency Psychiatric Medicine
   1993

Pocket Handbook of Primary Care Psychiatry
   1997

Various editions of the above books have been translated and published in French, German, Greek, Indonesian, Italian, Japanese, Polish, Portuguese, Spanish, and Turkish. In addition, an International Asian edition has been published in English.

By other publishers

Studies in Human Behavior, 1–5
   1972 (with A.M. Freedman)
Athenaeum
   1.   Diagnosing Mental Illness: Evaluation in Psychiatry and Psychology
   2.   Interpreting Personality: A Survey of Twentieth-Century Views
   3.   Human Behavior: Biological, Psychological, and Sociological
   4.   Treating Mental Illness: Aspects of Modern Therapy
   5.   The Child: His Psychological and Cultural Development
         Vol. 1:   Normal Development and Psychological Assessment
         Vol. 2:   The Major Psychological Disorders and their Treatment

Modern Group Books I–VI
   1972
E.P. Dutton
   I   Origins of Group Analysis
   II   Evolution of Group Therapy
   III   Groups and Drugs
   IV   Sensitivity Through Encounter and Motivation
   V   New Models for Group Therapy
   VI   Group Treatment of Mental Illness

The Human Animal
   1974 (with A.M. Freedman)
K.F.S. Publications
   Vol. 1: Man and His Mind
   Vol. 2: The Disordered Personality

About the Authors

HAROLD IRWIN KAPLAN, M.D., is currently professor of psychiatry at New York University (NYU) School of Medicine, an appointment dating back to 1980. Since that time he has been an attending psychiatrist at Tisch Hospital (the University Hospital of the NYU Medical Center) and Bellevue Hospital of the NYU Medical Center. He is codirector of NYU Medical Center's Continuing Medical Education Program in Psychiatry and is consultant psychiatrist at Lenox Hill Hospital in New York City. From 1958 to 1980, he was professor of psychiatry at New York Medical College and director of Psychiatric Education, heading the undergraduate, residency, and continuing education programs in psychiatry, and he was a visiting psychiatrist at Metropolitan Hospital in New York City. He received his Bachelor of Arts degree from New York University. He received his M.D. from New York Medical College in 1949 at the age of 21, interned at Jewish Hospital of Brooklyn, and served his psychiatric residency training at Kingsbridge Bronx Veterans Administration Hospital, New York's Mount Sinai Hospital, and at Jewish Board of Guardians (in child psychiatry). He has received awards for academic excellence in psychiatry from the Alumni Association of New York Medical College (1983), the Distinguished Service Award in Psychiatry from the Association of Psychiatric Outpatient Centers of America and the NYU Post-Graduate Medical School (1982), and a Founders Day Award for Scholastic Achievement from NYU (1988). During his tenure at New York Medical College, he was the principal investigator of 10 educational grants in psychiatry from NIMH, several specializing in the psychiatric training of women physicians. He was a member of the Preparatory Commission on Psychiatric Education for NIMH and the American Psychiatric Association during 1973–1975. IN 1957 he was certified in psychiatry by the American Board of Psychiatry and Neurology and has served as an Assistant and Associate Examiner of the American Board for 12 years. He received a Certificate of Commendation from the American Psychiatric Association for his work as chairman of their Committee on Education during 1973–1975. Professor Kaplan was certified in psychoanalysis in 1955 by New York Medical College. He has published many papers in numerous psychiatric journals and has authored and edited the books listed in this volume. He is a Life Fellow of the American Psychiatric Association, the American College of Physicians, the New York Academy of Medicine, and the American Orthopsychiatric Association. He is also a member of the Alpha Omega Alpha Honorary Medical Society and treasurer of the NYU-Bellevue Psychiatric Society. He presently makes his home in New York City, where is he is married to actress Nancy Barrett. He has three children, Jennifer, Peter Mark, and Phillip. He maintains an active general psychiatric practice in Manhattan, which includes individual and group psychotherapy, psychiatric consultation, psychoanalysis, and psychopharmacotherapy. In his leisure time he enjoys reading nonfiction, travel, and fine food.

BENJAMIN JAMES SADOCK, M.D., is currently professor and vice chairman of the Department of Psychiatry at the New York University (NYU) School of Medicine. He graduated from Union College in 1955 and received his M.D. from New York Medical College in 1959. After an internship at Albany Hospital, he completed his residency at Bellevue Psychiatric Hospital and then entered military service, where he served as Assistant Chief and Acting Chief of Neuropsychiatry at Sheppard Air Force Base, Texas. He held faculty and teaching appointments at Southwestern Medical School and Parkland Hospital in Dallas and at New York Medical College, St. Luke's Hospital, the New York State Psychiatric Institute, and Metropolitan Hospital in New York City. He joined the faculty of the NYU School of Medicine in 1980 and served in various positions: director of Medical Student Education in Psychiatry, codirector of the Residency Training Program in Psychiatry, and director of Graduate Medical Education. Since 1980, Dr. Sadock has been director of Student Mental Health Services, psychiatric consultant to the Admissions Committee, and codirector of Continuing Education in Psychiatry at the NYU School of Medicine. He is on the staff of Bellevue Hospital and Tisch Hospital (the University Hospital of the NYU Medical Center) and is consultant psychiatrist at Lenox Hill Hospital. Dr. Sadock became a Diplomate of the American Board of Psychiatry and Neurology in 1966 and served as an assistant and associate examiner for the Board for over a decade. He is a Fellow of the American Psychiatric Association, the American College of Physicians, and the New York Academy of Medicine. He is also a member of the Alpha Omega Alpha Honor Society. He is active in numerous psychiatric organizations and is president and founder of the NYU-Bellevue Psychiatric Society. Dr. Sadock was a member of the National Committee on Continuing Education in Psychiatry of the American Psychiatric Association, served on the Ad Hoc Committee on Sex Therapy Clinics of the American Medical Association, was delegate to the Conference on Recertification of the American Board of Medical Specialists, and was a representative of the American Psychiatric Association's Task Force on the National Board of Medical Examiners and the American Board of Psychiatry and Neurology. In 1985 he received the Academic Achievement Award from New York Medical College. He is author or editor of more than 100 publications, including the books listed in this volume, and is a book reviewer for psychiatry journals. He is married to Virginia Alcott Sadock, M.D., Clinical Professor of Psychiatry and Director of the Program in Human Sexuality and Sex Therapy at NYU Medical Center. They live in Manhattan and have an active private practice specializing in individual psychotherapy, group psychotherapy, sex and marital therapy, and pharmacotherapy. They have two children, James and Victoria. Dr. Sadock enjoys opera, skiing, and fly fishing in his leisure time.